Characterization and Production of Antibiotics

Characterization and Production of Antibiotics

Edited by Clancy Knightley

hayle
medical

New York

Hayle Medical,
750 Third Avenue, 9th Floor,
New York, NY 10017, USA

Visit us on the World Wide Web at:
www.haylemedical.com

ISBN: 978-1-64647-108-9

Cataloging-in-Publication Data

Characterization and production of antibiotics / edited by Clancy Knightley.
    p. cm.
Includes bibliographical references and index.
ISBN 978-1-64647-108-9
1. Antibiotics. 2. Antibiotics--Analysis. 3. Antibiotics industry. I. Knightley, Clancy.
RM267 .C43 2022
615.329--dc23

Table of Contents

Preface

An antibiotic is an antimicrobial substance which is used in the treatment and prevention of bacterial infections. It can either inhibit the growth of bacteria or kill them. It may be prescribed as a preventive measure to at-risk populations. These may include those with a weakened immune system or taking immunosuppressive drugs, or those undergoing surgery or affected by cancer. It is also used in surgical procedures for preventing infections of incisions, and in dental antibiotic prophylaxis for preventing bacteremia and subsequent infective endocarditis. Antibiotics can be classified as bactericidal and bacteriostatic. Bactericidals kill bacteria directly whereas bacteriostatics prevent bacteria from dividing. Antibiotics are also classified on the basis of target bacteria. They can be produced through synthetic and semi-synthetic methods. Evidence suggests that bacteria are increasingly developing resistance to antibiotics, which makes research, development and production of new antibiotics pertinent. This book brings forth some of the most innovative concepts and elucidates the unexplored aspects of antibiotics. It presents researches and studies performed by experts across the globe on the characterization and production of antibiotics. With state-of-the-art inputs by acclaimed experts of this field, this book targets students and professionals.

This book unites the global concepts and researches in an organized manner for a comprehensive understanding of the subject. It is a ripe text for all researchers, students, scientists or anyone else who is interested in acquiring a better knowledge of this dynamic field.

I extend my sincere thanks to the contributors for such eloquent research chapters. Finally, I thank my family for being a source of support and help.

Editor

Ribosomal Antibiotics: Contemporary Challenges

Tamar Auerbach-Nevo, David Baram, Anat Bashan, Matthew Belousoff, Elinor Breiner,
Chen Davidovich, Giuseppe Cimicata, Zohar Eyal, Yehuda Halfon, Miri Krupkin, Donna Matzov,
Markus Metz, Mruwat Rufayda, Moshe Peretz, Ophir Pick, Erez Pyetan, Haim Rozenberg,
Moran Shalev-Benami, Itai Wekselman, Raz Zarivach, Ella Zimmerman, Nofar Assis, Joel Bloch,
Hadar Israeli, Rinat Kalaora, Lisha Lim, Ofir Sade-Falk, Tal Shapira, Leena Taha-Salaime,
Hua Tang and Ada Yonath *

Department of Structural Biology, Weizmann Institute, Rehovot 76100, Israel; tauerba@its.jnj.com (T.A.-N.);
david@smzyme.com (D.B.); anat.bashan@weizmann.ac.il (A.B.); matthew.belousoff@monash.edu (M.B.);
elinor.breiner@weizmann.ac.il (E.B.); Chen.Davidovich@monash.edu (C.D.);
giuseppe.cimicata@gmail.com (G.C.); zohar.baram@weizmann.ac.il (Z.E.);
Yehuda.Halfon@weizmann.ac.il (Y.H.); Miri.Krupkin@weizmann.ac.il (M.K.);
Matzov.donna@weizmann.ac.il (D.M.); markusmetz.at@gmail.com (M.M.);
Rufayda.Mruwat@weizmann.ac.il (M.R.); moshe.peretz@weizmann.ac.il (M.P.); ophir.pick@gmail.com (O.P.);
erezpy@gmail.com (E.P.); Haim.Rozenberg@weizmann.ac.il (H.R.); benami.moran@gmail.com (M.S.-B.);
Itai.Wekselman@weizmann.ac.il (I.W.); zarivach@bgu.ac.il (R.Z.); Ella.Zimmerman@weizmann.ac.il (E.Z.);
nofar.assis@gmail.com (N.A.); joel.bloch@mol.biol.ethz.ch (J.B.); hadarisr@bgu.ac.il (H.I.);
rinat.kalaora@gmail.com (R.K.); lishaqjl@gmail.com (L.L.); ofir.sadefalk@gmail.com (O.S.-F.);
Tal.Shapira@weizmann.ac.il (T.S.); Leena.ta.salaime@gmail.com (L.T.-S.); hua2han2003@yahoo.com (H.T.)
* Correspondence: Ada.Yonath@weizmann.ac.il

Academic Editor: Claudio O. Gualerzi

Abstract: Most ribosomal antibiotics obstruct distinct ribosomal functions. In selected cases, in addition to paralyzing vital ribosomal tasks, some ribosomal antibiotics are involved in cellular regulation. Owing to the global rapid increase in the appearance of multi-drug resistance in pathogenic bacterial strains, and to the extremely slow progress in developing new antibiotics worldwide, it seems that, in addition to the traditional attempts at improving current antibiotics and the intensive screening for additional natural compounds, this field should undergo substantial conceptual revision. Here, we highlight several contemporary issues, including challenging the common preference of broad-range antibiotics; the marginal attention to alterations in the microbiome population resulting from antibiotics usage, and the insufficient awareness of ecological and environmental aspects of antibiotics usage. We also highlight recent advances in the identification of species-specific structural motifs that may be exploited for the design and the creation of novel, environmental friendly, degradable, antibiotic types, with a better distinction between pathogens and useful bacterial species in the microbiome. Thus, these studies are leading towards the design of "pathogen-specific antibiotics," in contrast to the current preference of broad range antibiotics, partially because it requires significant efforts in speeding up the discovery of the unique species motifs as well as the clinical pathogen identification.

Keywords: multi-drug resistance; microbiome; species-specific antibiotics susceptibility; novel degradable antibiotics

1. Introduction

The severe increase in antibiotic resistance and cross-resistance among pathogenic bacterial strains presents a significant health threat. Hence, focusing on the specific properties of antibiotics targets in pathogenic bacteria, and on the molecular mechanisms acquiring resistance to them, are of prime importance. So far, the main efforts to combat antibiotic resistance are based on attempts at the production of new antibiotics by various approaches, such as mining underexplored microbial niches or designing new chemical probes for improving the antibiotic performance of known molecular scaffolds, and, to a lesser extent, the development of novel therapeutic agents (for reviews, see [1]). Presently, most clinically useful antibiotics are either natural products, originated by microorganisms, or semi-synthetic compounds based on natural molecular scaffolds that are produced by microorganisms to aid their struggle for resources. Interestingly, antibiotic resistance genes have existed in microorganisms long before these compounds were discovered by humans and exploited for therapeutic and nutritional uses. For example, the Yanomami's gut bacteria have evolved a diverse array of antibiotic-resistance genes, even though this mountain tribe had never ingested antibiotics, nor animals raised in their presence [2].

Protein biosynthesis is a key life process in all organisms; hence, it is targeted by many antibiotics. This process, namely, the translation of the genetic code, involves decoding the genetic information and the creation of nascent proteins. Ribosomes, the universal flexible and dynamic giant multi-protein-RNA assemblies, perform both tasks in all living cells, including pathogenic bacteria. They are built of two structurally independent riboprotein subunits that associate upon initiation of protein biosynthesis. In all organisms, the small subunit accommodates the mRNA and provides the site for the decoding of the genetic information, and the large subunit contains the site for peptide bond formation, called the peptidyl transferase center (PTC), and the tunnel along which the nascent proteins progress until they emerge from the ribosome (Figure 1). Owing to their key role in life, many clinically useful antibiotics paralyze them. Diverse mechanisms have been developed by microorganisms to acquire resistance to antibiotics, and it seems that, for most of them, the microorganisms generated specific antibiotic resistance genes. Here, we focus solely on those that are correlated to ribosomal antibiotics. These include post-transcription modification in the ribosomal RNA (rRNA) by specific enzymes (e.g., those that methylate or ethylate the C8 position of rRNA nucleotides) or by substitution and deletion/insertion mutations in ribosomal proteins (rProtein) that are located in proximity to the antibiotic binding pockets).

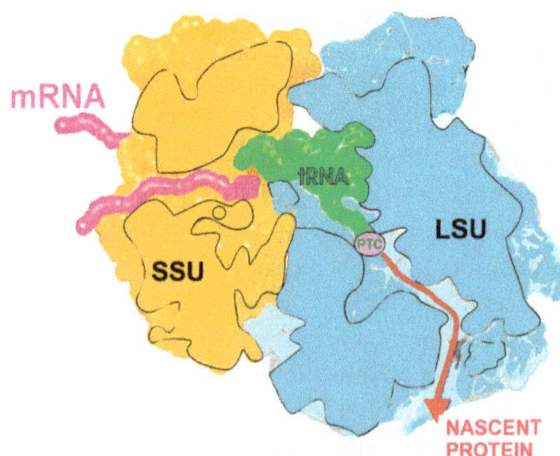

Figure 1. Overall structure of the bacterial ribosome showing the two subunits: the small (SSU) and the large (LSU), the mRNA, the PTC, and the nascent protein exit tunnel.

Concurrent with the determination of the high-resolution structures of bacterial ribosomes, intensive efforts have been made to identify molecular modes of antimicrobial action, in order to reveal the principles of their selectivity, to shed light on their synergism, and to elucidate the mechanisms of acquiring resistance. Consequently, the target site and the mode of action of at least one member of each family of ribosomal antibiotics have been located and described in detail, showing that they inhibit protein biosynthesis by targeting functional regions in the ribosomes (Figure 2). Examples of targets in ribosomes, which were found or verified by X-ray crystallography, are the decoding region, the PTC, the nascent chain exit tunnel, an intersubunit bridge, and the tRNA accommodating corridor [3–17].

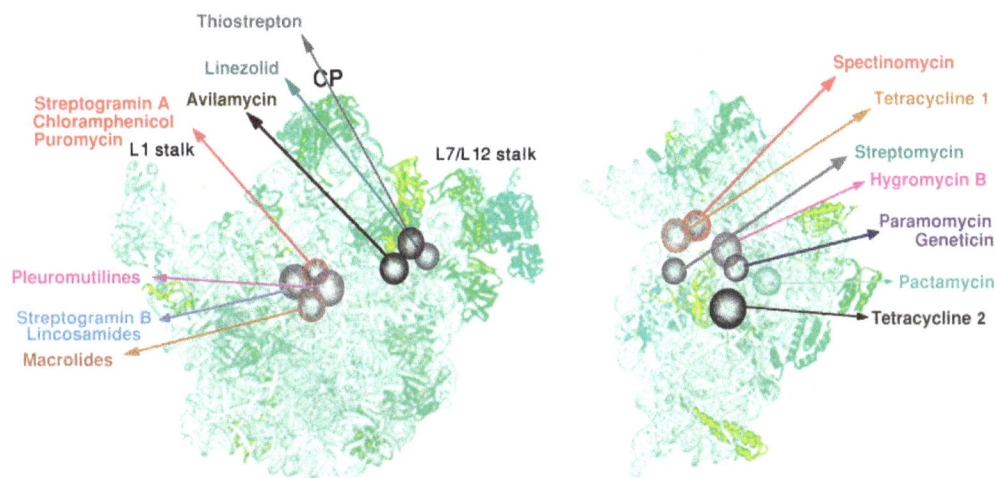

Figure 2. Main antibiotics binding sites shown on the skeletons of the large (**left**); and the small (**right**) ribosomal subunits.

Species specificity of pathogens to antibiotics can be reached by several cellular pathways, such as efflux pumps and membrane permeability properties. Here, we focus only on the structural bases of ribosomal antibiotics binding and their modes of action. The crystallographic structural information provided valuable insights into the common mechanisms of antibiotic function, resistance, and selectivity that are shared by most of the clinically relevant bacteria, but did not show the minor structural differences between different pathogenic bacteria [18] that may be exploited for addressing species-specific significant differences in antibiotic susceptibility. In this regard, the structures of complexes of antibiotics with ribosomes from two pathogenic bacteria, *Escherichia coli* [7,8,15] and *Staphylococcus aureus* (*S. aureus*) [16], were shown to be useful for identification of unique structural motifs. Thus, comparisons of ribosome structures from pathogens with their non-pathogenic mates shed light on the properties of antibiotic action and resistance, and consequently paved new paths for dealing with the current acute resistance issues. In addition, a careful analysis of their modes of inhibition shed light on vital regulatory pathways and on ribosomal inherent flexibility.

Looking into the future, it is clear that there is an immediate necessity for novel anti-bacterial agents based on the specific atomic structures of targets in the ribosomes of pathogenic strains. Until recently, such data could only be obtained through lengthy and demanding crystallographic studies. However, the current resolution revolution by single-particle cryo-electron microscopy provides opportunities for relatively fast structure determination, smaller amounts, and the elimination of crystals.

2. Main Findings

2.1. The Nascent Protein Exit Tunnel Seems to Be Involved in Cellular Regulation

Erythromycin, the first ribosomal antibiotic drug that was used in clinical therapy, and the semi-synthetic compounds that are based on its chemical scaffold (including macrolides, ketolides, azalides, and streptogramin B), bind with a high affinity to a pocket, made solely of ribosomal RNA (rRNA) located at the rims of the nascent protein exit tunnel. Thus, the main macrolides mode of action is interfering with the progression of the nascent proteins [3,4,6,9,19–24] in a fashion that is still not fully characterized [23,24]. Resistance to macrolides is commonly achieved by mutation, e.g., A2058G

(*E. coli* numbering is used throughout for rRNA nucleotides), or by modification, e.g., methylation, of the binding pocket's nucleotides [25–28].

The protein exit tunnel is lined by rRNA and small regions of three ribosomal proteins (rProteins), among which uL4 and uL22 form the narrowest constriction of the tunnel. Each of them possesses a long β-hairpin loop, the tips of which are located in proximity, albeit chemically rather distal, to the macrolides binding pocket. Early biochemical, genetic, and structural studies revealed that explicit interactions of specific nascent protein sequence motifs with the tunnel walls may lead to translation arrest, thereby regulating the expression level of some genes [29–40]. The crystal structures of troleandomycin bound to the large ribosomal subunit [40] and of erythromycin resistant mutant with a minute deletion in protein uL22 [41] indicated a motion of the tip of the uL22 hairpin loop across the tunnel that could be correlated with the regulatory properties of the exit tunnel [40–42]. Furthermore, 2058A->G laboratory alteration mediates ketolide resistance in combination with a deletion in protein uL22. Hence, it is likely that erythromycin resistance mechanism can be involved with interfering cellular regulation, beyond a simple tunnel blockage.

Interplay between macrolides binding and translation arrest was also shown to control expression of macrolide resistance genes. Remarkably, it was found that macrolides arrest translation of a truncated regulatory peptide, even when the nascent chain was too short to encounter the antibiotic (the first three amino acids) [43]. Additionally, it was shown that stalling by specific nascent peptides, a cellular mechanism used for the regulation of expression of some bacterial and eukaryotic genes, is sensitive to additional cellular signals, some of which are connected to antibiotics [36,40]. These results correlate well with biochemical and structural findings that alterations of ribosomal components that do not belong to binding pockets may also cause resistance, mainly by exploiting the inherent flexibility of ribosomal components for reshaping the binding pockets or their environments [42–44].

2.2. Inherent Flexity of Antibiotics Binding Pockets and of Their Surroundings

One of the intriguing questions in antibiotic action relates to their selectivity, even when bound to almost fully conserved regions. An example is the PTC , which is highly conserved yet provides a binding site for several useful antibiotics, such as the pleuromutilin [45], lincosamides, phenicols [3] or small macrolides (e.g., a mono-sugar macrolide with 12 members macrolactone ring) [46]. Furthermore, the PTC undergoes indigenous post-translational modification that confers resistance to an array of protein synthesis inhibitors [47]. Additionally, the PTC possesses significant functional flexibility. Thus, crystal structures of complexes of the large ribosomal subunit with several pleuromutilins indicated that all pleuromutilins bind to the same PTC pocket, albeit by creating somewhat different interactions networks, and are all associated with a shift in the flexible PTC nucleotide U2585 and with an induced fit that tightens the pocket on the bound pleuromutilin antibiotics. The binding selectivity and some resistance mechanisms of this highly conserved region exploit non-conserved remote residues (e.g., those located in the second shell around the binding pocket) that may affect the conformation of nucleotides in the immediate vicinity of the binding pocket [5,48–50].

Importantly, recent advances in pleuromutilin chemistry have yielded several new potential drugs; among them is BC-3205, a novel semisynthetic pleuromutilin derivative that was developed by Nabriva Therapeutics (Vienna, Austria) for intravenous or oral treatment of community-acquired bacterial pneumonia and skin infections. This compound is over 10 times more potent against *S. aureus* (SA) than most pleuromutilins and linezolid, and hence medically relevant. Interestingly, the crystal structure of the complex of the SA large ribosomal subunit (SA50S) indicated that this impressive improvement in potency is achieved by an addition of a single hydrogen bond between BC-3205 and the ribosome (Figure 3) [16].

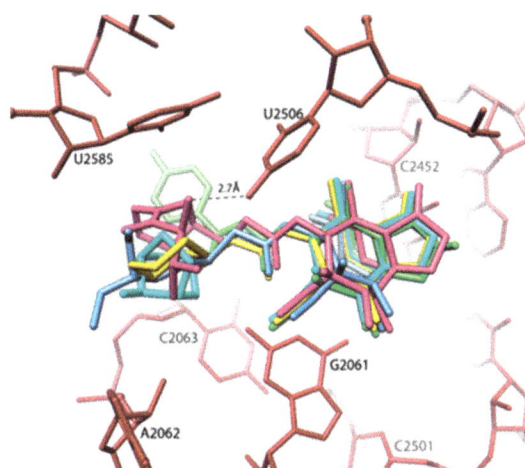

Figure 3. The pleuromutilins binding pocket in SA50S. Color code: SA rRNA-light brown, BC3205-violet, SB571579-green, Retapamulin-cyan, Tiamulin-slate, SB280080-yellow. The pleuromutilins antibiotics are superposed based on the locations of the rRNA of their binding pocket. The critical (additional) H = bond is shown.

2.3. Antibiotic Pairs and Synergism

A common resistance-acquiring mechanism is mutating the anchors between the antibiotic agent and its pocket. Hence, a potential approach to partially overcome (or reduce) resistance is to increase the number of anchors. This can be achieved by the use of pairs of antibiotics that bind to two different functional adjacent sites that can interfere synergistically with ribosomal function, although their synergy may occur independently of their individual effects on the translation [51]. Synercid™ is currently used as a synergetic pair against Gram-positive resistant strains, such as the methicillin-resistant *Staphylococcus aureus* (MSRA) and vancomycin-resistant *Enterococcus faecium* (VREF). This combined drug is made of a pair of semi-synthetic streptogramins, called dalfopristin (component A of Synercid™) and quinupristin (component B), which bind simultaneously to the PTC and to the macrolide binding pocket at the entrance to the exit tunnel, and exploit the inherent flexibility of these sites [52]. The synergistic effect of the streptogramins is driven by the streptogramin A (i.e., dalfopristin), which, upon binding to the 50S subunit, significantly increases the Kd of the streptogramin B (i.e., quinupristin) component. Importantly, the binding interactions network of streptogramin A is associated with a large shift of the essential flexible PTC nucleotide U2585, a motion that significantly alters the functional shape of the active site (Figure 4).

Although Synercid™ has been in use for a rather short period, resistance has already been reported. Hence, searches for additional synergetic pairs are being pursued. One of them is the lankamycin (LM)/lankacidin C (LC) pair, produced by a single organism, *Streptomyces rochei*, which uses dual genes harbored in a large plasmid. This dual production indicates a synergistic mode of action, which was found to display modest ability to inhibit cell growth as well as cell-free translation. In accordance with the biological results [52], the crystallographic structures of the large ribosomal subunit, in a complex with LM as well as with LM and LC together, indicate that their mechanisms for ribosomal inhibition are highly synergetic. It is based on LC binding to the PTC, thus preventing the proper placement of the aminoacyl end of the A-Site tRNA, whereas LM binds to the macrolides binding pocket and physically blocks the progression of the nascent peptides through the tunnel [38,53]. Both components of LM/LC and of Synercid™ bind to similar locations and significantly alter the functional shape of the PTC. Both indicate that flexible ribosomal nucleotides play a key role in drug binding. The stronger binding of LC aids the positioning of LM, thus allowing for synergistic inhibition of the ribosome function. Although the combination LM/LC is not as effective as Synercid™, their position within the ribosome provides clues to the development of more potent ribosomal interfering antibiotics.

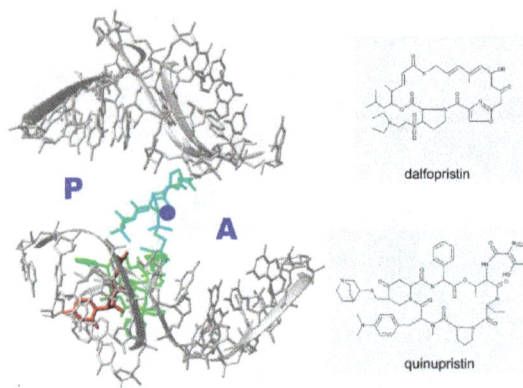

Figure 4. View into the PTC (rRNA backbone in grey), in which the approximate peptide bond formation position is marked by a blue circle, and the A- and P-sites tRNA 3'-ends are marked by A and P. Shown also are the locations of two components of Synercid™ (chemical formulas shown on the right side) within the PTC and in the tunnel's entrance (dalfopristin in cyan and quinupristin in green). Note the swung location, out of the active site of nucleotide U2585 (in red).

2.4. Species Specificity and Susceptibility to Antibiotics

Overall, the binding and functional modes of action of antibiotic drug are common to all eubacteria, including most of those comprising the microbiome. Therefore, an unintentional outcome of the currently preferred broad-spectrum antibiotic treatments is modifying the delicate composition of the microbiome, which was found to be exceedingly influential in issues related to several significant diseases. Since species specificity in antibiotic susceptibility of various pathogenic bacteria targeting the large ribosomal subunit has been reported [54,55], it is suggested that responsiveness to the species-specific differences in drug action should minimize the uncontrolled, wild alterations of the microbiome.

These expectations stimulated the structural studies on ribosomes from genuine pathogens and their careful comparisons to ribosomes from non-pathogenic species [16]. Consequently, the comparison between the structures of the large ribosomal subunit from non-pathogenic bacteria to those from *S. aureus* (SA) led to the identification of unique structural motifs that may be exploited for the design of advanced species-specific antibiotics [16]. Among others, considerable differences between the structures of ribosomes from non-pathogenic bacteria and that of *S. aureus* were detected in the stem loops of several rRNA helices (Figure 5). In parallel, differences were identified by structure and sequence alignments of ribosomal proteins, reflecting the ~50% sequence conservation between eubacterial rProteins. Among them is the medically important protein uL3 (Figure 6) [56,57], which contains a unique insertion segment of a few amino acids.

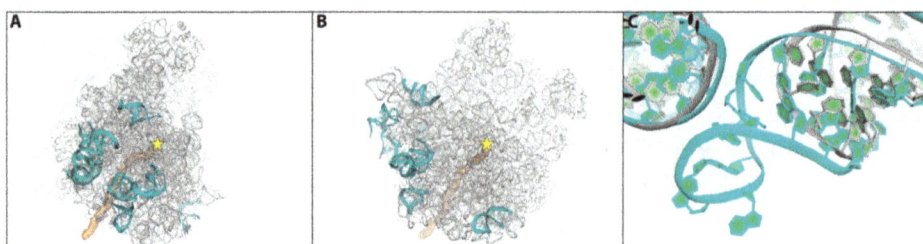

Figure 5. Left: The backbone of the large ribosomal subunit of SA50S is shown in gray from two views (face on (**A**) and a rotation of 90° (**B**)). The polypeptide exit tunnel is shown in gold and the PTC location is marked by a yellow star. The rRNA regions with fold variability compared with all other known structures on the SA50S surface are shown in cyan. Right (**C**): The stem loop of helix H63 in SA (cyan) and of *Deinococcus radiodurans* D50S (grey). Panel A & B are adapted from [16].

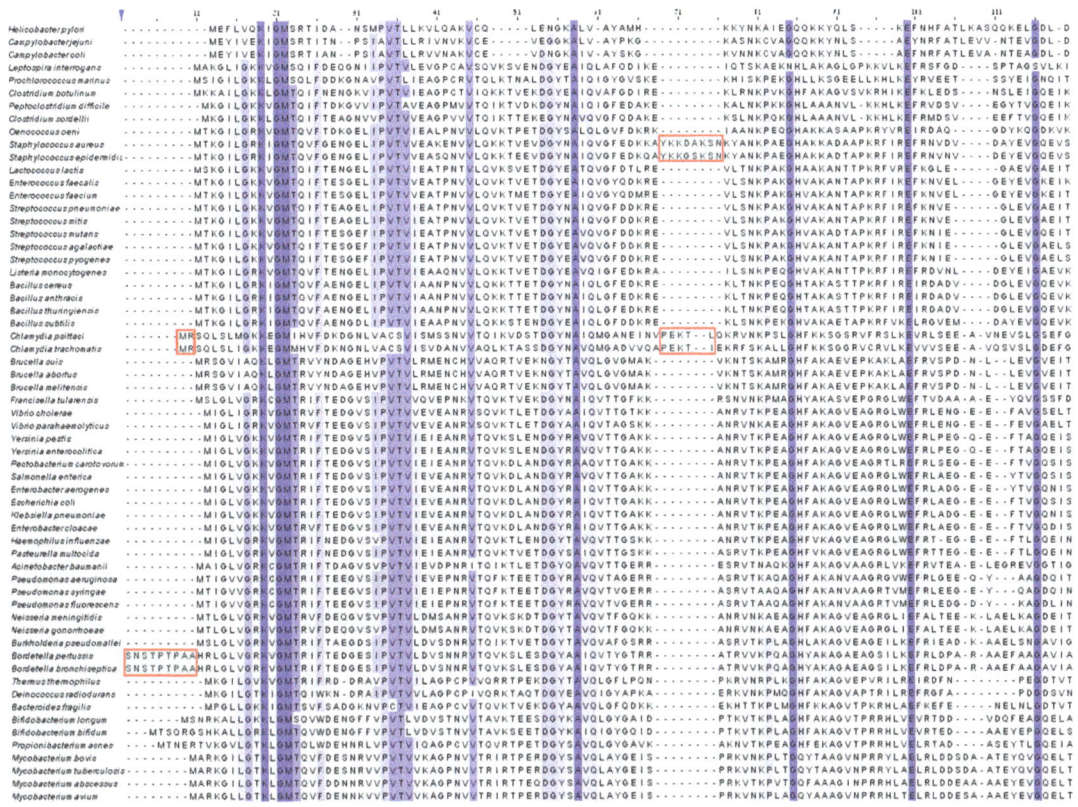

Figure 6. Multiple sequence alignment of protein uL3 from different bacterial species clearly showing its unique additional insertion (framed in red). The conserved sequences are highlighted in purple.

Consequently, it is suggested that species-specific structural motifs should be exploited as drug targets for better distinction between pathogens and the useful bacterial species in the microbiome, including the natural gut flora. This means aiming at the design of "pathogen-specific antibiotics" for each and every pathogen, in contrast to the current preference of broad-spectrum antibiotics. Furthermore, owing to the previous [16] and future identification of species-specific unique structural features, and to the recent indications of the importance of the content and variability of the microbiome, it is clear that the present goal in the field of ribosomal antibiotics should be to minimize antibiotic resistance alongside preserving the natural microbiome.

2.5. Ecological Aspects: Degradable Antibiotics

Many natural antibiotics are made of a scaffold, namely, an organic moiety core, to which one or more branches are covalently connected. Almost all of these scaffolds cannot be fully digested by humans or by animals (e.g., the macrolactone rings of erythromycin and of the various macrolides, ketolides and azalides; the central tricyclic mutilin ring of the pleuromutilins). Hence, their non-degradable metabolites, which are rather toxic, are reaching the environment, contaminating it, and thus increasing antibiotic resistance.

Some of the newly identified potential sites, such as the extended and exposed rRNA helices, can, in principle, be exploited for the design of species-specific potent degradable antibiotics. For pursuing this idea, preliminary studies showed that compounds such as complementary DNA or PNA can interact with these sites and hamper in vitro translation. The ongoing research is based on previous experiments that showed that, oligonucleotides could be used as ribosomal inhibitors as well as tools for structural and functional studies. For example, short DNA oligonucleotides were used as "antisense DNA" to probe rRNA accessibility and for locating specific functional regions [58], before the three-dimensional structures of the ribosomes were determined. Such oligonucleotides can also potentially serve as the basis for future antibacterial drugs. Furthermore, in principle, these sites can also be probed by peptides, as performed recently by using the first 16 residues of mammalian Bac7 [59], or by molecules containing nucleic acids alongside amino acids, which can be optimized in terms of chemical properties and length. Thus, it is suggested that novel antibiotic drugs from degradable chemical components be designed, because their usage should hardly cause ecological or environmental contamination and consequently should reduce antibiotic resistance.

3. Conclusions

The studies reported here highlighted the interplay between internal flexibility, motion complementarity, cellular regulation, and antibiotic resistance. Furthermore, although so far based on a single, albeit important, example, focusing on selected acute issues in current antibiotics usage led to several unexpected and less obvious results, some of which are briefly mentioned below.

- Minimal inhibitory concentration (MIC) values of known antibiotics can be optimized. For example, the additional of a single hydrogen bond between an antibiotic and its pocket improves the MIC dramatically (Figure 3). Flexibility is a common property of antibiotics binding pockets. For example, in synergetic antibiotics, alterations of rRNA conformation proximal to the macrolide's binding pockets can propagate towards the PTC. Additionally, it seems that there is an allosteric link between the tunnel and the catalytic center (PTC) of the ribosome.
- It is suggested that species-specific structural motifs should be exploited for the creation of novel antibiotics with a better distinction between pathogens and useful bacterial species in the microbiome. In fact, the next generation antibiotics should be degradable and species-specific. Thus, the aim of immediate research should be to minimize resistance to antibiotics while preserving the microbiome as well as reducing the contamination of the environment.
- The proposed design of "pathogen-specific antibiotics," which is a revolution in the current concepts of antibiotics, is of immediate need. "Pathogen-specific antibiotics" means antibiotic drugs specific for each and every pathogen. This strategy requires the clinically fast identification of pathogens that is already being addressed [60].
- The practical application of "pathogen-specific antibiotics" requires the swift determination of the structures of antibiotics targets (e.g., ribosomes) of all or most pathogens. For this aim, the recent exciting development of single particle 3D cryo-electron microscopy should be more suitable than X-ray crystallography, since it can be performed by the use of relatively small amounts and does not require crystals.

Acknowledgments: We thank Yael Posner, Shoshana Tel-Or, Miriam Lachever, Yaacov Halfon, and Maggie Kessler for experimental support, as well as the staff of beamlines at APS 19ID and 24ID at APS, and ID23-1, ID29, and ID23-2 at ESRF, for their assistance during data collection. Funding was provided by the Adams Foundation (to C.D. and M.K.) and the Clore Foundation (to M.S.B.), the U.S. National Institutes of Health (GM34360), the European Research Council (Grants ERC 322581-NOVRIB and POC 632167-PATRES), the Advanced Merieux Research Grant, and the Kimmelman Center for Macromolecular Assemblies. A.Y. holds the Martin S. and Helen Kimmel Professorial Chair.

Author Contributions: All authors contributed in one or more aspects of these studies, namely in the design of the biochemical experiments, in the sample preparation, in the collecting, merging, and interpolation of the crystallographic data and/or in the cryo 3D EM studies, in the construction of the electron density maps, in the tracing of the maps, in the comparisons between various structures, and in the identification of the species-specific structural motifs. The list comprises two sub-lists, each arranged alphabetically, among which the members of the first sub-list made major contributions.

References

1. Fischbach, M.A.; Walsh, C.T. Antibiotics for emerging pathogens. *Science* **2009**, *325*, 1089–1093. [CrossRef] [PubMed]

2. Gibbons, A. Resistance to antibiotics found in isolated Amazonian tribe. *Science AAAS* **2015**. [CrossRef]

3. Schlunzen, F.; Zarivach, R.; Harms, J.; Bashan, A.; Tocilj, A.; Albrecht, R.; Yonath, A.; Franceschi, F. Structural basis for the interaction of antibiotics with the peptidyl transferase centre in eubacteria. *Nature* **2001**, *413*, 814–821. [CrossRef] [PubMed]

4. Auerbach, T.; Bashan, A.; Harms, J.; Schluenzen, F.; Zarivach, R.; Bartels, H.; Agmon, I.; Kessler, M.; Pioletti, M.; Franceschi, F.; et al. Antibiotics targeting ribosomes: Crystallographic studies. *Curr. Drug Targets Infect. Disord.* **2002**, *2*, 169–186. [CrossRef] [PubMed]

5. Hansen, J.L.; Moore, P.B.; Steitz, T.A. Structures of five antibiotics bound at the peptidyl transferase center of the large ribosomal subunit. *J. Mol. Biol.* **2003**, *330*, 1061–1075. [CrossRef]

6. Pfister, P.; Jenni, S.; Poehlsgaard, J.; Thomas, A.; Douthwaite, S.; Ban, N.; Bottger, E.C. The structural basis of macrolide-ribosome binding assessed using mutagenesis of 23S rRNA positions 2058 and 2059. *J. Mol. Biol.* **2004**, *342*, 1569–1581. [CrossRef] [PubMed]

7. Schuwirth, B.S.; Borovinskaya, M.A.; Hau, C.W.; Zhang, W.; Vila-Sanjurjo, A.; Holton, J.M.; Cate, J.H. Structures of the bacterial ribosome at 3.5 A resolution. *Science* **2005**, *310*, 827–834. [CrossRef] [PubMed]

8. Dunkle, J.A.; Xiong, L.; Mankin, A.S.; Cate, J.H. Structures of the *Escherichia coli* ribosome with antibiotics bound near the peptidyl transferase center explain spectra of drug action. *Proc. Natl. Acad. Sci. USA* **2010**, *107*, 17152–17157. [CrossRef] [PubMed]

9. Bulkley, D.; Innis, C.A.; Blaha, G.; Steitz, T.A. Revisiting the structures of several antibiotics bound to the bacterial ribosome. *Proc. Natl. Acad. Sci. USA* **2010**, *107*, 17158–17163. [CrossRef] [PubMed]

10. Bulkley, D.; Johnson, F.; Steitz, T.A. The antibiotic thermorubin inhibits protein synthesis by binding to inter-subunit bridge B2a of the ribosome. *J. Mol. Biol.* **2012**, *416*, 571–578. [CrossRef] [PubMed]

11. Polikanov, Y.S.; Szal, T.; Jiang, F.; Gupta, P.; Matsuda, R.; Shiozuka, M.; Steitz, T.A.; Vazquez-Laslop, N.; Mankin, A.S. Negamycin interferes with decoding and translocation by simultaneous interaction with rRNA and tRNA. *Mol. Cell.* **2014**, *56*, 541–550. [CrossRef] [PubMed]

12. Roy, R.N.; Lomakin, I.B.; Gagnon, M.G.; Steitz, T.A. The mechanism of inhibition of protein synthesis by the proline-rich peptide oncocin. *Nat. Struct. Mol. Biol.* **2015**, *22*, 466–469. [CrossRef] [PubMed]

13. Amunts, A.; Fiedorczuk, K.; Truong, T.T.; Chandler, J.; Greenberg, E.P.; Ramakrishnan, V. Bactobolin A binds to a site on the 70S ribosome distinct from previously seen antibiotics. *J. Mol. Biol.* **2015**, *427*, 753–755. [CrossRef] [PubMed]

14. Harms, J.M.; Bartels, H.; Schlunzen, F.; Yonath, A. Antibiotics acting on the translational machinery. *J. Cell. Sci.* **2003**, *116*, 1391–1393. [CrossRef] [PubMed]

15. Noeske, J.; Wasserman, M.R.; Terry, D.S.; Altman, R.B.; Blanchard, S.C.; Cate, J.H. High-resolution structure of the *Escherichia coli* ribosome. *Nat. Struct. Mol. Biol.* **2015**, *22*, 336–341. [CrossRef] [PubMed]

16. Eyal, Z.; Matzov, D.; Krupkin, M.; Wekselman, I.; Paukner, S.; Zimmerman, E.; Rozenberg, H.; Bashan, A.; Yonath, A. Structural insights into species-specific features of the ribosome from the pathogen Staphylococcus aureus. *Proc. Natl. Acad. Sci. USA* **2015**, *112*, E5805–E5814. [CrossRef] [PubMed]

17. Krupkin, M.; Wekselman, I.; Eyal, Z.; Matzov, D.; Rozenberg, H.; Diskin-Posner, Y.; Zimmerman, E.; Yonath, B.A.A. The orthosomycins avilamycin and evernimicin block IF2 and A-tRNA binding to the large ribosomal subunit. In Proceedings of the Ribosome Structure and Function EMBO Meeting, Strasbourg, France, 6–10 July 2016.

18. Douthwaite, S. Designer drugs for discerning bugs. *Proc. Natl. Acad. Sci. USA* **2010**, *107*, 17065–17066. [CrossRef] [PubMed]

19. Berisio, R.; Harms, J.; Schluenzen, F.; Zarivach, R.; Hansen, H.A.; Fucini, P.; Yonath, A. Structural insight into the antibiotic action of telithromycin against resistant mutants. *J. Bacteriol.* **2003**, *185*, 4276–4279. [CrossRef] [PubMed]

20. Berisio, R.; Schluenzen, F.; Harms, J.; Bashan, A.; Auerbach, T.; Baram, D.; Yonath, A. Structural insight into the role of the ribosomal tunnel in cellular regulation. *Nat. Struct. Biol.* **2003**, *10*, 366–370. [CrossRef] [PubMed]

21. Schlunzen, F.; Harms, J.M.; Franceschi, F.; Hansen, H.A.; Bartels, H.; Zarivach, R.; Yonath, A. Structural basis for the antibiotic activity of ketolides and azalides. *Structure* **2003**, *11*, 329–338. [CrossRef]

22. Llano-Sotelo, B.; Dunkle, J.; Klepacki, D.; Zhang, W.; Fernandes, P.; Cate, J.H.; Mankin, A.S. Binding and action of CEM-101, a new fluoroketolide antibiotic that inhibits protein synthesis. *Antimicrob. Agents Chemother.* **2010**, *54*, 4961–4970. [CrossRef] [PubMed]

23. Johansson, M.; Chen, J.; Tsai, A.; Kornberg, G.; Puglisi, J.D. Sequence-dependent elongation dynamics on macrolide-bound ribosomes. *Cell Rep.* **2014**, *7*, 1534–1546. [CrossRef] [PubMed]

24. Kannan, K.; Kanabar, P.; Schryer, D.; Florin, T.; Oh, E.; Bahroos, N.; Tenson, T.; Weissman, J.S.; Mankin, A.S. The general mode of translation inhibition by macrolide antibiotics. *Proc. Natl. Acad. Sci. USA* **2014**, *111*, 15958–15963. [CrossRef] [PubMed]

25. Tu, D.; Blaha, G.; Moore, P.B.; Steitz, T.A. Structures of MLSBK antibiotics bound to mutated large ribosomal subunits provide a structural explanation for resistance. *Cell* **2005**, *121*, 257–270. [CrossRef] [PubMed]

26. Vester, B.; Douthwaite, S. Macrolide resistance conferred by base substitutions in 23S rRNA. *Antimicrob. Agents Chemother.* **2001**, *45*, 1–12. [CrossRef] [PubMed]

27. Vimberg, V.; Xiong, L.; Bailey, M.; Tenson, T.; Mankin, A. Peptide-mediated macrolide resistance reveals possible specific interactions in the nascent peptide exit tunnel. *Mol. Microbiol.* **2004**, *54*, 376–385. [CrossRef] [PubMed]

28. Blaha, G.; Gurel, G.; Schroeder, S.J.; Moore, P.B.; Steitz, T.A. Mutations outside the anisomycin-binding site can make ribosomes drug-resistant. *J. Mol. Biol.* **2008**, *379*, 505–519. [CrossRef] [PubMed]

29. Nakatogawa, H.; Ito, K. The ribosomal exit tunnel functions as a discriminating gate. *Cell* **2002**, *108*, 629–636. [CrossRef]

30. Gong, F.; Yanofsky, C. Rho's role in transcription attenuation in the TNA operon of *E. coli*. *Methods Enzymol.* **2003**, *371*, 383–391. [PubMed]

31. Woolhead, C.A.; Johnson, A.E.; Bernstein, H.D. Translation arrest requires two-way communication between a nascent polypeptide and the ribosome. *Mol. Cell.* **2006**, *22*, 587–598. [CrossRef] [PubMed]

32. Seidelt, B.; Innis, C.A.; Wilson, D.N.; Gartmann, M.; Armache, J.P.; Villa, E.; Trabuco, L.G.; Becker, T.; Mielke, T.; Schulten, K.; et al. Structural insight into nascent polypeptide chain-mediated translational stalling. *Science* **2009**, *326*, 1412–1415. [CrossRef] [PubMed]

33. Ito, K.; Chiba, S.; Pogliano, K. Divergent stalling sequences sense and control cellular physiology. *Biochem. Biophys. Res. Commun.* **2010**, *393*, 1–5. [CrossRef] [PubMed]

34. Chiba, S.; Ito, K. Multisite ribosomal stalling: A unique mode of regulatory nascent chain action revealed for MifM. *Mol. Cell.* **2012**, *47*, 863–872. [CrossRef] [PubMed]

35. Ramu, H.; Vazquez-Laslop, N.; Klepacki, D.; Dai, Q.; Piccirilli, J.; Micura, R.; Mankin, A.S. Nascent peptide in the ribosome exit tunnel affects functional properties of the A-site of the peptidyl transferase center. *Mol. Cell.* **2011**, *41*, 321–330. [CrossRef] [PubMed]

36. Vazquez-Laslop, N.; Klepacki, D.; Mulhearn, D.C.; Ramu, H.; Krasnykh, O.; Franzblau, S.; Mankin, A.S. Role of antibiotic ligand in nascent peptide-dependent ribosome stalling. *Proc. Natl. Acad. Sci. USA* **2011**, *108*, 10496–10501. [CrossRef] [PubMed]

37. Woolstenhulme, C.J.; Parajuli, S.; Healey, D.W.; Valverde, D.P.; Petersen, E.N.; Starosta, A.L.; Guydosh, N.R.; Johnson, W.E.; Wilson, D.N.; Buskirk, A.R. Nascent peptides that block protein synthesis in bacteria. *Proc. Natl. Acad. Sci. USA* **2013**, *110*, E878–E887. [CrossRef] [PubMed]

38. Belousoff, M.J.; Shapira, T.; Bashan, A.; Zimmerman, E.; Rozenberg, H.; Arakawa, K.; Kinashi, H.; Yonath, A. Crystal structure of the synergistic antibiotic pair, lankamycin and lankacidin, in complex with the large ribosomal subunit. *Proc. Natl. Acad. Sci. USA* **2011**, *108*, 2717–2722. [CrossRef] [PubMed]

39. Arenz, S.; Ramu, H.; Gupta, P.; Berninghausen, O.; Beckmann, R.; Vazquez-Laslop, N.; Mankin, A.S.; Wilson, D.N. Molecular basis for erythromycin-dependent ribosome stalling during translation of the ErmBL leader peptide. *Nat. Commun.* **2014**, *5*, 3501. [CrossRef] [PubMed]

40. Berisio, R.; Corti, N.; Pfister, P.; Yonath, A.; Bottger, E.C. 23S rRNA 2058A–>G alteration mediates ketolide resistance in combination with deletion in L22. *Antimicrob. Agents Chemother.* **2006**, *50*, 3816–3823. [CrossRef] [PubMed]

41. Wekselman, I.; Zimmerman, E.; Rozenberg, H.; Bashan, A.; Yonath, A. The structural basis for the mutated ribosomal protein L22 mediated resistance to erythromycin demonstrates the dynamics of the nascent protein exit tunnel. In Proceedings of the 7th FISEB Meeting, Eilat, Israel, 10–13 February 2014.

42. Gregory, S.T.; Dahlberg, A.E. Erythromycin resistance mutations in ribosomal proteins L22 and L4 perturb the higher order structure of 23S ribosomal RNA. *J. Mol. Biol.* **1999**, *289*, 827–834. [CrossRef] [PubMed]

43. Sothiselvam, S.; Liu, B.; Han, W.; Ramu, H.; Klepacki, D.; Atkinson, G.C.; Brauer, A.; Remm, M.; Tenson, T.; Schulten, K.; et al. Macrolide antibiotics allosterically predispose the ribosome for translation arrest. *Proc. Natl. Acad. Sci. USA* **2014**, *111*, 9804–9809. [CrossRef] [PubMed]

44. Pyetan, E.; Baram, D.; Auerbach-Nevo, T.; Yonath, A. Chemical parameters influencing fine-tuning in the binding of macrolide antibiotics to the ribosomal tunnel. *Pure Appl. Chem.* **2007**, *79*, 955–968. [CrossRef]

45. Poulsen, S.M.; Karlsson, M.; Johansson, L.B.; Vester, B. The pleuromutilin drugs tiamulin and valnemulin bind to the RNA at the peptidyl transferase centre on the ribosome. *Mol. Microbiol.* **2001**, *41*, 1091–1099. [CrossRef] [PubMed]

46. Auerbach, T.; Mermershtain, I.; Bashan, A.; Davidovich, C.; Rosenberg, H.; Sherman, D.H.; Yonath, A. Structural basis for the antibacterial activity of the 12-membered-ring mono-sugar macrolide methymycin. *Biotechnology* **2009**, *84*, 24–35.

47. Toh, S.M.; Mankin, A.S. An indigenous posttranscriptional modification in the ribosomal peptidyl transferase center confers resistance to an array of protein synthesis inhibitors. *J. Mol. Biol.* **2008**, *380*, 593–597. [CrossRef] [PubMed]

48. Schlunzen, F.; Pyetan, E.; Fucini, P.; Yonath, A.; Harms, J.M. Inhibition of peptide bond formation by pleuromutilins: The structure of the 50S ribosomal subunit from Deinococcus radiodurans in complex with tiamulin. *Mol. Microbiol.* **2004**, *54*, 1287–1294. [CrossRef] [PubMed]

49. Davidovich, C.; Bashan, A.; Auerbach-Nevo, T.; Yaggie, R.D.; Gontarek, R.R.; Yonath, A. Induced-fit tightens pleuromutilins binding to ribosomes and remote interactions enable their selectivity. *Proc. Natl. Acad. Sci. USA* **2007**, *104*, 4291–4296. [CrossRef] [PubMed]

50. Davidovich, C.; Bashan, A.; Yonath, A. Structural basis for cross-resistance to ribosomal PTC antibiotics. *Proc. Natl. Acad. Sci. USA* **2008**, *105*, 20665–20670. [CrossRef] [PubMed]

51. Noeske, J.; Huang, J.; Olivier, N.B.; Giacobbe, R.A.; Zambrowski, M.; Cate, J.H. Synergy of streptogramin antibiotics occurs independently of their effects on translation. *Antimicrob. Agents Chemother.* **2014**, *58*, 5269–5279. [CrossRef] [PubMed]

52. Harms, J.M.; Schlunzen, F.; Fucini, P.; Bartels, H.; Yonath, A. Alterations at the peptidyl transferase centre of the ribosome induced by the synergistic action of the streptogramins dalfopristin and quinupristin. *BMC Biol.* **2004**, *2*, 4. [CrossRef] [PubMed]

53. Auerbach, T.; Mermershtain, I.; Davidovich, C.; Bashan, A.; Belousoff, M.; Wekselman, I.; Zimmerman, E.; Xiong, L.; Klepacki, D.; Arakawa, K.; et al. The structure of ribosome-lankacidin complex reveals ribosomal sites for synergistic antibiotics. *Proc. Natl. Acad. Sci. USA* **2010**, *107*, 1983–1988. [CrossRef] [PubMed]

54. Wilson, D.N. On the specificity of antibiotics targeting the large ribosomal subunit. *Ann. N. Y. Acad. Sci.* **2011**, *1241*, 1–16. [CrossRef] [PubMed]

55. Kannan, K.; Mankin, A.S. Macrolide antibiotics in the ribosome exit tunnel: Species-specific binding and action. *Ann. N. Y. Acad. Sci.* **2011**, *1241*, 33–47. [CrossRef] [PubMed]

56. Meskauskas, A.; Petrov, A.N.; Dinman, J.D. Identification of functionally important amino acids of ribosomal protein L3 by saturation mutagenesis. *Mol. Cell Biol.* **2005**, *25*, 10863–10874. [CrossRef] [PubMed]

57. Pringle, M.; Poehlsgaard, J.; Vester, B.; Long, K.S. Mutations in ribosomal protein L3 and 23S ribosomal RNA at the peptidyl transferase centre are associated with reduced susceptibility to tiamulin in *Brachyspira* spp. Isolates. *Mol. Microbiol.* **2004**, *54*, 1295–1306. [CrossRef] [PubMed]

58. Weller, J.; Hill, W.E. Probing the initiation complex formation on *E. coli* ribosomes using short complementary DNA oligomers. *Biochimie* **1991**, *73*, 971–981. [CrossRef]

59. Seefeldt, A.C.; Graf, M.; Perebaskine, N.; Nguyen, F.; Arenz, S.; Mardirossian, M.; Scocchi, M.; Wilson, D.N.; Innis, C.A. Structure of the mammalian antimicrobial peptide Bac7(1–16) bound within the exit tunnel of a bacterial ribosome. *Nucleic Acids Res.* **2016**, *44*, 2429–2438. [CrossRef] [PubMed]

60. Lam, B.; Das, J.; Holmes, R.D.; Live, L.; Sage, A.; Sargent, E.H.; Kelley, S.O. Solution-based circuits enable rapid and multiplexed pathogen detection. *Nat. Commun.* **2013**, *4*, 2001–2003. [CrossRef] [PubMed]

2

Identification of *Staphylococcus aureus* Cellular Pathways Affected by the Stilbenoid Lead Drug SK-03-92 using a Microarray

William R. Schwan [1,2,*] ⓘ, Rebecca Polanowski [1,2], Paul M. Dunman [3], Sara Medina-Bielski [1,2], Michelle Lane [1,2], Marc Rott [1,2], Lauren Lipker [1,2], Amy Wescott [1,2], Aaron Monte [2,4], James M. Cook [5] ⓘ, Douglas D. Baumann [6], V.V.N. Phani Babu Tiruveedhula [5] ⓘ, Christopher M. Witzigmann [5], Cassandra Mikel [1,2] and Md Toufiqur Rahman [5] ⓘ

[1] Department of Microbiology, University of Wisconsin-La Crosse, La Crosse, WI 54601, USA; rpolanowski@uwlax.edu (R.P.); s.medinabielski@gmail.com (S.M.-B.); lanem7285@gmail.com (M.L.); mrott@uwlax.edu (M.R.); lipker.laur@uwlax.edu (L.L.); amywescott16@gmail.com (A.W.); cassandra.mm010@gmail.com (C.M.)

[2] Emerging Technology Center for Pharmaceutical Development, University of Wisconsin-La Crosse, La Crosse, WI 54601, USA; amonte@uwlax.edu

[3] School of Medicine and Dentistry, University of Rochester, Rochester, NY 14642, USA; paul_dunman@urmc.rochester.edu

[4] Department of Chemistry and Biochemistry, University of Wisconsin-La Crosse, La Crosse, WI 54601, USA

[5] Department of Chemistry and Biochemistry, University of Wisconsin-Milwaukee, Milwaukee, WI 53211, USA; capncook@uwm.edu (J.M.C.); tiruvee2@uwm.edu (V.V.N.P.B.T.); witzigm2@uwm.edu (C.M.W.); mdrahman@uwm.edu (M.T.R.)

[6] Department of Mathematics and Statistics, University of Wisconsin-La Crosse, La Crosse, WI 54601, USA; dbaumann@uwlax.edu

[*] Correspondence: wschwan@uwlax.edu

Academic Editor: Christopher C. Butler

Abstract: The mechanism of action for a new lead stilbene compound coded SK-03-92 with bactericidal activity against methicillin-resistant *Staphylococcus aureus* (MRSA) is unknown. To gain insight into the killing process, transcriptional profiling was performed on SK-03-92 treated vs. untreated *S. aureus*. Fourteen genes were upregulated and 38 genes downregulated by SK-03-92 treatment. Genes involved in sortase A production, protein metabolism, and transcriptional regulation were upregulated, whereas genes encoding transporters, purine synthesis proteins, and a putative two-component system (SACOL2360 (MW2284) and SACOL2361 (MW2285)) were downregulated by SK-03-92 treatment. Quantitative real-time polymerase chain reaction analyses validated upregulation of *srtA* and *tdk* as well as downregulation of the MW2284/MW2285 and purine biosynthesis genes in the drug-treated population. A quantitative real-time polymerase chain reaction analysis of *MW2284* and *MW2285* mutants compared to wild-type cells demonstrated that the *srtA* gene was upregulated by both putative two-component regulatory gene mutants compared to the wild-type strain. Using a transcription profiling technique, we have identified several cellular pathways regulated by SK-03-92 treatment, including a putative two-component system that may regulate *srtA* and other genes that could be tied to the SK-03-92 mechanism of action, biofilm formation, and drug persisters.

Keywords: stilbene; microarray; *Staphylococcus aureus*; gene regulation; drug mechanism of action; sortase; biofilm

1. Introduction

Staphylococcus aureus is a common inhabitant of the human body that also causes numerous infections, including skin and soft tissue infections as well as more serious infections, such as pneumonia and bacteremia [1].   Presently, around 60% of *S. aureus* clinical isolates are methicillin-resistant *S. aureus* (MRSA) [2], and this bacterium is a leading cause of nosocomial infections in the United States [3,4]. In 1997, community-associated methicillin-resistant *S. aureus* (CA-MRSA) strains emerged in the United States, causing infections in younger people, including necrotizing pneumonia [5–7]. Although skin infections caused by CA-MRSA are still prevalent, invasive MRSA infections have decreased [3,8]. In addition to methicillin resistance, CA-MRSA strains are becoming multidrug resistant at an alarming rate [9–11]. Heterogeneous vancomycin-intermediate *S. aureus* and vancomycin-resistant strains of *S. aureus* have led to vancomycin being less effective against some *S. aureus* infections [12–15]. Tolerance to vancomycin now has been reported to be as low as 3% and as high as 47% [16,17]. New drugs are needed to treat MRSA infections; however, most drugs currently in development are derivatives of drugs already being marketed [18,19]. *S. aureus* is one of the ESKAPE pathogens (*Enterococcus faecium, Staphylococcus aureus, Klebsiella pneumoniae, Acinetobacter baumannii, Pseudomonas aeruginosa* and *Enterobacter* species) targeted by the 10×20 initiative to develop 10 new, safe and effective antibiotics approved by 2020 [20].

In support of the 10×20 initiative, a new antibiotic identified as (E)-3-hydroxy-5-methoxystilbene with promising activity against *S. aureus* was identified from *Comptonia peregrina* (L.) Coulter ("sweet fern") [21].   A structure–activity relationship analysis identified our lead compound, (E)-3-(2-(benzo[b]thiophen-2-yl)vinyl)-5-methoxyphenol; for simplicity, SK-03-92. SK-03-92 was rapidly bactericidal (killing 90% of the population within an hour) against every Gram-positive species that was tested, including MRSA strains [22]. Importantly, a combined safety and pharmacokinetic study demonstrated that the SK-03-92 lead drug was safe in mice [23]. As with all antimicrobials, therapeutic treatment can result in residual bacteria not being killed by that antimicrobial, a phenomenon known as persistence [24–26]. Drug persisters are phenotypically different than the parent strain, but are not true drug resistant variants because the MICs of the drug persisters are the same as their parent strains [27,28]. Persisters are thought to be a major component of bacterial biofilms, allowing significant drug tolerance [29,30]. Many drugs used to treat *S. aureus* infections have drug persister population emerge that are recalcitrant to treatment. To gain insight into the mechanism of action of SK-03-92 and the mechanism of *S. aureus* persistence to SK-03-92 treatment, the effect of SK-03-92 on *S. aureus* cells was assessed by transcriptional profiling in the *S. aureus* strain MW2.

2. Results and Discussion

2.1. General Transcriptome Response of SK-03-92 Treatment

New drugs to treat *S. aureus* infections are urgently needed, and SK-03-92 holds considerable promise. SK-03-92 has a stilbenoid backbone [22] and is bactericidal within an hour; however, 10% of the population survives as drug persisters that can grow in media containing up to 32 µg/mL of SK-03-92 but with an MIC equivalent to untreated *S. aureus* cells. The mechanism of action for SK-03-92 is unknown. To ascertain the effects of SK-03-92 treatment on the transcriptome of *S. aureus*, total RNA was isolated from *S. aureus* strain MW2 cultures (Table 1) treated for 30 min with 8× the MIC of SK-03-92 and untreated MW2 cultures and an RNA microarray was performed. A total of 52 genes were dysregulated by the SK-03-92 drug treatment (Table 2), representing 2% of the total *S. aureus* transcriptome. This is remarkable because transcriptional profiling of other bactericidal compounds has shown a larger effect on the *S. aureus* transcriptome, including ortho-phenylphenol (24%) [31], amicoumacin A (20%) [32] and daptomycin (5% to 32%) [33,34]. Interestingly, the number of downregulated genes (73.1%) greatly surpassed the number of upregulated genes (26.9%).

An examination of genes affected by treatment with other stilbene type compounds demonstrates the disparity in their transcript profile compared to treatment with SK-03-92. Pterostilbene, another stilbenoid compound, in *Saccharomyces cerevisiae* showed 1189 genes that were dysregulated: 1007 upregulated (85%) and 182 downregulated (15%) [35]. Microarray analysis with resveratrol treated *Schizosaccharomyces pombe* showed 480 genes dysregulated, 377 genes that were upregulated and 103 that were downregulated [36]. RNA sequence analysis of resveratrol treated *S. aureus* cells demonstrated 444 dysregulated genes, 201 upregulated and 243 downregulated [37]. The majority of the genes in our study had a two- to four-fold difference in transcript abundance when comparing SK-03-92 treated vs. untreated *S. aureus* cultures. Very few genes dysregulated by SK-03-92 were previously shown to be dysregulated by resveratrol (e.g., downregulation of the *purD*, *purH*, *purL*, *lrgA*, and *sdhC* genes). Only three genes had a 10-fold or higher change in transcript levels, which included two genes annotated to be part of a putative two-component system (TCS) (*SACOL2360* (annotated as *MW2284* in MW2 strain) = 14.1-fold lower and *SACOL2361* (annotated as *MW2285* in MW2 strain) = 26.9-fold lower) as well as the *glpD* gene encoding glycerol-3-phosphate dehydrogenase (10-fold higher).

Table 1. Bacterial strains used in this study.

Bacterial Strain	Genotype	Reference
S. aureus		
MW2	USA400 wild-type	[7]
JE2	USA300 wild-type	[38]
NE272	JE2 *MW2284* mutant	[38]
NE671	JE2 *MW2285* mutant	[38]
NE1363	JE2 *srtB* mutant	[38]
NE1787	JE2 *srtA* mutant	[38]
L. monocytogenes		
EGD	Wild-type	[39]
EGD *srtA*	EGD *srtA* mutant	[39]
EGD *srtB*	EGD *srtB* mutant	[39]

Dysregulated genes tied to a potential mechanism of action for SK-03-92 included *glpD*, *adhE* (*SACOL0135*), *adhP* (*SACOL0660*), and *sdhC* (*SACOL1158*). GlpD funnels electrons into the respiratory chain via quinone or menaquinone reduction coupled to the oxidation of glycerol-3-phosphate to glycerone phosphate (dihydroxyacetone phosphate) [40], which can be enzymatically or non-enzymatically transformed into methylglyoxal (MG) [41]. Higher concentrations of MG are thought to halt bacterial growth by damaging proteins by acting as a protein glycating agent that mainly affects arginine residues [42,43]. In *Candida albicans*, ADH1 catalyzes the NAD+ linked oxidation of MG to pyruvate and disruption of the *adh1* gene in *C. albicans* caused accumulation of MG followed by inhibition of growth [44]. The dysregulation of *glpD* and *adh* genes suggests that MG was accumulating and glycation was occurring in SK-03-92-treated *S. aureus*. MG glycation of proteins, lipids, and DNA generate advanced glycation end products (AGEs) [43]. Importantly, GlpD has been implicated in drug persistence in *Escherichia coli* [45] and *S. aureus* [34].

A number of genes involved in metabolism were also dysregulated by SK-03-92 treatment, including the *gcvH* gene that encodes GcvH, which shuttles the methylamine group of glycine from the P-protein to the T-protein via a lipoyl group [46]. Genes associated with protein degradation and repair had altered transcript abundance in SK-03-92-treated *S. aureus*. Transcripts encoding a putative repair system for deglycation of Amadori protein adducts derived from ribose-5-P (*ptpA*) [47] showed altered abundance in SK-03-92-treated *S. aureus*, as did the transcript encoding the enzyme that produces ribose-5-P (*SACOL2605*). The formation of Amadori protein adducts occurs spontaneously via a dehydrogenation mechanism when ribose-5-P interacts with an amine, such as the lysine residues of proteins. Amadori glycated proteins undergo further spontaneous reactions to become AGEs. AGEs promote protein aggregation [47,48]. Since *ptpA* transcript abundance was increased 2.3-fold and the kinase transcript *SACOL2605* was decreased 9.6-fold, ribulosamine substrates produced were likely not being deglycated, and protein repair was not occurring. Phase-dark and phase-bright inclusions were observed microscopically in SK-03-92-treated *B. subtilis*, consistent with perturbation of proteostasis resulting in visible accumulation of protein aggregates [49]. Uncontrolled protein aggregation is toxic to cells [48].

Table 2. Microarray analysis of genes dysregulated in *S. aureus* MW2 cells treated with 8× the SK-03-92 MIC vs. untreated cells.

Locus	Fold-Difference	Description
Stress Response		
SACOL1759	−2.3	universal stress protein family
Transporter		
SACOL0086	−2.0	drug transporter, putative
SACOL0155	−5.7	cation efflux family protein
SACOL0178	−2.9	PTS system, IIBC components (*scrBC*)
SACOL0400	−2.6	ascorbate-specific PTS system subunit IIC (*ulaA*)
SACOL0454	−2.3	sodium:dicarboxylate symporter family protein
SACOL1018	−2.3	sodium:alanine symporter family protein
SACOL1872	−3.0	epidermin immunity protein F (*epiE*)
SACOL2146	−2.7	PTS system, mannitol-specific IIBC components (*mtlA*)
SACOL2333	−2.8	YnfA family protein
SACOL2573	−3.2	copper ion binding protein (*copZ*)
SACOL2664	−2.3	mannose-6-phosphate isomerase (*manA*)
SACOL2718	−4.6	2-oxoglutarate/malate translocator, sodium sulfate symporter
Signaling/Regulation		
SACOL2360	−14.1	LytTR family regulator protein
SACOL2361	−26.9	histidine kinase sensor membrane protein
SACOL2340	2.2	transcriptional regulator TetR-family
Cell Wall Associated		
SACOL0151	−2.7	UDP-*N*-acetylglucosamine 2-epimerase Cap5P (*cap5P*)
SACOL0247	−3.2	holin-like protein LrgA (*lrgA*)
SACOL0612	−2.1	glycosyl transferase, group 1 family protein
SACOL1071	−2.2	chitinase-related protein (*iraE*)
SACOL2554	−2.0	holin-like protein CidB (*cidB*)
SACOL2539	4.2	sortase A (*srtA*)
Anabolism/Nucleic Acids		
SACOL013	−2.1	5′ nucleotidase family protein
SACOL1078	−3.2	phosphoribosylformylglycinamidine synthase II (*purL*)
SACOL1082	−2.5	bifunctional purine biosynthesis protein (*purH*)
SACOL1083	−2.6	phosphoribosylamine-glycine ligase (*purD*)
SACOL2329	−3.5	ribose 5-phosphate isomerase (*rpiA*)
SACOL2111	2.2	thymidine kinase (*tdk*)
SACOL2377	2.3	conserved hypothetical protein
Anabolism/Proteostasis		
SACOL0085	−2.5	peptidase, M20.M25/M40 family
SACOL2605	−9.6	ribulosamine 3-kinase
SACOL0457	2.6	conserved hypothetical protein, heat induced stress
SACOL0590	2.4	30S ribosomal protein L7 Ae
SACOL0877	2.5	glycine cleavage system H protein (*gcvH*)
SACOL1907	2.4	ribosomal large subunit pseudouridine synthase (*rluD*)
SACOL1939	2.3	phosphotyrosine protein phosphatase (*ptpA*)
SACOL2596	2.6	metallo-dependent amidohydrolase

Table 2. *Cont.*

Locus	Fold-Difference	Description
Lipid Metabolism		
SACOL2091	−2.5	beta-hydroxyacyl-dehydratase FabZ (*fabZ*)
SACOL2459	−3.8	para-nitrobenzyl esterase (*pnbA*)
SACOL1142	10.0	aerobic glyerol-3-phosphate dehydrogenase (*glpD*)
Catabolism		
SACOL0135	−2.4	alcohol dehydrogenase, iron-containing (*adhE*)
SACOL0660	−3.4	alcohol dehydrogenase, zinc-containing (*adhA*)
SACOL1158	−2.5	succinate dehydrogenase, cytochrome b558 subunit (*sdhC*)
SACOL1604	−2.1	glucokinase (*glk*)
SACOL2338	−3.5	hypothetical protein (putative oxidoreductase)
SACOL1713	2.3	hypothetical protein, putative ammonia monooxygenase
Unknown		
SACOL0089	−4.4	myosin-reactive antigen, 67 kDa
SACOL2315	−3.8	conserved hypothetical protein
SACOL2338	−3.4	conserved hypothetical protein
SACOL2491	−2.9	conserved hypothetical protein
SACOL0742	3.1	conserved hypothetical protein
SACOL1789	2.4	conserved hypothetical protein

Three genes associated with purine synthesis were downregulated: *purD*, *purH*, and *purL*. Purine metabolism is a necessary part of DNA synthesis and energy production in *S. aureus* [50]. Genes involved in purine metabolism are often downregulated after treatment with a drug or plant extract [51–53]. In addition, one gene associated with pyrimidine synthesis, *tdk*, was upregulated. Thymidine kinase transfers the terminal phosphate from ATP to thymidine or deoxyuridine [54]. A decrease in the synthesis of purines coupled with an increase in phosphorylation of pyrimidines could result in a dramatic reorganization of the intracellular nucleotide pool. Moreover, less purine metabolism is often tied to drug persister populations [55,56]. Disruption of nucleotide metabolism in a library of *S. aureus* transposon insertion mutants caused a decrease in persister formation frequency when treated with rifampicin [57].

Consistent with the formation of persister strains, mRNA levels of genes linked to programmed cell death (PCD) were decreased in *S. aureus* cultures treated with SK-03-92. Specifically, the Cid/Lrg (holin/antiholin) system, which controls autolysis and affects the distribution of extracellular DNA in *S. aureus* during biofilm development [58–60]. This prokaryotic PCD is analogous to the bcl-2 pro-apoptotic effector and anti-apoptotic mediated apoptosis in eukaryotes [61,62].

Twelve putative transport genes were dysregulated encoding for proteins involved in anion transport, a cation efflux family protein, two phosphotransferase system (PTS) transporters, a sodium:alanine symporter, sodium:dicarboxylate symporter family protein, and a copper ion binding protein. The only true virulence factor genes affected by SK-03-92 treatment were the *SACOL0151 cap5P*, *epiE*, *SACOL2333* gene encoding a YnfA family protein putative transport small multidrug resistance family-3 protein [63], and the *srtA* gene encoding sortase A that will be described in more detail below [64]. Five genes identified by the microarray were annotated as hypothetical proteins with no known function (three downregulated and two upregulated).

2.2. Genes of a Putative TCS Are Significantly Downregulated by SK-03-92 Treatment

A surprising microarray result that was no known *S. aureus* global regulatory genes were shown to be affected by the drug treatment. Microarray analysis of daptomycin treated *S. aureus* demonstrated that the the *icaR* gene was dysregulated compared to untreated cells [34]. Our microarray showed that a *tetR*-family transcriptional regulator, SACOL2340, and two genes that comprise a putative TCS in *S. aureus* annotated as *MW2284* (14.1-fold downregulated) and *MW2285* in strain MW2 (26.3-fold downregulated) were downregulated. A bioinformatic analysis of the putative MW2284 and MW2285 proteins suggest that they comprise a putative two-component regulatory system where MW2284 (LytTR superfamily regulator protein) is the response regulator protein and MW2285 (membrane protein) is the sensor kinase protein. MW2284 was identified as a 440-bp ORF encoding a putative 14.7-kDa transcriptional regulator protein and MW2285 was identified as a 455-bp ORF encoding a putative 15.1-kDa histidine kinase sensor protein. The MW2285 ORF has a 3-bp overlap with the MW2284 ORF. BLASTP, PSI-BLAST, and BLASTN bioinformatics analyses [65] showed that MW2284 aligned with other two-component regulatory system regulator proteins and MW2285 aligned with other two-component regulatory system sensor proteins. Both proteins have homology with LytTR superfamily proteins involved in the regulation of bacterial genes [66]. LytTR proteins regulate virulence gene expression in a variety of bacterial species including *S. aureus*. The AgrA transcriptional regulator is one of these LytTR-type proteins [67]. Moreover, the MW2284 and MW2285 ORFs appeared to be conserved across a wide number of Gram-positive species, including all *Staphylococcus* and *Streptococcus* species, as well as *Bacillus, Clostridium, Lactobacillus, Listeria,* and *Leuconostoc*.

The same LytTR TCS dysregulated in SK-03-92-treated *S. aureus* was upregulated in purine synthesis deficient mutants in *S. aureus* [68]. The putative sensor kinase (MW2285) was upregulated in *purH* mutants and the response regulator (MW2284) was upregulated in *purA* mutants (adenylosuccinate synthetase involved in purine biosynthesis). The response regulator component transcript was also upregulated during anaerobic growth in another study [69]. A transposon mutant of the sensor kinase component has been previously shown to be viable, capable of producing a more robust biofilm, and had a lower LD50 than the parent strain [70,71]. The mechanistic link between defects in purine synthesis, persister formation, and the LytTR regulatory system remains unclear. Furthermore, RNAseq analysis of resveratrol treated *S. aureus* cells showed an almost 8-fold downregulation of the MW2284 gene, but no effect on the MW2285 gene [37].

2.3. Validation of Microarray Data by qRT-PCR

The microarray results were confirmed using qRT-PCR analyses on RNAs from 8× the MIC SK-03-92 treated MW2 cells vs. untreated MW2 cells. Transcription of the *srtA* gene was significantly upregulated almost 6-fold ($p < 0.006$, Figure 1) and the *tdk* gene was also upregulated 2.1-fold ($p < 0.03$) in SK-03-92 treated cells vs. untreated cells. On the other hand, several genes involved in purine biosynthesis (*purD, purH,* and *purL*) were shown to be significantly downregulated 2.2- to 2.4-fold ($p < 0.01$ to 0.04), whereas the MW2284 and MW2285 genes were downregulated 4- ($p < 0.01$) and 3-fold ($p < 0.003$), respectively, in the SK-03-92 treated samples. These results confirmed that treatment with the SK-03-92 lead compound caused dysregulation of the *srtA, tdk, purD, purH, purL,* MW2284, and MW2285 genes.

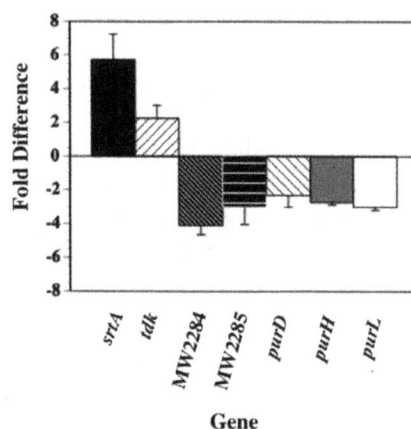

Figure 1. Quantitative reverse transcribed-polymerase chain reaction results of *S. aureus* MW2 cells treated with 8× the SK-03-92 MIC vs. untreated cells. The data represents the mean + standard deviation from at least three separate runs.

2.4. SK-03-92 Treatment Causes Alteration of Nucleotide Pool

Because three *pur* genes involved in purine synthesis and the *tdk* gene were dysregulated by SK-03-92 treatment, the rapid accumulation of the bacterial alarmone (p)ppGpp and the state of the intracellular nucleotide pool were examined using high-performance liquid chromatography (HPLC, Waters, Milford, MA, USA). Inhibition of isoleucyl tRNA synthetase by mupirocin has been shown to induce production of (p)ppGpp in *S. aureus* [72,73]. A highly phosphorylated ribonucleotide, (p)ppGpp, can be identified via rapid separation of the *S. aureus* nucleotide pool using anion-exchange HPLC, where (p)ppGpp elutes as a late peak, which can be detected by absorbance at 254 and 280 nm [74]. In control experiments, this late peak was not detected in untreated cells (Figure 2A), but was detected following treatment with mupirocin (Figure 2B). No (p)ppGpp was detected following treatment with SK-03-92 (Figure 2C). However, the composition and quantity (area under curve) of the nucleotide pool was altered in SK-03-92 treated *S. aureus* as compared to untreated cells (Figure 2A vs. Figure 2C), suggesting that dysregulation of *tdk* and the three purine biosynthesis genes by SK-03-92 treatment depleted the nucleotide pool.

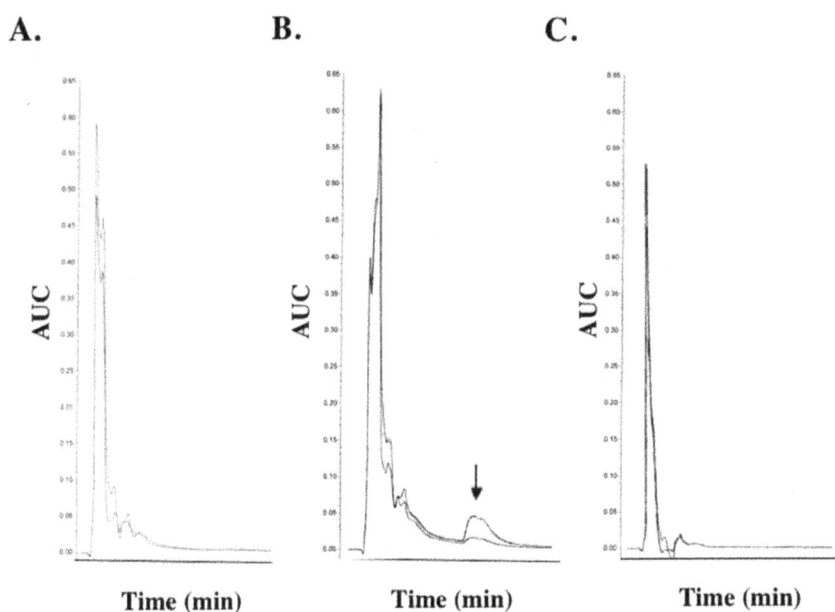

Figure 2. Absorbance (254 and 280 nm) of the formic acid extracted nucleotide pool of log-phase *S. aureus* ATCC 29213 after 20 min with either (**A**) no treatment, (**B**) 60 µg/mL mupirocin, or (**C**) 16 µg/mL SK-03-92. Arrow denotes the (p)ppGpp peak.

2.5. Biofilm Formation Increases as the Concentration of SK-03-92 Increases

With an increase in *srtA* transcript abundance shown by the qRT-PCR results, an increase in biofilm formation would be expected following SK-03-92 treatment. To further analyze the effects of the increase in *srtA* transcription, a biofilm assay in microtiter plates was performed after SK-03-92 drug treatment (Figure 3). Wild-type JE2 and MW2 cultures were tested following SK-03-92 drug treatment (range 0.5–0.64 µg/mL). The JE2 culture grown without drug showed an OD_{570} of 2.41, whereas the MW2 culture had an OD_{570} of 2.50.

The SK-03-92 drug had a biphasic effect on the wild-type strains. At low concentrations, the drug reduced biofilm formation as exhibited by the 0.5 and 1 µg/mL data points that were significant for both strains that were tested ($p < 0.05$). As concentrations of SK-03-92 increased, the OD570 readings increased, plateauing at 32 µg/mL for both strains. Strain MW2 showed significant increases in biofilm formation going from 0 µg/mL to 8–64 µg/mL SK-03-92 concentration ($p < 0.05$). A similar finding was observed when *Candida* species grown as a biofilm were exposed to varying concentrations of echinocandin [75]. *Candida* treated with low drug concentrations killed the fungal cells but at concentrations higher than the MIC showed there was an increase in the cell density of the biofilms. Echinocandin acting on the *Candida* species has the same effect as our SK-03-92 drug, triggering upregulation of a specific gene that increases biofilm formation.

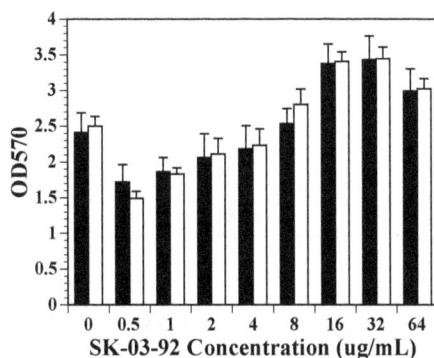

Figure 3. The effects of SK-03-92 drug concentration on 24 h biofilm formation (OD_{570}) for *S. aureus* strains JE2 (black column) and MW2 (white column). All experiments represent the mean + standard deviation of at least 10 runs done in triplicate.

Under normal growth conditions, biofilm formation is not necessary for a cell, but under stressful environmental conditions, such as exposure to the SK-03-92 drug, biofilm formation would greatly benefit the *S. aureus* population. Formation of a biofilm would benefit cells by allowing for the formation of persister cell populations [76]. When biofilms form, the cells at the base of the biofilm slow or stop most cell metabolism and go into a dormant state, allowing the organisms to survive in the presence of a drug, for example SK-03-92. In addition, cells in a biofilm often undergo quorum sensing, which also can lead to the emergence of persister cells [77].

2.6. A Sortase A Mutant Has a Lower MIC against SK-03-92 Than Wild-Type

Since the putative MW2284/MW2285 TCS appears to repress transcription of the *srtA* gene, this regulatory effect could be tied to the mechanism of action of the SK-03-92 drug. Sortase A was first described in *S. aureus* in 1999 [64]. The protein covalently anchors surface proteins (e.g., fibronectin-binding protein, fibrinogen-binding protein, protein A, clumping factors, collagen adhesion protein) to the cell wall of *S. aureus* and other Gram-positive bacteria [77]. An LPXTG motif [78–80] is common among these anchored proteins and many are important for phase I of biofilm formation that allows attachment to biotic or abiotic surfaces [81]. A mutation of the *srtA* gene caused less expression of several cell wall anchored surface proteins [82,83]. Moreover, *srtA* mutants are attenuated compared to the wild-type strain in a variety of murine models of infection [82,84,85].

Because *srtA* and *MW2284/MW2285* transcription were affected by SK-03-92 treatment, MICs were performed using the SK-03-92 lead compound on an *srtA* mutant (NE1787), *srtB* mutant (control, NE1363), *MW2284* mutant (NE671), and *MW2285* mutant (NE272) compared to the wild-type strain JE2 [38]. The *srtB*, *MW2284*, and *MW2285* mutants had MICs that were equal to the wild-type strain (Table 3). However, the *srtA* mutant had an MIC that was 2-fold lower than the wild-type strain. When a *Listeria monocytogenes srtA* mutant was tested [39], the MIC for the *srtA* strain was 8-fold lower than the wild-type strain. A *L. monocytogenes srtB* mutant had the same MIC as the wild-type bacteria.

Table 3. MIC results for *S. aureus* and *L. monocytogenes* mutants and wild-type strains against SK-03-92.

Strain	Genotype	MIC
S. aureus		
JE2	Wild-type	1 [a]
NE272	*MW2285*	1
NE671	*MW2284*	1
NE1363	*srtB*	1
NE1787	*srtA*	0.5
L. monocytogenes		
EGD	Wild-type	1
EGD *srtA*	*srtA*	0.125
EGD *srtB*	*srtB*	1

[a] Mean + standard deviation from three separate runs.

Presumably, SK-03-92 treatment causes downregulation of the *MW2285* gene with an effect that would be similar to a mutation in the MW2285 gene. The regulatory effect could be derepression of *srtA* transcription. Either event would create more SrtA protein that in turn would allow greater extracellular presentation of proteins on the surface of *S. aureus* cells. This result may suggest that something tethered to the cell walls by sortase A that is conserved in both species may be tied to the mechanism of action of the SK-03-92 drug, and we are exploring this possibility.

2.7. Mutations in the MW2284/MW2285 Two-Component Regulatory Genes Cause an Upregulation of the srtA Gene

Since the microarray results showed significant upregulation of the *srtA* gene and downregulation of the *MW2284* and *MW2285* genes, we hypothesized that the MW2284 gene product, a putative transcriptional regulator protein, may be repressing the *srtA* gene. To confirm that the putative two-component regulatory system (MW2284/MW2285) may be involved in repressing the *srtA* gene, we obtained transposon mutant strains from the Nebraska Transposon Mutant Library [38] with insertion mutations in the *MW2284* and *MW2285* genes. A qRT-PCR analysis was then undertaken on RNA isolated from the NE272 (*MW2285* mutation) and NE671 (*MW2284* mutation) strains compared to the wild-type strain JE2, targeting the *srtA* gene. The results showed that mutations in both the *MW2284* and *MW2285* genes led to a 9.2-fold ($p < 0.005$) and 8.1-fold ($p < 0.0008$) upregulation of *srtA* transcription, respectively, suggesting that this putative two-component regulatory system may be repressing transcription of the *srtA* gene (Figure 4).

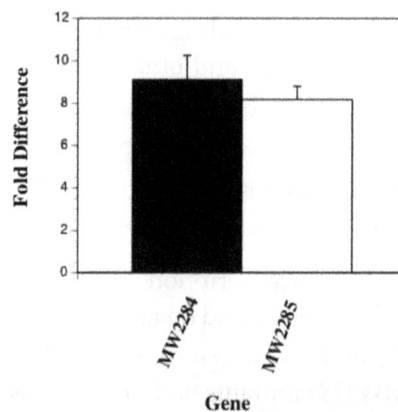

Figure 4. Quantitative reverse transcribed-polymerase chain reaction results of *S. aureus srtA* transcription in wild-type bacteria compared to MW2284 and MW2285 mutants. The data represents the mean + standard deviation from three separate runs.

3. Experimental Section

3.1. SK-03-92 Synthesis

SK-03-92 was synthesized as described previously [22].

3.2. Bacterial Strains and Growth Conditions

The *S. aureus* MW2 strain [7] used for the initial microarray and confirmatory qRT-PCRs (Table 1) was obtained from Jean Lee (Brigham and Young Hospital, Boston, MA, USA). *S. aureus* strains JE2 (wild-type), NE671 (MW2284), and NE272 (MW2285) were obtained from the Network on Antimicrobial Resistance in *Staphylococcus aureus* (NARSA) strain repository (Table 1), representing part of the Nebraska Transposon Mutant Library [38]. Strain JE2 is a plasmid-cured derivative of a USA300 CA-MRSA [86]. Phillip Klebba (Kansas State University, Manhattan, KS, USA) [39] provided the *Listeria monocytogenes* wild-type strain EGD as well as the isogenic *srtA* and *srtB* mutant strains. All strains were grown in brain heart infusion broth (Becton Dickinson, Franklin Lakes, NJ, USA) or trypticase soy broth (Becton Dickinson) shaken 250 rpm at 37 °C. The transposon mutant strains had 5 μg/mL of erythromycin (Sigma-Aldrich, St. Louis, MO, USA) added to the media.

3.3. RNA Extractions

Total RNA was isolated from *S. aureus* MW2 cells grown to exponential growth phase (OD$_{600}$ approximately 0.5) either treated with dimethyl sulfoxide (DMSO) or 8× the MIC of SK-03-92 dissolved in DMSO using TRizol extraction (Life Technologies, Carlsbad, CA, USA) according to manufacturer's instructions with an additional lysostaphin treatment step to help lyse the *S. aureus* cell walls. The RNA samples were digested with DNase I (New England Biolabs, Ipswich, MA, USA) followed by phenol and chloroform extractions to remove the protein. RNAs were run on 0.8% agarose gels to confirm concentration and integrities of the RNAs. To assess DNA contamination of the samples, PCRs were performed on the RNA samples using SaFtsZ1 and SaFtsZ2 primers (see Table 4). The PCR conditions for amplification with the SaFtsZ1/SaFtsZ2 primers was as follows: 94 °C, 1 min; 55 °C, 1 min; and 72 °C, 1 min for 35 cycles.

Table 4. Oligonucleotide primers used in this study.

Primer	Gene	Sequence
SaFtsZ1	*ftsZ*	5′-GGTGTAGGTGGTGGCGGTAA-3′
SaFtsZ2		5′-TCATTGGCGTAGATTTGTC-3′
GuaBF1	*guaB*	5′-GCTCGTCAAGGTGGTTTAGGTG-3′
GuaBR1		5′-TAAGACATGCACACCTGCTTCG-3′
SrtA1	*srtA*	5′-TCGCTGGTGTGGTACTTATC-3′
SrtA2		5′-CAGGTGTTGCTGGTCCTGGA-3′
MW2284A	*MW2284*	5′-CAATGCAAATGAGACGGAATCT-3′
MW2284B		5′-GAAGAATAGGTGTAGTGTGCAT-3′
MW2285A	*MW2285*	5′-GTATGTTATTTGCAGACGGCAA-3′
MW2285B		5′-AAAGGCAAGAATCCGACATACG-3′
SA2043A	*tdk*	5′-CTTGTTCACTGACAGCCATCA-3′
SA2043B		5′-ACGCACGACTTAACTAATGTTG-3′
SaPurD1	*purD*	5′-CAGCCGCTAATTGATGGATTA-3′
SaPurD2		5′-AGCACTTCTGGCTGCTTCAAT-3′
SaPurH1	*purH*	5′-CCAGAAATAATGGATGGCCGT-3′
SaPurH2		5′-TGCCGGATGTACAATTGTTGT-3′
SaPurL1	*purL*	5′-GTTATGTGGAGTGAACATTGC-3′
SaPurL2		5′-AGCCCCAATAGAGACAATGTC-3′

3.4. Microarray

Total RNAs from cells treated with DMSO or 8× the MIC of SK-03-92 were converted to cDNAs, biotinylated, and hybridized to *S. aureus* GeneChips following the manufacturer's recommendations (Affymetrix, Santa Clara, CA, USA). Agilent GeneSpring G× 7.3 software (Santa Clara, CA, USA) was used to gauge transcript differences and a two-fold or higher difference in the transcript level for one population over the other was considered significant. Nucleic acid sequences with a ≥2-fold change in transcriptional abundance were mapped to the *S. aureus* COL genome (taxid: 93062) via BLASTN, BLASTX, or PSI-BLAST analysis [65] through the National Center for Biotechnology Information (NCBI, Bethesda, MD, USA) website and their putative products were annotated.

3.5. cDNA Synthesis

The cDNAs were synthesized from 5 µg of total RNA from SK-03-92 treated or untreated *S. aureus* MW2 using a First-Strand Synthesis kit (Life Technologies) according to manufacturer's instructions.

3.6. Real Time-Quantitative Polymerase Chain Reaction (qRT-PCR)

All of the qRT-PCRs were performed using the LightCycler FastStart DNA MasterPLUS SYBR Green kit according to manufacturer's instructions (Roche, Indianapolis, IN, USA). Primers used in this study were based off of the MW2 sequenced genome [87] and synthesized by Integrated DNA Technologies (Coralville, IA, USA) that are shown in Table 4. A LightCycler 1.5 machine (Roche) or a CFX96 machine (BioRad, Hercules, CA, USA) were used throughout the study. The *guaB* and *ftsZ* housekeeping genes were used as standardization controls. Each RT-qPCR run followed the minimum information for publication of quantitative real-time PCR experiments guidelines [88]. The qRT-PCRs were done at least three times under the following conditions: 94 °C, 20 s; 55 °C, 30 s; and 72 °C, 1 min for 35 cycles. The level of target gene transcripts in MW2 cells was compared to the *guaB* and *ftsZ* genes. Crossover points for all genes were standardized to the crossover points for *ftsZ* and *guaB* in each sample using the $2^{-\Delta\Delta CT}$ formula [89].

3.7. HPLC

High-performance liquid chromatography was used to detect the presence of (p)ppGpp in the intracellular nucleotide pools of mid-log phase *S. aureus* cells following treatment with SK-03-92, mupirocin (positive control), or dimethyl sulfoxide (negative control) [90–92]. SK-03-92 was added at 16 µg/mL to 100 mL mid-log (OD_{600} = 0.4–0.6) culture in cation-adjusted Mueller Hinton broth and incubated for 20 min with shaking at 37 °C. Mupirocin was added at 60 µg/mL. Cells were collected after a 20 min incubation by centrifugation at 10,000× *g* for 10 min at 4 °C. The supernatant was discarded and the cell pellet suspended in 12 mL of ice cold 0.4 M formic acid (pH 3.5). After 30 min on ice, the cell extract was centrifuged at 10,000× *g* for 10 min at 4 °C to remove cell debris. The supernatant was evaporated under vacuum and filtered (0.2 µm pore size). Filtered cell extract was stored at −20 °C until use. Fifty microliters of filtered cell extract were loaded on a Hypersil SAX column (Thermo Fisher Scientific, Waltham, MA, USA) (5 µm, 4.6 × 250 mm) at a flow rate of 1.0 mL/min in 0.45 M potassium phosphate 0.05 M magnesium sulfate buffer (pH 3.5) using a Waters 600E pump and 996 photodiode array detector (Waters, Milford, MA, USA). Absorbance of the separated nucleotide pool was monitored at 254 and 280 nm.

3.8. Biofilm Assay

To determine the effect of SK-03-92 treatment on the ability of *S. aureus* to form a biofilm, a biofilm assay was performed [93]. The *S. aureus* parent strains MW2 and JE2 were treated with SK-03-92 at concentrations of 0.5–64 µg/mL and those plates were compared to wells with bacteria not treated with the drug. After drying, the remaining dried crystal violet dye stained biofilm material was extracted with 160 µL 33% glacial acetic acid per well and the OD_{570} was measured for each well. The total biofilm assay was performed a minimum of 10 times for each strain to achieve statistical significance.

3.9. MICs

In vitro minimum inhibitory concentration (MIC) determinations were performed on the *S. aureus* strains using SK-03-92 according to the Clinical and Laboratory Standards Institute guidelines [94]. All MICs were done a minimum of three times.

3.10. Statistical Analysis

A two-tailed Student's *t*-test was run for the qRT-PCR comparisons and an ANOVA analysis was used for the biofilm assays to assess probabilities. *p*-values < 0.05 were considered significant.

4. Conclusions

Drug treatment with the stilbenoid compound SK-03-92 caused more genes to be transcriptionally downregulated than upregulated compared to other bactericidal and stilbenoid compounds (e.g., pterostilbene and resveratrol). The methoxy substitution on the main benzene ring at position 5 is likely to be responsible for this effect. A putative TCS, MW2284/MW2285, is clearly downregulated by SK-03-92 treatment. Is the TCS the prime target of the SK-03-92 lead compound and could targeting this TCS be the mechanism of action for SK-03-92 in Gram-positive bacteria? We hypothesize that one of the SK-03-92 targets is this putative TCS. Knockouts of both *MW2284* and *MW2285* showed substantial upregulation of the *srtA* gene that encodes sortase A. Sortase A may present something on the exterior of the *S. aureus* cell that causes rapid cell lysis. Furthermore, the MW2284 and MW2285 ORFs lie just upstream of the MW2286 ORF, which is thought to encode a malate:quinone oxidoreducatase gene important in the electron transport chain. If the MW2284/MW2285 TCS positively regulates this gene, then a mutation in either gene or treatment of *S. aureus* with a SK-03-92 drug may, in turn, cause downregulation of this gene as well as *sdhC* and *glpD* that would disrupt the electron transport chain in *S. aureus*. Evidence presented in this study also suggests the existence of a conserved bacterial pathway, involving PCD and persister formation, which is triggered by protein glycation and aggregation that may be responsible for the killing mechanism of SK-03-92. Could this putative TCS be tied to these phenomena? Further study may help us determine if the SK-03-92-induced *S. aureus* cell lysis is caused by a disruption of the electron transport chain, regulation of a conserved prokaryotic PCD pathway, or a combination of both of these events.

Acknowledgments: We thank Phillip Klebba, Jean Lee, and the NARSA for several *S. aureus* and *L. monocytogenes* strains used in this study. We also thank Greg Somerville for reviewing the paper. This work was funded by an ARG-WiTAG grant to W.R.S., a WiSys grant to W.R.S. and A.M., a National Institute of Neurological Disorders and Stroke grant NS076517 to J.M.C., a University of Wisconsin-La Crosse (UWL) Undergraduate Research Grant to M.L., a UWL College of Science and Allied Health supply grant to L.L., WisCAMP scholarships to M.L. and S.M.B., and a McNair Scholarship to M.L.

Author Contributions: W.R.S. conceived the experiments, wrote the paper, designed some of the primers, and ran data analysis: P.M.D. ran the microarray analysis and initial microarray annotation; A.M., J.M.C., V.V.N.P.B.T., C.W., and M.T.R. synthesized the SK-03-92 lead compound used in the study; S.M.B., M.L., L.L., and A.B. isolated the RNA samples, designed primers, and ran qRT-PCR; A.W. performed the biofilm assays, D.B. ran the biofilm statistical analysis; and R.P. and M.R. completed the HPLC and some bioinformatic analysis of the microarray results.

References

1. Suaya, J.A.; Mera, R.M.; Cassidy, A.; O'Hara, P.; Amrine-Madsen, H.; Burstin, S.; Miller, L.G. Incidence and cost of hospitalizations associated with *Staphylococcus aureus* skin and soft tissue infections in the United States from 2001 to 2009. *BMC Infect. Dis.* **2014**, *14*, 296. [CrossRef] [PubMed]

2. Klein, E.Y.; Sun, L.; Smith, D.L.; Laxminarayan, R. The changing epidemiology of methicillin-resistant *Staphylococcus aureus* in the United States: A national observational study. *Am. J. Epidemiol.* **2013**, *177*, 666–674. [CrossRef] [PubMed]

3. Hidron, A.I.; Edwards, J.R.; Patel, J.; Horan, T.C.; Sievert, D.M.; Pollock, D.A.; Fridkin, S.K.; National Healthcare Safety Network Team; Participating National Healthcare Safety Network Facilities. NHSN annual update: Antimicrobial-resistant pathogens associated with healthcare-associated infections: Annual summary of data reported to the National Healthcare Safety Network at the Centers for Disease Control and Prevention, 2006–2007. *Infect. Control Hosp. Epidemiol.* **2008**, *29*, 996–1011. [PubMed]

4. Maree, C.L.; Daum, R.; Boyle-Vavra, S.; Matayoshi, K.; Miller, L. Community associated methicillin-resistant *Staphylococcus aureus* isolates causing healthcare-associated infections. *Emerg. Infect. Dis.* **2007**, *13*, 236–242. [CrossRef] [PubMed]

5. Herold, B.C.; Immergluck, L.C.; Maranan, M.C.; Lauderdale, D.S.; Gaskin, R.E.; Boyle-Vavra, S.; Leitch, C.D.; Daum, R.S. Community-acquired methicillin-resistant *Staphylococcus aureus* in children with no identified predisposing risk. *JAMA* **1998**, *279*, 593–598. [CrossRef] [PubMed]

6. Lina, G.; Piémont, Y.; Godail-Gamot, F.; Bes, M.; Peter, M.O.; Gauduchon, V.; Vandenesch, F.; Etienne, J. Involvement of Panton-Valentine leukocidin-producing *Staphylococcus aureus* in primary skin infections and pneumonia. *Clin. Infect. Dis.* **1999**, *29*, 1128–1132. [CrossRef] [PubMed]

7. Center for Disease Control and Prevention.   Four pediatric deaths from community-acquired methicillin-resistant *Staphylococcus aureus*—Minnesota and North Dakota, 1997–1999. *Morbid. Mortal. Wkly. Rep.* **1999**, *52*, 88.

8. Dantes, R.; Mu, Y.; Belflower, R.; Aragon, D.; Dumyati, G.; Harrison, L.H.; Lessa, F.C.; Lynfield, R.; Nadle, J.; Petit, S.; et al. National burden of invasive methicillin-resistant *Staphylococcus aureus* infections, United States, 2011. *JAMA Intern. Med.* **2013**, *173*, 1970–1978. [PubMed]

9. Pate, A.J.; Terribilini, R.G.; Ghobadi, F.; Azhir, A.; Barber, A.; Pearson, J.M.; Kalantari, H.; Hassen, G.W. Antibiotics for methicillin-resistant *Staphylococcus aureus* skin and soft tissue infections: The challenge of outpatient therapy. *Am. J. Emerg. Med.* **2014**, *32*, 135–138. [CrossRef] [PubMed]

10. Pendleton, J.N.; Gorman, S.P.; Gilmore, B.F. Clinical relevance of the ESKAPE pathogens. *Expert Rev. Anti-Infect. Ther.* **2013**, *11*, 297–308. [CrossRef] [PubMed]

11. Stryjewski, M.E.; Corey, G.R. Methicillin-resistant *Staphylococcus aureus*: An evolving pathogen. *Clin. Infect. Dis.* **2014**, *58*, S10–S19. [CrossRef] [PubMed]

12. Bae, I.G.; Federspiel, J.J.; Miró, J.M.; Woods, C.W.; Park, L.; Rybak, M.J.; Rude, T.H.; Bradley, S.; Bukovski, S.; de la Maria, C.G.; et al. Heterogeneous vancomycin-intermediate susceptibility phenotype in bloodstream methicillin-resistant *Staphylococcus aureus* isolates from an international cohort of patients with infective endocarditis: prevalence, genotype, and clinical significance. *J. Infect. Dis.* **2009**, *200*, 1355–1366. [CrossRef] [PubMed]

13. Gomes, D.M.; Ward, K.E.; LaPlante, K.L. Clinical implications of vancomycin heteroresistant and intermediately susceptible *Staphylococcus aureus*. *Pharmacotherapy* **2015**, *35*, 424–432. [CrossRef] [PubMed]

14. Moise, P.A.; North, D.; Steenbergen, J.N.; Sakoulas, G. Susceptibility relationship between vancomycin and daptomycin in *Staphylococcus aureus*: Facts and assumptions. *Lancet Infect. Dis.* **2009**, *9*, 617–624. [CrossRef]

15. Sader, H.S.; Jones, R.N.; Rossi, K.L.; Rybak, M.J. Occurrence of vancomycin-tolerant and heterogeneous vancomycin-intermediate strains (hVISA) among *Staphylococcus aureus* causing bloodstream infections in nine USA hospitals. *J. Antimicrob. Chemother.* **2009**, *64*, 1024–1028. [CrossRef] [PubMed]

16. Jones, R.N. Microbiological features of vancomycin in the 21st century: Minimum inhibitory concentration creep, bactericidal/static activity, and approved breakpoints to predict clinical outcomes or detect resistant strains. *Clin. Infect. Dis.* **2006**, *42*, S13–S24. [CrossRef] [PubMed]

17. Traczewski, M.M.; Katz, B.D.; Steenbergen, J.N.; Brown, S.D. Inhibitory and bactericidal activities of daptomycin, vancomycin, and teicoplanin against methicillin-resistant *Staphylococcus aureus* isolates collected from 1985–2007. *Antimicrob. Agents Chemother.* **2009**, *53*, 1735–1738. [CrossRef] [PubMed]

18. Bassetti, M.; Righi, E. Development of novel antibacterial drugs to combat multiple resistant organisms. *Langenbecks Arch. Surg.* **2015**, *400*, 153–165. [CrossRef] [PubMed]

19. Coates, A.R.M.; Halls, G.; Hu, Y. Novel classes of antibiotics or more of the same? *Br. J. Pharmacol.* **2011**, *163*, 184–194. [CrossRef] [PubMed]

20. Infectious Diseases Society of America. The 10×20 initiative: Pursuing a global commitment to develop 10 new antibacterial drugs by 2020. *Clin. Infect. Dis.* **2010**, *50*, 1081–1083.

21. Kabir, M.S.; Engelbrecht, K.; Polanowski, R.; Krueger, S.M.; Ignasiak, R.; Rott, M.; Schwan, W.R.; Stemper, M.E.; Reed, K.D.; Sherman, D.; et al. New classes of Gram-positive selective antibacterials: Inhibitors of MRSA and surrogates of the causative agents of anthrax and tuberculosis. *Bioorg. Med. Chem. Lett.* **2010**, *18*, 5745–5749. [CrossRef] [PubMed]

22. Schwan, W.R.; Kabir, M.S.; Kallaus, M.; Krueger, S.; Monte, A.; Cook, J.M. Synthesis and minimum inhibitory concentrations of SK-03-92 against *Staphylococcus aureus* and other gram-positive bacteria. *J. Infect. Chemother.* **2012**, *18*, 124–126. [CrossRef] [PubMed]

23. Schwan, W.R.; Kolesar, J.M.; Kabor, M.S.; Elder, E.J., Jr.; Williams, J.B.; Minerath, R.; Cook, J.M.; Witzigmann, C.M.; Monte, A.; Flaherty, T. Pharmacokinetic/toxicity properties of the new anti-staphylococcal lead compound SK-03-92. *Antibiotics* **2015**, *4*, 617–626. [CrossRef] [PubMed]

24. Cohen, N.R.; Lobritz, M.A.; Collins, J.J. Microbial persistence and the road to drug resistance. *Cell Host Microbe* **2013**, *13*, 632–642. [CrossRef] [PubMed]

25. Conlon, B.P. *Staphylococcus aureus* chronic and relapsing infections: Evidence of a role for persister cells: An investigation of persister cells, their formation and their role in *S. aureus* disease. *Bioessays* **2014**, *36*, 991–996. [CrossRef] [PubMed]

26. Lechner, S.; Lewis, K.; Bertram, R. *Staphylococcus aureus* persisters tolerant to bactericidal antibiotics. *J. Mol. Microbiol. Biotechnol.* **2012**, *22*, 235–244. [CrossRef] [PubMed]

27. Lewis, K. Persister cells. *Annu. Rev. Microbiol.* **2010**, *64*, 357–372. [CrossRef] [PubMed]

28. Keren, I.; Shah, D.; Spoering, A.; Kaldalu, N.; Lewis, K. Specialized persister cells and the mechanism of multidrug tolerance in *Escherichia coli*. *J. Bacteriol.* **2004**, *186*, 8172–8180. [CrossRef] [PubMed]

29. Spoering, A.L.; Lewis, K. Biofilms and planktonic cells of *Pseudomonas aeruginosa* have similar resistance to killing by antimicrobials. *J. Bacteriol.* **2001**, *183*, 6746–6751. [CrossRef] [PubMed]

30. Stewart, P.S.; Costerton, J.W. Antibiotic resistance of bacteria in biofilms. *Lancet* **2001**, *358*, 135–138. [CrossRef]

31. Jang, H.; Nde, C.; Toghrol, F.; Bentley, W.E. Microarray analysis of toxicogenomic effects of ortho-phenylphenol in *Staphylococcus aureus*. *BMC Genomics* **2008**, *9*, 411. [CrossRef] [PubMed]

32. Lama, A.; Pané-Farré, J.; Chon, T.; Wiersma, A.M.; Sit, C.S.; Vederas, J.C.; Hecker, M.; Nakano, M.M. Response of methicillin-resistant *Staphylococcus aureus* to amicoumacin A. *PLoS ONE* **2012**, *7*, e34037. [CrossRef] [PubMed]

33. Muthaiyan, A.; Silverman, J.A.; Jayaswal, R.K.; Wilinson, B.J. Transcriptional profiling reveals that daptomycin induces the *Staphylococcus aureus* cell wall stress stimulon and gene responsive to membrane depolarization. *Antimicrob. Agents Chemother.* **2008**, *52*, 980–990. [CrossRef] [PubMed]

34. Lechner, S.; Prax, M.; Lange, B.; Huber, C.; Eisenreich, W.; Herbig, A.; Nieselt, K.; Bertram, R. Metabolic and transcriptional activities of *Staphylococcus aureus* challenged with high-doses of daptomycin. *Int. J. Med. Microbiol.* **2014**, *304*, 931–940. [CrossRef] [PubMed]

35. Pan, Z.; Agarwal, A.K.; Xu, T.; Feng, Q.; Baerson, S.R.; Duke, S.O.; Rimando, A.M. Identification of molecular pathways affected by pterostilbene, a natural dimethylether analog of resveratrol. *BMC Med. Genomics* **2008**, *20*, 1–7. [CrossRef] [PubMed]

36. Wang, Z.; Gu, Z.; Shen, Y.; Wang, Y.; Li, J.; Lv, H.; Huo, K. The natural product resveratrol inhibits yeast cell separation by extensively modulating the transcriptional landscape and reprogamming the intracellular metabolome. *PLoS ONE* **2016**, *11*, e0150156. [CrossRef]

37. Qin, N.; Tan, X.; Jiao, Y.; Liu, L.; Zhao, W.; Yang, S.; Jia, A. RNA-Seq-based transciptome analysis of methicillin-resistant *Staphylococcus aureus* biofilm inhibition by ursolic acid and resveratrol. *Sci. Rep.* **2014**, *4*, 5467. [CrossRef] [PubMed]

38. Fey, P.D.; Endres, J.L.; Yajjala, V.K.; Widhelm, T.J.; Boissy, R.J.; Bose, J.L.; Bayles, K.W. A genetic resource for rapid and comprehensive phenotype screening of nonessential *Staphylococcus aureus* genes. *mBio* **2013**, *4*, e00537012. [CrossRef] [PubMed]

39. Xiao, Q.; Jiang, X.; Moore, K.J.; Shao, Y.; Pi, H.; Dubail, I.; Charbit, A.; Newton, S.M.; Klebba, P.E. Sortase independent and dependent systems for acquisition of haem and haemoglobin in *Listeria monocytogenes*. *Mol. Microbiol.* **2011**, *80*, 1581–1597. [CrossRef] [PubMed]

40. Yeh, J.I.; Chinte, U.; Du, S. Structure of glycerol-3-phosphate dehydrogenase, an essential monotopic membrane enzyme involved in respiration and metabolism. *Proc. Nat. Acad. Sci. USA* **2008**, *105*, 3280–3285. [CrossRef] [PubMed]

41. Ramasamy, R.; Yan, S.F.; Schmidt, A.M. Methylglyoxal comes of AGE. *Cell* **2006**, *124*, 258–260. [CrossRef] [PubMed]

42. Ackerman, R.S.; Cozzarelli, N.R.; Epstein, E.W. Accumulation of toxic concentrations of methylglyoxal by wild-type *Escherichia coli* K-12. *J. Bacteriol.* **1974**, *119*, 357–362. [PubMed]

43. Rabbani, N.; Thornalley, P.J. Methylglyoxal, glyoxalase 1 and the dicarbonyl proteome. *Amino Acids* **2012**, *42*, 1133–1142. [CrossRef] [PubMed]

44. Kwak, M.; Ku, M.; Kang, S. NAD⁺-linked alcohol dehydrogenase 1 regulates methylglyoxal concentration in *Candida albicans*. *FEBS Lett.* **2014**, *588*, 1144–1153. [CrossRef] [PubMed]

45. Spoering, A.L.; Vulić, M.; Lewis, K. GlpD and PlsB participate in persister cell formation in *Escherichia coli*. *J. Bacteriol.* **2006**, *188*, 5136–5144. [CrossRef] [PubMed]

46. Stauffer, L.T.; Steiert, P.S.; Steiert, J.G.; Stauffer, G.V. An *Escherichia coli* protein with homology to the H-protein of the glycine cleavage enzyme complex from pea and chicken liver. *DNA Seq.* **1991**, *2*, 13–17. [CrossRef] [PubMed]

47. Gemayel, R.; Fortpied, J.; Rzem, R.; Vertommen, D.; Veiga-da-Cunha, M.; van Schaftingen, E. Many fructosamine 3-kinase homologues in bacteria are ribulosamine/erythrulosamine 3-kinases potentially involved in protein deglycation. *FEBS J.* **2007**, *274*, 4360–4374. [CrossRef] [PubMed]

48. Polanowski, R.; Rott, M.; University of Wisconsin-La Crosse, La Crosse, WI, USA. unpublished data. 2016.

49. *Performance Standards for Antimicrobial Susceptibility Testing, 16th Informational Supplement*; NCCLS document M100-S16; Clinical and Laboratory Standards Institute: Wayne, PA, USA, 2006.

50. Bednarska, N.G.; Schymkowitz, J.; Rousseau, F.; van Eldere, J. Protein aggregation in bacteria: The thin boundary between functionality and toxicity. *Microbiology* **2013**, *159*, 1795–1806. [CrossRef] [PubMed]

51. Wood, R.C.; Steers, E. Study of the purine metabolism of *Staphylococcus aureus*. *J. Bacteriol.* **1959**, *77*, 760–765. [PubMed]

52. Subramanian, D.; Natarajan, J. Network analysis of *S. aureus* response to ramoplanin reveals modules for virulence factors and resistance mechanisms and characteristic novel genes. *Gene* **2015**, *574*, 149–162. [CrossRef] [PubMed]

53. Cuaron, J.A.; Dulal, S.; Song, Y.; Singh, A.K.; Montelongo, C.E.; Yu, W.; Nagarajan, V.; Jayaswal, R.K.; Wilkinson, B.J.; Gustafson, J.E. Tea tree oil-induced transcriptional alterations in *Staphylococcus aureus*. *Phytother. Res.* **2013**, *27*, 390–396. [CrossRef] [PubMed]

54. Shen, F.; Tang, X.; Wang, Y.; Yang, Z.; Shi, X.; Wang, C.; Zhang, Q.; An, Y.; Cheng, W.; Jin, K.; et al. Phenotype and expression prolife analysis of *Staphylococcus aureus* biofilms and planktonic cells in response to licochalcone A. *Appl. Microbiol. Biotechnol.* **2015**, *99*, 359–373. [CrossRef] [PubMed]

55. Blakely, R.L.; Vitols, E. The control of nucleotide biosynthesis. *Annu. Rev. Biochem.* **1968**, *37*, 201–224. [CrossRef] [PubMed]

56. Fung, D.K.; Chan, E.W.; Chin, M.L.; Chan, R.C. Delineation of a bacterial starvation stress response network which can mediate antibiotic tolerance development. *Antimicrob. Agents Chemother.* **2010**, *54*, 1082–1093. [CrossRef] [PubMed]

57. Maisonneuve, E.; Gerdes, K. Molecular mechanisms underlying bacterial persisters. *Cell* **2014**, *157*, 539–548. [CrossRef] [PubMed]

58. Yee, R.; Cui, P.; Shi, W.; Feng, J.; Zhang, Y. Genetic screen reveals the role of purine metabolism in *Staphylococcus aureus* persistence to rifampicin. *Antibiotics* **2015**, *4*, 627–642. [CrossRef] [PubMed]

59. Ranjit, D.K.; Endres, J.L.; Bayles, K.W. *Staphylococcus aureus* CidA and LrgA proteins exhibit holin-like properties. *J. Bacteriol.* **2011**, *193*, 2468–2476. [CrossRef] [PubMed]

60. Sadykov, M.R.; Bayles, K. The control of death and lysis in staphylococcal biofilms: A coordination of physiological signals. *Curr. Opin. Microbiol.* **2012**, *15*, 211–215. [CrossRef] [PubMed]

61. Yang, S.J.; Rice, K.C.; Brown, R.J.; Patton, T.G.; Liou, L.E.; Park, Y.H.; Bayles, K.W. A LysR-type regulator, CidR, is required for induction of the *Staphylococcus aureus* cidABC operon. *J. Bacteriol.* **2005**, *187*, 5893–5900. [CrossRef] [PubMed]

62. Bayles, K.W. Bacterial programmed cell death: Making sense of a paradox. *Nat. Rev. Microbiol.* **2014**, *12*, 63–69. [CrossRef] [PubMed]

63. Tanouchi, Y.; Lee, A.J.; Meredith, H.; You, L. Programmed cell death in bacteria and implications for antibiotic therapy. *Trends Microbiol.* **2013**, *21*, 265–270. [CrossRef] [PubMed]

64. Sarkar, S.K.; Bhattacharyya, A.; Mandal, S.S. YnfA, a SMP family efflux pump is abundant in *Escherichia coli* isolates from urinary infection. *Indian J. Med. Microbiol.* **2015**, *33*, 139–142. [PubMed]

65. Mazmanian, S.K.; Liu, G.; Ton-That, H.; Schneewind, O. *Staphylococcus aureus* sortase, an enzyme that anchors surface proteins to the cell wall. *Science* **1999**, *285*, 760–763. [CrossRef] [PubMed]

66. Altschul, S.F.; Madden, T.L.; Schäffer, A.A.; Zhang, J.; Zhang, Z.; Miller, W.; Lipman, D.J. Gapped BLAST and PSI-BLAST: A new generation of protein database search programs. *Nucleic Acids Res.* **1997**, *25*, 3389–3402. [CrossRef] [PubMed]

67. Nikolskaya, A.N.; Galperin, M.Y. A novel type of conserved DNA-binding domain in the transcriptional regulators of the AlgR/AgrA/LytR family. *Nucleic Acids Res.* **2002**, *30*, 2453–2459. [CrossRef] [PubMed]

68. Nicod, S.S.; Weinzierl, R.O.; Burchell, L.; Escalera-Maurer, A.; James, E.H.; Wigneshweraraj, S. Systematic mutational analysis of the LytTR DNA binding domain of *Staphylococcus aureus* virulence gene transcription factor AgrA. *Nucleic Acids Res.* **2014**, *42*, 12523–12536. [CrossRef] [PubMed]

69. Lan, L.; Cheng, A.; Dunman, P.M.; Missiakas, D.; He, C. Golden pigment production and virulence gene expression are affected by metabolisms in *Staphylococcus aureus*. *J. Bacteriol.* **2010**, *192*, 3068–3077. [CrossRef] [PubMed]

70. Fuchs, S.; Pané-Farré, J.; Kohler, C.; Hecker, M.; Engelmann, S. Anaerobic gene expression in *Staphylococcus aureus*. *J. Bacteriol.* **2007**, *189*, 4275–4289. [CrossRef] [PubMed]

71. Kadurugamuwa, J.L.; Sin, L.; Albert, E.; Yu, J.; Francis, K.; DeBoer, M.; Rubin, M.; Bellinger-Kawahara, C.; Parr, T.R., Jr.; Contag, P.R. Direct continuous method for monitoring biofilm infection in a mouse model. *Infect. Immun.* **2003**, *71*, 882–890. [CrossRef] [PubMed]

72. Xiong, Y.Q.; Willard, J.; Kadurugamuwa, J.L.; Yu, J.; Francis, K.P.; Bayer, A.S. Real-time in vivo bioluminescent imaging for evaluating the efficacy of antibiotics in a rat *Staphylococcus aureus* endocarditis model. *Antimicrob. Agents Chemother.* **2005**, *49*, 380–387. [CrossRef] [PubMed]

73. Reiß, S.; Pané-Farré, J.; Fuchs, S.; François, P.; Liebeke, M.; Schrenzel, J.; Lidequist, U.; Lalk, M.; Wolz, C.; Hecker, M.; Engelmann, S. Global analysis of the *Staphylococcus aureus* response to mupirocin. *Antimicrob. Agents Chemother.* **2012**, *56*, 787–804. [CrossRef] [PubMed]

74. Anderson, K.L.; Roberts, C.; Disz, T.; Vonstein, V.; Hwang, K.; Overbeck, R.; Olson, P.D.; Projan, S.J.; Dunman, P.M. Characterization of the *Staphylococcus aureus* heat shock, cold shock, stringent, and SOS responses and their effects on log-phase mRNA turnover. *J. Bacteriol.* **2006**, *188*, 6739–6756. [CrossRef] [PubMed]

75. Fischer, M.; Zimmerman, T.P.; Short, S.A. A rapid method for the determination of guanosine 5′-diphosphate-3′-diphosphate and guanosine 5′triphosphate-3′-diphosphate by high performance liquid chromatography. *Anal. Biochem.* **1982**, *121*, 135–139. [CrossRef]

76. Melo, A.; Colombo, A.; Arthington-Skaggs, B. Paradoxical growth effect of caspofungin observed on biofilms and planktonic cells of five different *Candida* species. *Antimicrob. Agents Chemother.* **2007**, *51*, 3081–3088. [CrossRef] [PubMed]

77. Wood, T.; Knabels, S.; Kwan, B. Bacterial persister cell formation and dormancy. *Appl. Environ. Microbiol.* **2013**, *79*, 7116–7121. [CrossRef] [PubMed]

78. Marraffini, L.A.; DeDent, A.C.; Schneewind, O. Sortases and the art of anchoring proteins to the envelopes of Gram-positive bacteria. *Microbiol. Mol. Biol. Rev.* **2006**, *70*, 192–221. [CrossRef] [PubMed]

79. Fischetti, V.A.; Pancholi, V.; Schneewind, O. Conservation of a hexapeptide sequence in the anchor region of surface proteins from gram-positive bacteria. *Mol. Microbiol.* **1990**, *4*, 1603–1605. [CrossRef] [PubMed]

80. Boekhorst, J.; de Been, M.W.; Kleerebezem, M.; Siezen, R.J. Genome-wide detection and analysis of cell wall-bound proteins with LPxTG-like sorting motifs. *J. Bacteriol.* **2005**, *187*, 4928–4934. [CrossRef] [PubMed]

81. Ton-That, H.; Liu, G.; Mazmanian, S.K.; Faull, K.F.; Schneewind, O. Purification and characterization of sortase, the transpeptidase that cleaves surface proteins of *Staphylococcus aureus* at the LPXTG motif. *Proc. Natl. Acad. Sci. USA* **1999**, *96*, 12424–12429. [CrossRef] [PubMed]

82. Foster, T.J.; Hook, M. Surface protein adhesins of *Staphylococcus aureus*. *Trends Microbiol.* **1998**, *6*, 484–488. [CrossRef]

83. Mazmanian, S.K.; Liu, G.; Jensen, E.R.; Lenoy, E.; Schneewind, O. *Staphylococcus aureus* mutants defective in the display of surface proteins and in the pathogenesis of animal infections. *Proc. Natl. Acad. Sci. USA* **2000**, *97*, 5510–5515. [CrossRef] [PubMed]

84. Sibbald, M.J.J.; Yang, X.-M.; Tsompanidou, E.; Qu, D.; Hecker, M.; Becher, D.; Buist, G.; Maarten van Dijl, J. Partially overlapping substrate specificities of staphylococcal group—A sortases. *Proteomics* **2012**, *12*, 3049–3062. [CrossRef] [PubMed]

85. Jonsson, I.M.; Mazmanian, S.K.; Schneewind, O.; Bremell, T.; Tarkowski, A. The role of *Staphylococcus* aureus sortase A and sortase B in murine arthritis. *Microbes Infect.* **2003**, *5*, 775–780. [CrossRef]

86. Weiss, W.J.; Lenoy, E.; Murphy, T.; Tardio, L.; Burgio, P.; Projan, S.J.; Schneewind, O.; Alksne, L. Effect of *srtA* and *srtB* gene expression on the virulence of *Staphylococcus aureus* in animal infection. *J. Antimicrob. Chemother.* **2004**, *53*, 480–486. [CrossRef] [PubMed]

87. Voyich, J.M.; Braughton, K.R.; Sturdevant, D.E.; Whitney, A.R.; Saïd-Salim, B.; Porcella, S.F.; Long, R.D.; Dorward, D.W.; Gardner, D.J.; Kreiswirth, B.N.; et al. Insights into mechanisms used by *Staphylococcus aureus* to avoid destruction by human neutrophils. *J. Immunol.* **2005**, *175*, 3907–3919. [CrossRef] [PubMed]

88. Baba, T.; Takeuchi, F.; Kuroda, M.; Yuzawa, H.; Aoki, K.; Oguchi, A.; Nagai, Y.; Iwama, N.; Asano, K.; Naimi, T.; et al. Genome and virulence determinants of high virulence community-acquired MRSA. *Lancet* **2002**, *359*, 1819–1827. [CrossRef]

89. Bustin, S.S.; Benes, V.; Garson, J.A.; Hellemans, J.; Huggett, J.; Kubista, M.; Mueller, R.; Nolan, T.; Pfaffl, M.W.; Shipley, G.L.; et al. The MIQE guidelines: Minimum information for publication of quantitative real-time PCR experiments. *Clin. Chem.* **2009**, *55*, 611–622. [CrossRef] [PubMed]

90. Livak, K.J.; Schmittgen, T.D. Analysis of relative gene expression data using real-time quantitative PCR and the $2^{-\Delta\Delta CT}$ Method. *Methods* **2001**, *25*, 402–408. [CrossRef] [PubMed]

91. Ochi, K. Occurrence of the stringent response in *Streptomyces* sp. and its significance for the initiation of morphological and physiological differentiation. *J. Gen. Microbiol.* **1986**, *132*, 2621–2631. [PubMed]

92. Ochi, K. Metabolic initiation of differentiation and secondary metabolism by *Streptomyces griseus*: Significance of the stringent response (ppGpp) and GTP content in relation to A factor. *J. Bacteriol.* **1987**, *169*, 3608–3616. [CrossRef] [PubMed]

93. Wilson, J.M.; Oliva, B.; Cassels, R.; O'Hanlon, P.J.; Chopra, I. SB 205952, a novel semisynthetic monic acid analog with at least two modes of action. *Antimicrob. Agents Chemother.* **1995**, *39*, 1925–1933. [CrossRef] [PubMed]

94. Stepanovic, S.; Vukovic, D.; Pavlovic, M.; Svabic-Vlahovic, M. Influence of dynamic conditions on biofilm formation by staphylococci. *Eur. J. Clin. Microbiol. Infect. Dis.* **2001**, *20*, 502–504. [CrossRef] [PubMed]

3

Identification and Antimicrobial Susceptibility Testing of Anaerobic Bacteria: Rubik's Cube of Clinical Microbiology?

Márió Gajdács [1,*], **Gabriella Spengler** [1] **and Edit Urbán** [2]

[1] Department of Medical Microbiology and Immunobiology, Faculty of Medicine, University of Szeged, 6720 Szeged, Hungary; spengler.gabriella@med.u-szeged.hu

[2] Institute of Clinical Microbiology, Faculty of Medicine, University of Szeged, 6725 Szeged, Hungary; urban.edit@med.u-szeged.hu

* Correspondence: gajdacs.mario@med.u-szeged.hu

Academic Editor: Leonard Amaral

Abstract: Anaerobic bacteria have pivotal roles in the microbiota of humans and they are significant infectious agents involved in many pathological processes, both in immunocompetent and immunocompromised individuals. Their isolation, cultivation and correct identification differs significantly from the workup of aerobic species, although the use of new technologies (e.g., matrix-assisted laser desorption/ionization time-of-flight mass spectrometry, whole genome sequencing) changed anaerobic diagnostics dramatically. In the past, antimicrobial susceptibility of these microorganisms showed predictable patterns and empirical therapy could be safely administered but recently a steady and clear increase in the resistance for several important drugs (β-lactams, clindamycin) has been observed worldwide. For this reason, antimicrobial susceptibility testing of anaerobic isolates for surveillance purposes or otherwise is of paramount importance but the availability of these testing methods is usually limited. In this present review, our aim was to give an overview of the methods currently available for the identification (using phenotypic characteristics, biochemical testing, gas-liquid chromatography, MALDI-TOF MS and WGS) and antimicrobial susceptibility testing (agar dilution, broth microdilution, disk diffusion, gradient tests, automated systems, phenotypic and molecular resistance detection techniques) of anaerobes, when should these methods be used and what are the recent developments in resistance patterns of anaerobic bacteria.

Keywords: anaerobic bacteria; susceptibility testing; methodology; antimicrobial resistance; MALDI-TOF MS; *Bacteroides fragilis* group; *Clostridium* spp. taxonomy; metronidazole; β-lactams

1. Introduction

Anaerobic bacteria have been implicated in a wide range of infectious processes. As an integral part of the human microbiome, these microorganisms can be found in different anatomical sites and they can be responsible for a plethora of infections that may be serious or life-threatening [1–4]. For this reason, anaerobes are often categorized by the body site(s) where they occur, the infections they are associated with, although they are most frequently classified by their microscopic morphology (rods or cocci) and their Gram-staining (for a summary of the most important genera of anaerobic bacteria, see Table 1) [3,5,6]. Infections caused by anaerobes can also be divided according to the origin of the microorganisms. Exogenous anaerobic infections are predominantly caused by Gram-positive spore-forming bacilli (*Clostridium* spp.; *C. difficile* being an exception to this rule), these microorganisms are the causative agents of serious infections like visceral gas gangrene, lockjaw, myonecrosis and botulism. These infections are monobacterial in almost all cases and the effects of bacterial toxins are the prime causes of these pathologies [1,7]. In these cases—although microbiological evaluation is still recommended—diagnosis is mostly reached based on the characteristic clinical symptoms—on the other hand, the overwhelming majority of anaerobic infections are of polymicrobial nature, due to multiple causative agents, involving both obligate aerobes, facultative and obligate anaerobes, in addition, the vast majority of these organisms originate from the normal flora of the skin and mucous membranes [1,2]. These infections commonly involving anaerobes including but not limited to: actinomycosis, root canal and other odontogenic infections, chronic otitis media, chronic sinusitis, aspiration pneumonia, peritonitis and appendicitis, endometritis, salpingitis, necrotising fasciitis, osteomyelitis, septic arthritis, anaerobic cellulitis, infections of wounds and ulcers, abscesses of the head and neck region, lungs, intra-abdominal organs, liver, fallopian tube, ovary and adjacent pelvic organs etc. The most frequent causative agents of these infections are Gram-negative (e.g., *Bacteroides fragilis* group, *Porphyromonas* spp., *Prevotella* spp. and *Fusobacterium* spp.) and Gram-positive (non-spore forming) bacilli (e.g., *Actinomyces* spp., *Propionibacterium* spp., *Eubacterium* spp., *Bifidobacterium* spp.) as well as Gram-positive cocci (e.g., *Anaerococcus* spp., *Atopobium* spp., *Finegoldia* spp., *Peptostretococcus* spp., *Sarcina* spp.) [2,4,8]. The involvement of anaerobic infections varies based on the anatomical site but their significance should not be underrated, as they are present in around 5–10% of bacteraemia, 89% of brain abscesses, 93% of post-surgery abdominal infections, 76% of thoracic empyemas, 95% of diabetic foot infections, 52% in chronic sinusitis, 30–40% of all bite wound infections and 63% in septic abortions [2,4,6,9–13]. Their importance was further underlined when their roles in the pathomechanism of bacterial vaginosis (BV) and pelvic inflammatory disease (PID) were explained [14,15], also with the emergence of antibiotic-associated diarrhoea (AAD) and toxic megacolon caused by toxin producing *Clostridium difficile* (especially the hyper virulent ribotype 027), a significant nosocomial pathogen which is very hard to eradicate, both from a hospital hygiene perspective and therapeutic setting [16–19]. The clinical significance of anaerobes and the interest concerning these bacteria is steadily increasing, with new species described in various infectious processes almost every day, especially in immunocompromised patients [20].

Table 1. Summary of the most important genera of anaerobic bacteria [3,6].

Gram-Positives		Gram-Negatives	
Cocci	**Rods**	**Cocci**	**Rods**
Anaerococcus	*Actinomyces*	*Acidaminococcus*	*Bacteroides*
Atopobium	*Bifidobacterium*	*Megasphera*	*Bilophila*
Coprococcus	*Clostridium*	*Veillonella*	*Butyrivibrio*
Finegoldia	*Eubacterium*		*Centipeda*
Gaffkya	*Lactobacillus*		*Desulfonomonas*
Gallicola	*Propionibacterium*		*Fusobacterium*
Parvimonas			*Leptotrichia*
Murdochiella			*Mitsuokella*
Peptococcus			*Mobiluncus*
Peptostreptococcus			*Porphyromonas*
Peptoniphilus			*Prevotella*
Ruminococcus			*Selenomonas*
Sarcina			*Succinimonas*
			Succinivibrio
			Sutterella
			Wolinella

A range of factors are known to increase the likelihood of anaerobic (mixed) infections, most of which are related to either processes that damage the mucous membranes or conditions reducing the oxygen levels of tissues. Some of these predisposing factors include diabetes, angiopathies of different origin, malignancies, animal and human bites, wounds contaminated with soil, burns, trauma, surgical interventions (both minor and major), foreign bodies, immunosuppression due to AIDS or drug therapy (corticosteroids, cytotoxic agents), procedures involving fine needle aspiration among others [2,4]. In some cases, other infections can be predisposing factors as well (e.g., the correlation between the causative agent of infectious mononucleosis (Epstein-Barr virus; EBV) and Lemiere's syndrome (necrobacillosis caused by *Fusobacterium necrophorum*) [21,22]. Aminoglycoside monotherapy is also associated with the selection and overgrowth of anaerobes (since these microorganisms are intrinsically resistant), which may lead to secondary infections in a healthy or immunocompromised host [23].

In the recent years, considerable changes occurred in the taxonomy of anaerobic bacteria thanks to the developments in molecular methods (DNA hybridization, G + C nucleotide content analysis) and sequencing technologies (next generation sequencing). Anaerobic Gram-negative bacilli (AGNB) were mostly affected, although other genera experienced some changes as well, e.g., in the case of the genus *Peptostreptococcus* (several species were reclassified to other genera, e.g., *Anaerococcus, Finegoldia, Parvimonas, Peptoniphylus*) or the proposal to change *Clostridium difficile* to *Clostridioides difficile* to name a few under the umbrella of Gram-positive anaerobes [24–31]. There is debate however, on the role of these changes in the healthcare setting and whether clinicians should familiarise themselves with the new nomenclature [3,25].

Anaerobic bacteria are significant constituents of the normal microbiome of humans, so much so that they outnumber aerobic microorganisms 10:1–1000:1 in the normal flora of the skin and gut, additionally, they are important in keeping the physiological homeostasis of the oral cavity and the genito-urinary tract of females [3]. These bacteria are passed from mother to the new-born during vaginal birth, becoming an important part of our microbiota in the very early stages of life [32,33].

The colon accommodates the largest population of bacteria in the human body (10^{10}–10^{12}/g), with most of these organisms being anaerobes [33]. Some hypothesize that we should consider the microbiota of our gastro-intestinal tract as an "organ" by itself, critical in maintaining health and preventing various diseases [34]. There are also reports drawing parallels between the state of the gut microbiome and obesity [35], type I diabetes [36], several types of cancer [37–40], psychiatric disorders and depression [41–43], attention deficit hyperactivity disorder [44] and even autism [45]. It has been described that commensal anaerobes have a critical role in regulating the immune functions of the large intestine, protecting us against their pathogenic counterparts, contributing to colonisation resistance (e.g., the metabolising of bile salts to prevent the overgrowth and spore formation of *C. difficile*) [34]. From another point of view, the composition of the microbiota is also significant due to inter-species and intra-species horizontal gene transfer (HGT) of various resistance determinants [46,47].

2. Cultivation and Identification of Anaerobes

Anaerobic bacteria (according to a definition by Syndey M. Finegold) are microorganisms that are unable to grow on solid media in an atmosphere containing 18% O_2 and 10% CO_2 [2]. They vary in their level of tolerance towards atmospheric oxygen and toxic oxygen species (i.e., hydrogen peroxide [H_2O_2], superoxide anion [O_2^-], hydroxyl radical [OH^*] and singlet oxygen [O_2^*]), based on the presence or absence of the enzymes required to eliminate them (superoxide dismutase; SOD, catalase and peroxidase) [2,5,48,49]. Obligate anaerobes (e.g., *C. perfringens*) do not tolerate the effects of oxygen exposure (damage through oxidation of lipids, inactivation of enzymes and direct effects on the genetic material of these microorganisms). On the other hand, aerotolerant anaerobes (e.g., *Cutibacterium/formerly known as Propionibacterium/acnes*) possess superoxide dismutase and peroxidase, therefore oxygen does not have a detrimental effect on them (note: strain-to-strain differences in aerotolerance is common even among strict anaerobes) [48,50]. The tolerance of these bacteria to oxygen is further influenced by certain environmental conditions (*C. perfringens* can withstand higher oxygen levels at lower pH, e.g., in an abscess). Microaerophilic bacteria (e.g., *Helicobacter pylori, Campylobacter jejuni*) and anaerobes should be discussed separately. Although their growth requires lower levels of oxygen than atmospheric levels (in addition to this, some of these microbes are capnophilic, which means they thrive in higher levels of CO_2) but they ultimately need it for survival, since they do not have the ability to ferment, in contrast to anaerobic bacteria using fermentation as a primary source of ATP and cellular energy [51,52].

When it comes to the cultivation of anaerobes in a clinical microbiology laboratory, accepting only the samples appropriate for such purposes is of utmost importance. Specimen collection should be done using suitable equipment, while making sure that the sample is not contaminated with the resident flora of the body site in question. If sample processing is taking place somewhere else (e.g., is sent to a reference laboratory) adequate precautions need to be met for the use of anaerobic transport media and storage. The following specimen types should be considered for cultivation: samples taken from normally sterile body sites (e.g., blood cultures, cerebrospinal fluid samples, synovial fluid, samples from the chest and abdominal cavity), surgical discharge (or sample taken from the surgical site), samples from deep wounds (e.g., animal bites), abscesses of different anatomical localisation (liver, brain, lungs), perioral and gingival samples, samples from diabetic foot ulcers, respiratory secretions taken with a double-lumen device, urine samples (taken only with suprapubic aspiration) and faecal samples (in the suspected case of C. difficile infection). The best specimens for anaerobic cultivation are those taken using a needle and a syringe. Any other sample type received should not be accepted for anaerobic processing since they do not meet the requirements (risk of oxygen exposure: false negative result; contaminants: false positive results and/or cultivation of microorganisms with no clinical significance) [5,6,49,53–55].

Adequate laboratory conditions are necessary for the cultivation and diagnosis of anaerobic bacteria, the most important of which is a suitable method to anaerobiosis (stable anaerobic environment for cultivation) and the availability of pre-reduced anaerobically sterilised (PRAS) media. Some *physical* (McIntosh-Filde's jar), *chemical* (e.g., basic pyrogallol to bind atmospheric oxygen) and *biological* (Fortner's method; co-cultivation with a strong aerobic metabolism in a split Petri-dish, e.g., *Serratia marcescens*) methods are now only of historical significance. Depending on the size of the clinical laboratory and the number of incoming isolates, GasPak sachets, anoxomat systems or anaerobic chambers (glove boxes) are used, although the availability of some of these is limited to anaerobic reference laboratories [5,6,49,53,56].

Anaerobic bacteria are fastidious microorganisms, culturing them requires nutrition-rich media and some of these include components that allow for the selective growth of these bacteria. Examples include liquid enrichment media like Holman-broth (chopped meat and carbohydrates) and thioglycolate-broth and a variety of pre-reduced anaerobically sterilised solid media (anaerobic blood agar, Brucella blood agar supplemented with 5% lysed horse blood, 5 µg/mL hemin and 1 µg/mL Vitamin K1 [BBA], Schaedler blood agar [SCS], Bacteroides-bile-esculin agar [BBE], kanamycin-vancomycin leaked blood agar [KVLB or LKV], phenylethyl alcohol agar [PEA], cycloserine-cefoxitine fructose agar [CCFA], colistin-nalidixic acid media [CNA], egg-yolk agar [EYA]) [5,49,57].

A variety of methods can be used for the identification of anaerobic isolates, from presumptive identification (based on growth characteristics, colony morphology, susceptibility to given antibiotics, presence or absence of fluorescence, classical biochemical tests and spot-tests) to commercial kits (e.g., Vitek 2 ANI card, API 20A, RapidID 32A: bioMérieux, Fr., MicroScan, BBLCrystal Anaerobe ID: Beckton Dickinson, UK) [49,58]. When it comes to the biochemical ID, it is important to be aware of the enzymes we target in an assay. Reactions involving *constitutive* enzymes can be included in rapid identification kits, while in the case of *inducible* enzymes, the presence of the substrate and additional time for the reaction is required. An additional method, specific for these bacteria, is available: using gas-liquid chromatography (GLC), a rapid, accurate and reliable identification method of anaerobes is possible, based on the alcohols, organic acids and short-chain fatty acids they produce [59]. This method can also be used to differentiate between aerobic and anaerobic infections (e.g., from a haemoculture), many laboratories however, do not possess the instruments required to carry out this assay [60,61]. For further reading on the phenotypic methods concerning anaerobic bacteria, see the *Wadsworth-KTL Anaerobic Bacteriology Manual*, which is considered as a reference in the phenotypic identification of these microorganisms [5].

The introduction of molecular methods, array-based systems and novel technological advancements in clinical microbiology, such as whole-genome sequencing (WGS) and matrix-assisted laser desorption/ionization time-of-flight (MALDI-TOF) mass spectrometry (which utilizes the spectra of conserved ribosomal proteins for identification) has revolutionised the detection and correct identification of anaerobic bacteria. Although the development of databases containing bacterial spectra, required for identification is still underway (with projects like the 'European Network for Rapid Identification of Anaerobes' [ENRIA] leading the charge), MALDI-TOF MS changed the face of diagnostic bacteriology in the last decade, both in the case of aerobes and anaerobes [62–71]. Whole-genome sequencing is a novel technology used for culture-independent diagnostic testing (CIDT). WGS is considered the "golden standard" of bacterial species identification, based on the complete sequencing of their genetic material and then, comparing the data to reference genomic libraries based on bioinformational methods. Nevertheless, while there are some commercial MALDI-TOF MS systems available, specifically for all purposes (including anaerobes and fungi) of routine clinical microbiology (e.g., VITEK MS: bioMérieux, Fr., MALDI Biotyper or Microflex LT of Bruker-Daltonics, Gr.) [72,73], sequencing technologies are-in most cases-still in their developmental/experimental phase (and not necessarily well characterized for anaerobes) [29,62,74–76]. Besides the growing interest in the research related to anaerobic bacteria, the description and verification of new species has also been facilitated by the introduction of these new technologies-although such research is limited to reference laboratories with the appropriate facilities [20,77,78].

Compared to the processing time of aerobic bacteria or facultative anaerobes the workup of anaerobic isolates usually takes much longer. For this reason, continuous communication between the clinicians and the diagnostic lab is crucial. The laboratory should supply any clinically relevant information in a precise and timely manner, while the feedback of the physicians is also important, since based on the information about the symptoms and the clinical picture, the lab can narrow down (or include more specific tests) the list of the possible causative agents. If anaerobic bacteria were present at the infection site and we failed to detect them, it can often lead to inappropriate therapeutic choices and clinical failure [8].

3. Examples of Clinically Relevant Anaerobic Bacteria

3.1. Members of the Bacteroides Fragilis Group

Anaerobic Gram-negatives include some of the most important human pathogens among the group of anaerobic bacteria. The group is included in the phylum *Bacteroidetes* (together with pathogens like *Capnocytophaga canimorsus*, *Porphyromonas gingivalis*, *Prevotella melaninogenica* and *Tannerella forsythia*) [6,50]. Together with the taxonomy of other anaerobic species, the classification of *Bacteroidetes* has undergone major changes due to findings of studies related to molecular, sequencing and other related metagenomic studies. The most profound changes can be seen in the genus *Bacteroides*, in which mostly Gram-negative, bile-resistant bacilli remained (Table 2). Species that were saccharolytic, bile-sensitive (pigmented [formerly known as *B. melaninogenicus*] or nonpigmented) were relocated to the genus *Prevotella*, while the asaccharolytic, pigmented species to the genus *Porphyromonas* [24]. The previous classification of the group was as an order of subspecies (e.g., *B. thetaiotaomicron* was previously known as *B. fragilis* ssp. *thetaiotaomicron*) but later was reclassified based on studies related to the DNA homology of the respective species. The members of the *Bacteroides* spp. are important constituents of the faecal bacteria flora of adult humans, they have an active role in the metabolism of bile salts, nitrogen-containing substrates and various carbohydrates and polysaccharides (e.g., arabinogalactan, starch, pectin, xylan) [6,23,50].

The antibiotic resistance levels among anaerobes is the best characterized in *Bacteroides* isolates and according to the relevant literature, the species of the genus have the highest levels of antibiotic resistance and the most numerous number of antibiotic resistance mechanisms among all human pathogenic anaerobic bacteria (described in detail in Section 5) [79,80]. It is important to note that resistance levels of these bacteria are in inverse relationship with their incidence and clinical significance: *P. distasonis* and *B. thetaiotaomicron* (13–23% of *Bacteroides* isolates) exhibit the highest levels of resistance, while the strains of *B. fragilis* is generally the most susceptible species in the *B. fragilis* group.

B. fragilis is a pleomorphic (with varying sizes of 1.5–6 μm), non-pigmented, non-motile, encapsulated, Gram-negative rod. The species is catalase-positive (which is not common for anaerobe bacteria), indole-negative and the clinical isolates are growing well in the presence of 20% bile (bile resistant). They do not produce fluorescence under UV-light and they are resistant to vancomycin, kanamycin and colistin antibiotic disks, which can be used for their presumptive identification. *B. fragilis* is the most frequently isolated member of this group and although they only represent 2–5% of the species isolated from the fecal flora, it accounts for >50% of the clinical isolates of the *Bacteroides* genus and is responsible for around 80% of infections caused by the genus [50].

Certain strains termed enterotoxigenic *B. fragilis* (ETBF) produce a metalloprotease enterotoxin, which is coded by the *bft* genes on the *B. fragilis* pathogenicity island (BfPAI). The disease was first described in new-born lambs and calves, nowadays it is acknowledged as a significant cause of a self-limiting diarrheal disease in adults. Certain reports drew the conclusions that colonisation with enterotoxigenic *B. fragilis* is also associated with higher risk for colorectal cancer and irritable bowel syndrome (IBS), however there is still debate over the conclusions of these results. The proper diagnosis of enterotoxigenic *B. fragilis* infection is laborious, detection of the toxin genes (*bft*1–3) by polymerase chain reaction or the determination of the biological activity of the BFT protein in a cell culture assay (for this purpose, only those cell lines can be used, which have the ability to polarize in vitro, e.g., HT-29, Caco-2, HCT-8, MDCK, etc.) is needed. Animal models have also been described to verify the presence of the enterotoxin of *B. fragilis*, however the use of these models is only appropriate in a research setting [50,81,82]. A very important virulence factor of these bacteria is the presence of the capsule (consisting of two, well characterised polysaccharides), the significance of which in abscess formation was proven earlier in animal studies [83]. Additional virulence determinants of this species include the presence of various fimbriae and adhesions, which help the bacteria to adhere to matrix proteins of the host [50]. The most significant role of *B. fragilis* as an infectious agent is thought to be in anaerobic bacteraemia, where the associated mortality is estimated to be around 19% (60% if left untreated) [84,85].

B. fragilis is frequently termed as the "anaerobic *Escherichia coli*" due to the many parallels in the characteristics of these microbes: (i) both are bile-resistant Gram-negative rods; (ii) both colonise the colon and have integral roles as a part of the microbiota; (iii) both have the proclivity to become multidrug resistant pathogens through a variety of resistance mechanisms (iv) some strains produce enterotoxin (enterotoxigenic *B. fragilis* vs. enterotoxigenic *E. coli*) and capsule (in the case of extra-intestinal pathogenic *E. coli* strains). The presence of this species was associated with pathogen synergy, it has been described that the presence of *B. fragilis* and *E. coli* in mixed intra-abdominal infections enhanced the anti-complement environment of the infection site through bacterial virulence factors [86].

Table 2. Species of the *Bacteroides fragilis* group [50].

Bacteroides				Parabacteroides
B. acidifaciens	B. eggerthii	B. massiliensis	B. sartorii	P. chartae
B. barnesiae	B. faecis	B. nordiia	B. stercoris	P. distasonis
B. caccae	B. finegoldii	B. oleiciplenus	B. thetaiotaomicron	P. goldsteinii
B. cellulosilyticus	B. fluxus	B. ovatus	B. uniformis	P. gordonii
B. chinchillae	B. galacturonicus	B. plebeius	B. vulgatus	P. johnsonii
B. clarus	B. gallinarium	B. propionifaciens	B. xylanisolvens	P. merdae
B. coagulans	B. graminisolvens	B. pyogenes	B.xylanolyticus	
B. coprocola	B. helcogenes	B. rodentium	B. zoogleoformans	
B. coprophilus	B. heparinolyticus	B. salanitronis		
B. dorei	B. intestinalis	B. salyersiae		

3.2. Members of the Clostridium Genus

Anaerobic bacteria were traditionally classified into the *Clostridium* spp. based on the following characteristics: (i) their staining result was Gram-positive (ii) being strict anaerobic (iii) formation of characteristic endospores (their position is useful in species identification; *C. tetani* has round, terminal spores, *C. botulinum* and *C. difficile* forms oval, subterminal spores, *C. perfringens* has central spores with oval shape, i.e., in the appropriate environment) (iv) inability to reduce sulphates (SO_4^{2-}) into sulphites (SO_3^{2-}) [6,7]. Nevertheless, the classification of these bacteria based on these phenotypic criteria has become difficult, since some species do not form spores or only do in specific conditions (e.g., *C. perfringens*, *C. ramosum*), some are uncharacteristically tolerant to atmospheric oxygen (e.g., *C. tertium*, *C. histolyticum*), while others consistently present as Gram-negative after staining (*C. ramosum*, *C. clostridiforme*). Due to these discrepancies, it's not surprising that the reclassification of multiple species to various other genera (e.g., *Butyrivibrio*, *Dendrosporobacter*, *Enterocloster*, *Eubacterium*, *Faecalicatena*, *Lacriformis*, *Sedimentibacter*) has been proposed, based on 16S rRNA gene sequencing data [87,88].

Species of the *Clostridium* spp. are transient or permanent members of the normal flora of the gastro-intestinal tract and skin of animals and humans alike. Their spores naturally occur in the soil, their presence is facilitated with the use of manure as fertilizer. It is important to point out that many clinical specimens could contain *Clostridium* spp. as accidental contaminants, not involved in the disease process. It is up to the clinician to decide, whether the presence of these bacteria has any clinical significance, based on the symptoms of the patient, the presence of other microorganisms of pathogenic potential, frequency of isolation of the species and local epidemiology. The adequate management of clostridial infections involves administering antibiotic therapy (e.g., penicillin, vancomycin, metronidazole), with tissue debridement, where it is necessary. In some cases (like tetanus) toxoid immunization and antitoxin therapy are also important tools for clinicians [1,2,6,7].

The pre-requisite for clostridial wound infections is trauma to host tissue, to lower the oxidation-reduction potential and provide an environment suitable for anaerobic growth, followed by accidental contamination of the wound. Clostridial wound infections usually are polymicrobial in nature, because the sources of wound contamination (faeces, soil) is polymicrobial, involving a variety of other bacterial isolates (e.g., *Bacillus* spp., *Bacteroides* spp., *Escherichia* spp., *Proteus* spp., *Staphylococcus* spp.) [6,7]. All clostridial species involved in human diseases (see Table 3.) produce some kind of protein exotoxin (e.g., tetanus toxin, botulinum toxin) which plays an important role in the corresponding pathologies. Based on the pathogenesis of the disease caused by these microorganisms, they can be divided into the group of *histotoxic clostridia* (or gas-gangrene clostridia: *C. perfringens*, *C. novyi*, *C. septicum*, *C. histolyticum*) and neurotoxic clostridia (lockjaw/tetanus: *C. tetani*; botulism: *C. botulinum*, *C. baratii*, *C. butyricum*). Toxin-producing *C. difficile* strains represent an additional group, as the causative agents of antibiotic-associated diarrhoea (AAD), pseudomembranous colitis and toxic megacolon [6,7].

Various strains of *C. perfringens* produce potent necrotizing and haemolytic toxins and enzymes, based on this quality, these strains can be classified into types A-E. All types produce the α-toxin (the principal virulence factor of this species), which is a lecithinase that destroys the membranes of red and white blood cells and of surrounding tissue cells. The production of α-toxin can be detected by the Nagler-reaction, using egg-yolk agar (EYA). Other toxins of *C. perfringens* have a haemolytic, necrotizing and cardiotoxic effect. Among its other enzymes, the most important are collagenase, hyaluronidase and deoxyribonuclease. Some of the type A strains produce a heat-labile enterotoxin during sporulation (often occurring in the small intestine, at a relatively high pH), binds to the membrane of the epithelial cells of the small intestine, causing diarrhoea. The activity of this toxin is greatly increased by digestion with trypsin [6,7,89]. Tetanospasmine (or tetanus toxin, which is a typical AB-type exotoxin), the most important virulence factor of *C. tetani*, is released by dissolution the microbial cell. The toxin can reach the spinal cord, partially through the blood stream and the lymphatic system but mainly and typically by retrograde axonal transport through the peripheral neurons. The active A subunit, which is a zinc-endopeptidase, inhibits the release of inhibitory neurotransmitters (glycine and γ-aminobutyric acid) from inhibitory neurons. Thus, the proliferation of acetylcholine generates a continuous activation resulting in spastic, convulsive paralysis (causing the characteristic symptoms of the disease) [6,7].

The botulinum toxin (or botulotoxin) is the exotoxin of *C. botulinum*. It is produced as a consequence of lysogenic conversion, seven different (A-G) structurally different variants are known, of which the A, B, E and F-type toxins have been reported in human diseases. For any symptom to occur, whether or not it is caused by preformed toxins (classical food poisoning) or the effect of toxins produced by the microorganism in the body (infant and wound-botulism), the botulinum toxins is responsible. Botulinum toxin is a very powerful poison and in contrast to other toxins, protein-digesting enzymes of the intestinal tract do not hydrolyse it but it is heat-labile, meaning that the proper treatment of the food (at 80 °C for at least 10 min) inactivates it. In many respects, it is similar to the tetanus toxin (it is also an AB-type zinc-endopeptidase). However, unlike tetanus toxin, the botulinum toxin does not migrate retrograde to the neuronal cell, after entering the neuromuscular junctions through endocytosis. The toxin cleaves the protein required for acetylcholine release in the presynaptic neuron, the release of acetylcholine is thus omitted and in the absence of the neurotransmitter, the distinct symptoms of flaccid paralysis can be observed [6,7,90].

Similarly to other members of the genus, exotoxins are responsible for the symptoms of *C. difficile* infection as well. The A-toxin is an enterotoxin, which causes injury to intestinal cell-cell connections with subsequent increase in the permeability of the intestinal epithelium and fluid secretion. It also enhances the migration white blood cells, inducing a local inflammatory reaction. B-toxin is a cytotoxin that damages the cytoskeleton of the cells by disorganizing intracellular actin filaments. The two toxins have a synergistic effect but the A-toxin negative strains seem to be just as capable of causing illness and even causing hospital epidemics. The third toxin is the so-called binary toxin (or CDT), the exact mode of action of which is unknown, although it has been recognized that strains producing binary toxin are associated with higher mortality and produce A and B toxins in much larger quantities than CDI-negative strains [6,17,18].

Table 3. Illnesses caused by human pathogenic species of the *Clostridium* genus [6,7,17,18,87–90].

Pathogen	Disease
C. argentinense C. baratii **C. botulinum** C. butyricum	Botulism
C. bifermentans C. fallax C. histolyticum C. novyi **C. perfringens** C. sordelii	Soft tissue infections (gas gangrene, suppurative myonecrosis, cellulitis) Food poisoning Enteritis necrotisans Endometritis Sepsis
C. tetani	Tetanus
C. difficile	Antibiotic-associated diarrhoea Pseudomembranous colitis Toxic megacolon
C. clostridioforme C. innocuum C. sporogenes C. tertium	Opportunistic infections

The bacteria in bold represent the most prevalent species in the group.

4. Antimicrobial Susceptibility Testing of Anaerobes

4.1. General Considerations

According to the international guidelines, the susceptibility testing of anaerobic bacteria is very expensive, time-consuming and requires experienced laboratory staff, testing every patient's isolate received in a routine laboratory is not warranted. There are some diagnostic institutions (e.g., in low-income countries, with no technical capabilities) where even the cultivation of these microorganisms is a challenge. In these cases, isolates are usually sent to higher-tier facilities or a national anaerobic reference laboratory. Based on current recommendations, susceptibility testing should be performed in the following cases: (i) infections of a serious and life-threatening nature (e.g., in endocarditis, bacteraemia, abscesses involving the brain) [2,10,84]; (ii) relapsing infections or infections that did not respond to empirical therapy at all; (iii) when the antibiotic therapy needs to take place for an extended time period (e.g., infections involving bones, joints, implanted devices or grafts) [12,13]; (iv) there is limited or no available data on the susceptibilities of the given organism; (v) there is a known pattern of resistance against the antimicrobial agent by the microorganism [79]; (vi) the causative agent is a particularly virulent anaerobe (see Table 4) with unpredictable resistance [8,23]; (vii) the microorganism was isolated in pure culture and/or from a normally sterile body site (see Section 2) [8,23]. Besides the abovementioned points, susceptibility testing should be performed wherever it is possible, for epidemiological purposes and to guide the choice of the therapeutic agents [8,91,92]. This aspect of surveillance (both locally and globally) needs to be reiterated, since recommendations on first-line agents of therapy is usually based on similar data (Table 5). For example, due to the high level of resistance, cefoxitin and cefotetan are not advised as first-line drugs and clindamycin has been completely removed from such recommendations (although it can still be used in various oral infections and aspiration pneumonia), with beta-lactam/beta-lactamase inhibitor combinations emerging as first line drugs next to metronidazole [1,93]. It is also important to realise that different susceptibility testing methods are appropriate for various needs and end points, e.g., whether it is performed in a diagnostic laboratory of a hospital, for epidemiological/surveillance purposes in a reference laboratory or in a research institution [94].

Table 4. List of anaerobic bacteria where routine susceptibility testing is recommended [23].

Bacteroides fragilis group
Bilophila wadsworthia
Clostridium innocuum
Clostridium perfringens
Clostridium ramosum
Fusobacterium spp.
Prevotella spp.
Sutterella wadsworthensis
novel clinically important anaerobes (where surveillance data is not available)

Table 5. Antimicrobial agents that should be included in the routine susceptibility testing on anaerobic isolates [11,23,92].

Obligatory [a]	Accessory [b]
5-nitroimidazole group drugs [c]	cefoxitin
penicillins	moxifloxacin
beta-lactam-beta-lactamase inhibitore combination [d]	tigecycline
clindamycin	Vancomycin [f]
Carbapenems [e]	Fidaxomycin [f]

[a] Accurate if the bacteria have no intrinsic resistance to the agent; [b] If the agent has the appropriate indications by the FDA/EMA for the infection in question; [c] Including metronidazole, tinidazole, secnidazole, onidazole; [d] Including amoxicillin/clavulanic acid, ticarcillin/clavulanic acid, ampicillin/sulbactam, piperacillin/tazobactam; [e] Including imipenem, meropenem, ertapenem and doripenem; [f] Relevant in the case of *Clostridium difficile*.

Some organisations govern the standards and practices for the antimicrobial susceptibility testing of bacteria: the Clinical Laboratory Standards Institute (CLSI; previously NCLLS) [95], the European Committee for Antimicrobial Susceptibility Testing (EUCAST; operating as a standing committee in the European Society of Clinical Microbiology and Infectious Diseases) [96], the British Society for Antimicrobial Chemotherapy (BSAC; which has since harmonized its criteria with EUCAST standards [97,98]) and the Deutsches Institut für Normung (DIN; German Institute for Standardization) [99]. The ESCMID Study Group for Anaerobic Infections (ESGAI) [100] and the Anaerobe Society of Americas (ASA) [101] play an equally important role in the facilitation of proper practice in the case of these bacteria.

Since there is no specified testing method for anaerobes by EUCAST, the standard procedures established by CLSI (currently M11-A8) are most frequently used [102]. According to this document, broth microdilution and agar dilution are the reference methods for this group of bacteria, although different methods are also accepted if their uniformity is confirmed with the reference method. CLSI also recommends that at least 100, randomly selected isolates of a given genera should be tested for their resistance patterns, to acquire adequate information on the regional (hospital) patterns of resistance [102]. Irrespective of the method used for the susceptibility testing on anaerobic bacteria, these all share the following: (i) without the proper (stable) level of anaerobiosis during the incubation period, the results cannot be interpreted [103]; (ii) since the generation time of these bacteria is longer than their aerobic counterparts, results of the susceptibility testing can only be interpreted after 48–72 h (or more); (iii) extensive quality control and staff experience is required [94]; (iv) breakpoints determined by CLSI and EUCAST do not always match, making interpretation of the susceptibility results difficult [102,103].

4.2. Disk Diffusion Method (Kirby-Bauer Method)

Disk diffusion susceptibility testing is an easy-to-perform and cost-effective technique developed by EUCAST, their standardized methods and clinical breakpoints were embraced by clinical microbiology laboratories in Europe as well as in other parts of the globe [104]. Due to the popularity of this method, several studies (by EUCAST or otherwise) aiming at the evaluation of the suitability of this technique for the use in routine anaerobic bacteriology (mainly aiming at *B. fragilis* group isolates and "fast-growing" anaerobic strains) were performed [105,106]. Although some of these studies showed promising results in reproducibility (the inhibition zone diameters correlated well with the MICs in the case of metronidazole, imipenem, moxifloxacin and tigecycline), in other cases intermediate (I) and susceptible (S) isolates had overlaps in their inhibition zone diameters (in the case of beta-lactam/beta-lactamase inhibitor combinations and cefoxitin) [107]. Since the criteria for the use of this method has only been determined on aerobic bacteria so far, antimicrobial susceptibility testing of anaerobes using the disk diffusion method is not recommended in the routine lab yet and it is only used in a research setting or for preliminary screening for the antibacterial activity of different bioactive compounds [105]. However, "identification" disks containing specific antibiotics (usually colistin, kanamycin, metronidazole, penicillin and vancomycin are used) and sodium polyanethole sulfonate (SPS) are routinely used in the clinical microbiology laboratories for the presumptive identification of these bacteria [5].

4.3. Broth Microdilution Method

Broth microdilution assay is usually carried out using 96-well microtiter plates, where two-fold serial dilutions of the antibiotics are made. Commercial and in-house preparations are both available and the latter is more appropriate for the particular needs of the laboratory (various drugs can be tested in different concentrations), using only small volumes of reagents and media (Brucella broth supplemented with 5% lysed horse blood, 5 µg/mL hemin and 1 µg/mL Vitamin K1; according to CLSI recommendations) in the process. The results can be interpreted visually or with the help of a photometer. The results of the broth microdilution method are reported in Minimum Inhibitory

Concentration (MIC) values, or the lowest concentration of antibiotics that stopped bacterial expansion. The commercially available standard broth microdilution panels are the breakpoint panels, in which only one or a few concentrations of each antimicrobial agent are tested in a single panel. Unfortunately, this method is not an all-round solution for anaerobic bacteriology, since apart from *Bacteroides* spp. the growth of other species is not consistent in broth (homogenous growth cannot be attained, which leads to reporting false susceptibility, spore-forming bacteria with no visible growth can also be falsely reported as susceptible). Another significant drawback of this method is that it can only be performed in an anaerobic glove box (for the appropriate level of anaerobiosis to be maintained), therefore its use in the clinical microbiology lab is limited [108].

4.4. Agar Dilution Method

Agar-dilution method is currently the *gold standard* for the antimicrobial susceptibility testing of anaerobic bacteria. During this procedure, nutrient agar plates (Brucella Agar supplemented with 5% laked sheep blood, 5 µg/mL hemin and 1 µg/mL Vitamin K1; according to CLSI recommendations) are made with various antibiotics incorporated in the media in different concentrations, following with the inoculation of the plates with a standardized number (inocula of 0.5 McFarland standard from a pure culture incubated for 48 h) of bacterial cells, usually with the help of a Steers-Foltz replicator device. After incubation of the plates for 48–72 h in anaerobic atmosphere, the plates are read and compared visually. Based on this method, the lowest concentration of antibiotic that inhibited the growth of the given bacterial strain is the MIC. Agar-dilution is an labour-intensive method recommended for anaerobic reference laboratories [23,102].

4.5. Gradient Tests (E-Test, Spiral Gradient Test)

Gradient tests such as the E-test are the most frequently used in hospital laboratories for performing anaerobic susceptibility testing. During the procedure, a plastic/paper strip (containing a pre-determined amount of antibiotic in a gradient fashion and a corresponding scale for MIC determination) is placed on the plate, after inoculation with the sample. It is recommended to dry the agar plates before applying the strips, to prevent excess moisture to change the characteristic concentration gradient. The zone of inhibition will present itself in an elliptical shape (hence the 'E' in the name of the test), the MIC should be read at the point where the zone of inhibition intersects the strip. The MIC reading of the E-test is independent of the number of colony forming units (CFU) of the inoculated sample, therefore the results should be considered reliable, and there is good correlation with the reference method. E-test can be used for the detection of heteroresistance (e.g., in the case of imipenem resistance of *B. fragilis* or in the case of metronidazole resistance of *C. difficile* and *B. fragilis*) as well [109,110]. It is easy to perform and it is especially useful for the testing of a small number of isolates or only one antibiotic in laboratories without a steady flow of numerous anaerobic isolates.

The spiral gradient endpoint (SGE) technique is a special susceptibility testing method, which entails the use of a special agar plate, on which an apparatus deposits a specific amount of antibiotic stock solution in a spiral pattern [111]. By doing so, the concentration of the antibiotic is decreasing from the centre of the plate, creating a concentration gradient. After the inoculation of the plate with the relevant bacteria in a radial manner (thus, a single plate can be inoculated with multiple isolates and their susceptibilities to a single antibiotic can be determined simultaneously), the extent of growth is marked and the distance of the colonies from the centre of the plates is recorded. This data is then entered into a software (usually supplied by the manufacturer) which takes into account the physico-chemical characteristics of the antibiotic when determining the MIC related to the isolate in question. The emergence of resistant mutants can also be detected with this technique (colonies growing beyond the endpoint can be observed), while clumping of the bacteria was described (making interpretation difficult) when high-density inocula was used [112]. This method is becoming more and more popular because it's easy-to-use and it showed favourable results, when compared with the results of agar dilution, however it is similarly high-priced to the reference method [111,113]. The lack of commercially available designs based on this method and the additional need to calculate the MIC from the observed results are some of the other drawbacks of this method [23].

4.6. Examples of Resistance Detection Using Phenotypic and Genotypic Methods

Some rapid tests are available for the detection of β-lactamase enzyme production of bacteria. Such methods, e.g., nitrocefin disks are practical due to the ease-of-use and the express results they provide.   These colorimetric assays (a positive result is read if the disk changes to an orange or red colour in 5–60 min) are particularly useful if penicillin or ampicillin is the desired therapy [114].   During the interpretation of the results, it should be kept in mind that a negative result does not rule out resistance due to other mechanisms (e.g., changes in permeability due to poring loss or efflux pumps, modifications of PBPs) [115].   Performing this test is unnecessary on *B. fragilis* isolates, as the overwhelming majority produces β-lactamase enzymes [50].   Novel methods such as chromogenic media also present practical solutions for the use in the routine laboratory. An attempt for the development of such media was the *Bacteroides chromogenic agar* (BCA), in which 3,4-cyclohexenoesculetin-β-D-glucoside was included in the media instead of esculin to target the β-glucosidase activity of *B. fragilis*.   In a precipitation reaction between the hydrolysed substrate with iron salts added to the media, an insoluble black precipitate appears, which allows for the differentiation of *B. fragilis* colonies from a polymicrobial isolate.   Additionally, supplementation of BCA media with the appropriate concentrations of meropenem or metronidazole allows for the rapid detection of resistant strains of *B. fragilis* (e.g., from faeces), although this method is not yet routinely used in diagnostic laboratories [116].

Detection of resistance genes using polymerase chain reaction is a reliable method of identifying various antibiotic resistance determinants (for example: *nim* genes responsible for metronidazole resistance, *erm* genes conferring resistance to the macrolide-lincosamide-streptogramin (MLS) group of antimicrobials, the *cfiA* gene of carbapenem resistance, *gyr* and *parC* implicated in quinolone resistance, *cat* gene of chloramphenicol resistance, various *tet* genes making the microorganism resistant to tetracycline etc.) [23,117].   The end point would be the development of a multiplex PCR or a similar complex system, which would hopefully be able to identify multiple genes of resistance at once [117]. However, the development of similar methods is hindered by the fact that the presence of the resistance determinant genes in the genome does not automatically confer resistance to the antibiotics in question. This phenomenon has been well defined in the case of *B. fragilis* group isolates, harbouring "silent" *cfiA* or *cepA* genes (requiring specific insertion sequence (IS) elements to be activated), thus their genotypic resistance did not reflect their phenotypic resistance (i.e., their in vitro antimicrobial susceptibility patterns) [23,117,118].

Various experimental studies were conducted to test the potential future applications of matrix-assisted laser desorption/ionization time-of-flight (MALDI-TOF) mass spectrometry in the detection of various resistance determinants in anaerobes.   In these studies, *B. fragilis* was predominantly used as a test organism for the detection of carbapenem resistance (as one of the most worrying resistance trends) from standard laboratory strains and later from clinical samples, such as blood cultures [118–120].   There is great interest in MALDI-TOF MS-based resistance determination, due to the superior speed of communicating the results, not to mention that these tests could be implemented on the mass spectrometry devices already purchased (with the addition of the appropriate database for detection). The detection of beta-lactamase production is also possible with the use of this technology. The hydrolysis of beta-lactam antibiotics by these enzymes results in a molecular mass shift, which can be detected by a MALDI-TOF MS-based assay, although due to its time-consuming nature, this method is not yet widely used [121–123].

Whole-genome sequencing for the prediction of antimicrobial resistance is a novel and emerging research area, the development of which is further facilitated by the emergence of reasonably-priced WGS systems [124–127]. Detection of known antibiotic resistant determinant genes from the bacterial strain isolated from the patients allows for a culture-independent method to predict the susceptibility pattern of microorganisms. This makes WGS a useful tool for surveillance purposes, even in the case of drugs that are usually not included in classical (phenotypic) susceptibility testing routines (e.g., in drug development). [74,128,129]. Additionally, resistant phenotypes caused by dissimilar genetic backgrounds can be differentiated [124,125]. According to recent studies on selected species groups, the concordance rate between the presence of antibiotic resistance genes and the actual antibiogram (phenotype) of the microorganism is between 72–99%, although the use of this method is still in its experimental stages, due to the lack of properly developed reference libraries of bacterial resistance determinants (seeing that only the resistance genes included in the web-based databases will be recognized-a common disadvantage of molecular diagnostic methods) [129,130].

5. Antibiotic Resistance in Anaerobic Bacteria: The Importance of Surveillance

Nowadays the treatment of infections caused by anaerobic bacteria (or a mixed infection having an anaerobic component) rests upon the following antimicrobials: penicillins (ampicillin/ticarcillin), beta-lactam-beta-lactamase inhibitor combinations (amoxicillin/clavulanic acid, ticarcillin/clavulanic acid, ampicillin/sulbactam, piperacillin/tazobactam), cefoxitin and cefotetan (cephamycins), clindamycin, tigecycline, moxifloxacin, macrolides (azithromycin, clarithromycin), chloramphenicol and metronidazole [1,23,93,131].

Some data available on the resistance trends of anaerobes (apart from hospital-level or regional surveillance studies conducted where resources were available) is restricted to the studies published by anaerobic reference laboratories or major trans-national collaborations [23,132–136]. Although the variations between different geographical regions are notable, common tendencies can be observed.

While three decades ago the antibiotic susceptibility pattern of anaerobic bacteria was straightforward, nowadays we cannot so easily predict the efficiency of the chosen empirical therapy [91]. Clinicians can no longer "expect" certain drugs to work in anaerobic infections because they showed potent activity before [137]. Though not at the same speed as some other microorganisms (e.g., carbapenem-resistant *Acinetobacter baumannii*, *Pseudomonas aeruginosa* or members of the *Enterobacteriaceae* [138]) resistance has steadily increased among anaerobes during the last 30 years.

With the use of broad-spectrum antimicrobials in addition to the suitable surgical measures, the issue of emerging resistance of anaerobic bacteria was maybe less obvious [93,131]. But if we observe the data from the (inter)national surveillance reports from Europe (Table 6) [139–147] and the United States (Table 7) [95,135,144–147], the same trends can be discovered: steadily growing resistance to all classes of antimicrobial agents, with some of them rendered completely useless. Several publications report the emergence of multidrug resistant anaerobic Gram-negative bacteria (especially within the *B. fragilis* group isolates), harbouring multiple resistance genes or with a combination of intrinsic and acquired resistance mechanisms [80,85,147–151]. In these cases, the bacteria were usually termed multidrug resistant if they were resistant to 3–4 antibiotic classes besides metronidazole (due to *nim* nitroimidazole resistance genes) and the carbapenems (a metallo-β-lactamase encoded by *cfiA/ccrA* genes) [79]. Mobile genetic elements (plasmids containing resistance determinants, insertion sequence elements, transposons) have a significant role in the spread of the multidrug resistant phenotype in anaerobes.

The significance of the abovementioned tendencies is further underlined by the fact, that treatment failure has been described in empirical treatment in cases of anaerobic bacteraemia, as result of a multidrug resistant *B. fragilis* infection [9,84,152–155]. What makes this problem even more insidious is the fact that the correlation between the presence of multidrug resistant anaerobic bacterial strains and clinical failure is hard to prove. Mixed infections that include anaerobic bacteria often improve by drainage or surgical debridement [2]. The well-being of the patient (chronic diseases, immunosuppression) and the effect of the administered antibiotics on the aerobic component of the infection could further influence clinical outcome. Lastly, if the specimen collection and processing of the anaerobic isolate was not appropriate, the suspected microorganism cannot be cultivated, even if there is strong clinical suspicion of its presence [63].

Table 6. Resistance trends of clinical *Bacteroides* isolates in Europe between 1990–2010 (expressed as the percentage of resistant isolates) [94,135,145].

Europe	AMP	AMX/CLA	PIP/TAZ	FX	IMP	CLI	TET	MET	CIP	MXF
Breakpoints (mg/L)	**32/64**	**8**	**128**	**32/64**	**4/16**	**4/8**	**4**	**8/32**	**4**	**8**
1990	16.0%	1.0%	-	3.0%	0.3%	9.0%	64.0%	0.0%	56.0%	-
2000	99.3%	-	1.0%	6.0%	0.7%	15.0%	-	0.5%	-	9.0%
2010	98.2%	10.4%	10.3%	17.2%	1.2%	32.4%	-	0.5%	-	13.6%

AMP: ampicillin; AMX/CLA: amoxicillin/clavulanic acid; PIP/TAZ: piperacillin/tazobactam; FX: cefoxitin; IMP: imipenem; CLI: clindamycin; TET: tetracycline; MET: metronidazole; CIP: ciprofloxacin; MXF: moxifloxacin.

Table 7. Resistance trends of clinical *Bacteroides* isolates in the United States between 1990–2009 (expressed as the percentage of resistant isolates) [139–142].

USA	AMP	AMP/SUL	PIP/TAZ	FX	IMP	CLI	TET	MET	CIP	MXF
Breakpoints (mg/L)	**-**	**32**	**128**	**16/64**	**8/16**	**4/8**	**-**	**16**	**-**	**8**
1990	-	-	-	11.0%	0.0%	5.0%	-	0.0%	-	-
1997/2004	-	2.6%	0.5%	10.3%	0.4%	25.6%	-	0.0%	-	34.5%
2009 [a]	-	6.5%	0.8%	10.9%	0.6%	35.2%	-	-	-	50.1%

AMP: ampicillin; AMP/SUL: ampicillin/sulbactam; PIP/TAZ: piperacillin/tazobactam; FX: cefoxitin; IMP: imipenem; CLI: clindamycin; TET: tetracycline; MET: metronidazole; CIP: ciprofloxacin; MXF: moxifloxacin.
[a] calculated from the average of the resistance percentages of the individual *Bacteroides* strains investigated.

A summary of some of the important resistance mechanisms (and their genetic determinants) is presented in Table 8. While the growing problem of resistance stems from the fact that resistance is gradually developing against drugs that once were efficacious in treatment (analogous to the trends observed in other bacteria, e.g., *Enterobacteriaceae*) it is important to be aware that anaerobes–owing to their biological nature–are inherently resistant to some antimicrobials. For example, all anaerobic bacteria are resistant to the aminoglycosides, since the antibiotic cannot reach its target molecule (30S subunit of the ribosome). The uptake of an aminoglycoside drug by a bacterial cell is a two-step process, requiring the presence of oxygen- or nitrogen-dependent electron transport chains, a mechanism that all anaerobes lack, therefore making the impact of this antibiotic class limited. Anaerobes exhibit similar innate resistance towards fosfomycin, trimethoprim, aztreonam and all 1st and 2nd generation quinolones through a variety of processes, therefore using these drugs in therapy would be ill-advised [156–158]. Other instances of intrinsic resistance are species dependent, like in the case of metronidazole resistance of various Gram-positive anaerobes (*Actinomyces* spp., *Lactobacillus* spp., Bifidobacterium spp., *Propionibacterium* spp.), the macrolide and rifampin resistance in *Fusobacterium nucleatum* and *F. mortiferum* and the resistance against cephalosporins in *C. difficile*.

Clindamycin was considered the gold standard for the treatment of anaerobic infections some 40–50 years ago but with the emergence of high levels of resistance among *C. difficile* (~70%), *B. fragilis* group (30–40%), *Prevotella* spp. (10–40%), other related anaerobic Gram-negative bacteria (~10%) and *Peptostreptococcus* spp (~10%), this drug lost its significance as a first-line drug. Clindamycin resistance of chromosomal origin is linked to tetracycline resistance determinants, although their presence in plasmids and conjugative transposons was also described. Several studies showed that *macrolides* (azithromycin, clarithromycin) are potent agents against some anaerobic bacteria, although their bacteriostatic effects hinder their usefulness in serious infections. Resistance to the macrolide-lincosamide-streptogramine-group of antimicrobials manifest uniformly (which can be attributed to various *erm* genes): due to the methylation of two specific adenine residues of the 23S rRNA, the effective binding of the drugs to ribosome is prevented [159–163].

Chloramphenicol was a drug-of-choice for the treatment of serious anaerobic infections (especially if the central nervous system was involved), nowadays is an infrequently used drug, due to its considerable toxicity and serious reversible (haemolytic anaemia, optic neuritis, bone marrow suppression) and irreversible (fatal aplastic anaemia) side effects. Resistance against chloramphenicol is mostly plasmid-mediated, by inactivation of the active drug through acetylation or nitro-reduction [164,165].

Quinolones were generally considered ineffective against anaerobic bacteria due to their bacteriostatic effects and the poor drug penetration to the target sites, together with the low affinity for the target enzymes, owing to point mutations in the *gyrA-B* (Topoisomerase II) and *parC* genes (Topoisomerase IV). Additionally, quionolone resistance determining regions (QRDR; like that found in *E. coli*) were observed in several anaerobic species, with an increased expression of efflux proteins. These quinolone resistance mechanisms were mostly observed in *B. fragilis* group, *C. perfringens* and *C. difficile* isolates [166–169]. Moxifloxacin is a new drug in this group of antimicrobials, with FDA approval for complicated skin and skin structure infections, with promising anti-anaerobe activity.

Resistance against *β-lactam antibiotics* is very common among anaerobes (predominantly due to the production of β-lactamase enzymes), although there are significant variations to the levels of resistance between these bacteria. Almost 100% of *B. fragilis* isolates are resistant to penicillin G, since they constitutively produce a chromosomally-encoded penicillinase enzyme; this is around 50% in the case of *Prevotella* spp. and between 8–17% for *Porphyromonas* spp. While *Cl. perfringens* isolates are ~100% susceptible to penicillin G (ampicillin), resistance has emerged in non-perfringens clostridia (e.g., *Cl. clostidiforme, Cl. butyricum, Cl. ramosum*) [170]. The production of a class 2e cephalosporinase (encoded by the *cepA* and *cfxA* genes; *B. fragilis*) confers resistance against cefoxitin and cefotetan; this enzyme is inhibited by β-lactamase enzyme inhibitors (clavulanic acid, sulbactam, tazobactam). Cephamycins such as cefoxitin (with a 7α-methoxyl side chain) and cefotetan (with an N-methylthiotetrazole side chain) can still be considered appropriate therapy for anaerobic infections (in contrast to cephalosporins) but consulting regional epidemiological data about resistance levels is recommended. An emerging issue is the appearance of a Zn^{2+}-metallo-β-lactamase enzyme (essentially a carbapenemase, encoded by the *cfiA/ccrA* genes; it is inhibited by EDTA) in *B. fragilis*. These isolates are resistant against the carbapenem antibiotics, which are usually preserved as last-resort drugs in serious, life threatening infections. It has been described that more *Bacteroides* isolates harbour these resistance genes than the number of isolates with a phenotypic resistance. The probable cause of this phenomenon is that these genes are not expressed in levels ("silent genes"), where they could exhibit decreased susceptibility carbapenems. However, with a one-step mutation, or with the insertion of an IS element, the strain can easily mutate to become resistant. Reduced permeability of the drugs through the outer membrane in some *Fusobacterium* spp., *Porphyromonas* spp. and *Bacteroides* spp. can also lead to decreased susceptibility. PBP alterations (leading to reduced binding affinity of these drugs) were described in several Gram-positive anaerobic cocci. It can be said that, for now, β-lactam antibiotics (especially beta-lactam/beta-lactamase inhibitor combinations and carbapenems) still represent the frontline of treatment in mixed aerobic-anaerobic infections [23,93]. Penicillin G is still a useful drug in our disposal and its use is appropriate if the strain in question is susceptible. Beta-lactam-beta-lactamase inhibitor combinations (with resistance levels of 0.5–10%) and carbapenems (0–2%) should be considered safe choices for empiric therapy [151,171–181]. The importance of surveillance is extremely important related to this group of drugs, with the number of resistant strains steadily growing and with the emergence of multidrug resistant anaerobes (note: some carbapenem and metronidazole resistance elements share mobile genetic elements) [79,149]. Such a pathogen of increasing importance is *Sutterella wadsworthiensis*, with increasing resistance rates to piperacillin/tazobactam, cefoxitin, clindamycin and metronidazole [182,183].

Metronidazole resistance is common in various Gram-positive anaerobic rods (*Actinomyces* spp., *Propionibacterium* spp., *Lactobacillus* spp.), while the prevalence of resistant Gram-positive cocci and Gram-negatives is usually very low (<1%). Metronidazole (and other related drugs) are a part of the 5-nitroimidazole group drugs and are one of the most important agents for the treatment of anaerobic infections. Metronidazole is a pro-drug: for the desired antimicrobial activity, it must be reduced for the release of toxic nitroso-residues (PFOR; pyruvate: ferredoxin oxidoreductase and the nitroreductase enzymes) that are extremely reactive (able to damage DNA, proteins and membranes of bacteria). Some consider metronidazole an example for the "ideal antibiotic model" [184]. Resistance to this drug is conferred by the *nim* genes (*nimA-J*) coding for a nitroimidazole-reductase: this transforms the pro-drug to a non-toxic amino-imidazole, with no antimicrobial activity. These *nim* genes share around 70% homology (*B. fragilis* group), apart from *nimI* (*Prevotella* spp.). *nimB* has been associated with moderate to high level metronidazole resistance. Other mechanisms of reduced susceptibility include lower levels of the PFOR enzyme (a significant decrease of the reducing power of the microorganisms) and the induction of lactate dehydrogenase (LDH) activity. These resistance determinants are predominantly found in the chromosome but their presence has been described in transferable plasmids and IS elements as well, with some experts fearing the rapid dissemination of these genes [149,150,185–194].

Tetracycline resistance is very common in anaerobic isolates (>95% of *Bacteroides* spp., >50% of *Prevotella* spp., *Fusobacterium* spp. and *Clostridium* spp.) to the point that the use of these drugs is not advised. Among the resistance mechanisms, drug efflux (*tetA-E*, *tetK-L*), ribosomal protection (*tetM*, *tetQ*, *tetW*) and oxidation (*tetX*) can be found. The *tet* genes are induced by sub-inhibitory tetracycine exposure, stimulating the spread of resistance trough conjugative transposons [160,170,195–197]. Tigecycline (the tert-butylglycamido-derivative of minocycline) is a novel drug in this antibiotic class, having FDA approval for soft tissue and intra-abdominal infections.

Efflux pumps are important determinants of antimicrobial resistance both in aerobic and anaerobic bacteria, their over-expression can often be associated with therapeutic failure. These transmembrane proteins can bind and expel various substrates and xenobiotics (such as antibiotics) before they could reach their target site or protein. Several efflux pumps have been characterized among anaerobic bacteria: the BexA of *B. thetaiotaomicron* (a transporter of the multi-antimicrobial extrusion protein [MATE] superfamily) the bmeABC1–16 (members of the resistance-nodulation-cell division [RND] superfamily, analogous to the AcrAB-TolC tripartite efflux systems of *E. coli*) and TetA-E efflux transporters (members of the major facilitator superfamily [MFS] superfamily) of *B. fragilis*, bcrABD (an ATP-binding cassette [ABC] transporter) of *Cl. perfringens* and XepCAB (member of the RND superfamily) of *P. gingivalis* [198–201]. Experimental studies have shown that knocking out one or more of these efflux proteins has a remarkable effect on the MICs of several antibiotics, although due to the redundancy of these proteins in the bacterial genome, other transporter mechanisms usually compensate for the loss of the selected transporter. An emerging therapeutic strategy is the use of efflux pump inhibitors (EPI) as adjuvant compounds, although these compounds were only tested extensively in laboratory conditions so far [198,202].

(Since this is not the main topic of our review, the information on the various modes of antibiotic resistance among anaerobes presented above is a brief summary of the available literature. For further reading on this topic, see [11,23,93,200,203]).

Table 8. Examples for antimicrobial resistance mechanisms exhibited by anaerobes [11,23,93,200,203].

Antibiotic Class	Mechanism of Resistance	Genes or Enzymes Implicated	Examples of Microorganisms
Aminoglycosides	Lack of O- or N-based electron transport systems; Unable to reach target ribosome subunit (30S)		All anaerobes
β-lactams	β-lactamase enzymes:		
	Penicillinases		*Clostridium* spp. *Fusobacterium* spp., *Prevotella* spp., *Porphyromonas* spp.
	Cephalosporinases	*cepA, cfxA*	*B. fragilis* gp
	Metallo-β-lactamases	*cfiA, ccrA*	*B. fragilis* gp.
	Reduced affinity to target molecule	PBP1–2 alterations	Anaerobic Gram-positive cocci, *B. fragilis* gp.
		PBP3 (aztrenonam)	All anaerobes
	Loss of porin channels		*B. fragilis* gp.

Table 8. *Cont.*

Antibiotic Class	Mechanism of Resistance	Genes or Enzymes Implicated	Examples of Microorganisms
Chloramphenicol	Inactivation		
	Acetylation	cat	*B. fragilis* gp.
	Nitro-reduction		*B. fragilis* gp.
Clindamycin	Methylation of the 23S rRNA	*ermF, ermG, ermS*	*B. fragilis* gp.
		ermB, ermF, ermG, ermFG,	*Prevotella* spp.
		ermF	*Porphyromonas* spp.
		ermB, ermQ	*Cl. difficile*
		ermP, ermQ	*Cl. perfringens*
	Inactivation		*B. fragilis* gp.
Macrolides	Methylation of the 23S rRNA	*ermA, ermB, ermF, ermG, ermQ, ermTM*	*F. magna, P. tetradius, P. anaerobius*
Metronidazole	Intrinsic		Gram-positive anaerobic bacteria
	Reduction of the drug by nitroimidazole reductase	*nimA-H*	*B. fragilis* gp., *Veillonella* spp.
		nimI	*Prevotella* spp.
	Reduced uptake of the drug		*B. fragilis* gp.
	Increase in LDH activity		*B. fragilis* gp.
Quinolones	Mutations in target enzymes		
	DNA-gyrase (Topoisomerase II)	*gyrA, gyrB*	*B. fragilis, Cl. perfringens, Cl. difficile*
	Topoisomerase IV	*parC*	*Cl. difficile*
Tetracyclines	Ribosomal protection	*tet(Q)*	*B. fragilis* gp.
		tet(M), tet(W)	*Fusobacterium* spp.
		tet(M), tet(Q), tet(W)	*Prevotella* spp.
	Ribosomal modification	*tetA(P), tetB(P)*	*Clostridium* spp.
	Efflux pumps	*tetA-E*	*B. fragilis* gp.
		tetK-L	*Peptostreptococcus* spp., *Veillonella* spp.
	Enzymatic degradation (oxidative)	*tetX*	*B. fragilis* gp.

6. Conclusions

Anaerobic microorganisms are now widely accepted as significant pathogens in human diseases, as such, the proper diagnosis and treatment of these infections are important healthcare priorities. The emergence of antimicrobial resistance in anaerobic bacteria is a discernible phenomenon, which deserved the attention of people working in diagnostic microbiology and infectious disease treatment. Microbiology laboratories should perform antimicrobial susceptibility testing to the best of their abilities, taking into account the number of incoming anaerobic isolates, as well as monetary considerations of the given institution. This incentive is important to broaden the information on regional, national and global patterns of resistance of anaerobes. Based on the plethora of literature available, the slow but steady increase of metronidazole and carbapenem resistance isolates is a cause for concern, especially if we observe what happened to the efficiency of other agents (like clindamycin) in the previous 20–30 years.

Acknowledgments: This study was supported by the European Union and the State of Hungary, co-financed by the European Social Fund in the framework of TÁMOP 4.2.4. A/2-11-1-2012-0001 'National Excellence Program.' G.S. was supported by the János Bolyai Research Scholarship of the Hungarian Academy of Sciences. M.G. was supported by the UNKP-17-3 New National Excellence Program of the Ministry of Human Capacities. M.G. has received input for the study/project through ESCMID's mentorship program by E.U. The authors would like to thank the "Top 35 of Antibiotics Travel Awards 2017" for the opportunity to publish in the Journal.

Author Contributions: M.G. did the literature review and formulated the initial draft of the manuscript. M.G., G.S. and E.U. discussed the initial draft and produced together the final version of the manuscript.

Abbreviations

AAD	antibiotic associated diarrhoea
ABC	ATP-binding cassette
AGNB	anaerobic Gram-negative bacilli
AIDS	acquired immunodeficiency syndrome
AMX/CLA	amoxicillin-clavulanic acid
AMP/SUL	ampicillin-sulbactam
ASA	Anaerobe Society of the Americas
AST	antimicrobial susceptibility testing
ATP	adenosine-triphosphate
BBA	Brucella blood agar
BBE	Bacteroides bile esculin agar
BfPAI	*Bacteroides fragilis* pathogenicity island
BL-BLIC	beta-lactam-beta-lactamase inhibitor combination
BSAC	British Society for Antimicrobial Chemotherapy
BV	bacterial vaginosis
Caco-2	Human epithelial colorectal adenocarcinoma
CCFA	Cefoxitin-cycloserine fructose agar
CNA	Colistin-nalidixic acid agar
CIDT	culture-independent diagnostic testing
CIP	ciprofloxacin
CLI	clindamycin
CLSI	Clinical and Laboratory Standards Institute
DIN	Deutsches Institut für Normung
DNA	deoxyribonucleic acid
EBV	Epstein-Barr virus
EDTA	ethylenediaminetetraacetic acid
EPI	efflux pump inhibitor
EMA	European Medicines Agency
ENRIA	European Network for Rapid Identification of Anaerobes
ESGAI	ESCMID Study Group for Anaerobic Infections
ETBF	enterotoxigenic *Bacteroides fragilis*
EUCAST	European Committe for Antimicrobial Susceptibility Testing
EYA	Egg-yolk agar
FDA	Food and Drug Administration of the United States
FX	cefoxitin
GLC	gas-liquid chromatography
IBS	irritable bowel syndrome
HCT-8	human ileocecal carcinoma
HGT	horizontal gene transfer
HT-29	human colon adenocarcinoma cell line
ID	identification
IS	insertion sequence
IMP	imipenem
KVLB	Kanamycin-vancomycin laked blood agar
LDH	lactate-dehydrogenase
MALDI-TOF MS	matrix-assisted laser desorption/ionization time-of-flight mass spectrometry
MATE	Multi-antimicrobial extrusion protein

MDCK	Madin Darby Canine Kidney cell line
MDR	multidrug resistant
MET	metronidazole
MIC	minimal inhibitory concentration
MLS	Macrolide-lincosamide-streptogramin B
MXF	moxifloxacin
NCLLS	National Committee for Clinical Laboratory Standards
PBP	penicillin-binding protein
PCR	polymerase chain reaction
PEA	Phenyletyl alcohol agar
PFOR	pyruvate:ferredoxin oxidoreductase
PID	pelvic inflammatory disease
PIP/TAZ	piperacillin-tazobactam
PRAS	pre-reduced anaerobically sterilised
QRDR	quionole resistance determining regions
RND	Resistance nodulation and division
rRNA	ribosomal ribonucleic acid
SCFA	short-chained fatty acid
SGE	spiral gradient endpoint
SOD	superoxide-dismutase
SCS	Schaedler blood agar
SPS	sodium polyanethol sulfonate
TET	tetracycline
WGS	whole-genome sequencing

References

1. Nagy, E. Anaerobic Infections Update on Treatment Considerations. *Drugs* **2010**, *70*, 841–858. [CrossRef] [PubMed]

2. Finegold, S.M. Anaerobic Infections: General Concepts. In *Principles and Practice of Infectious Diseases*; Mandell, G.L., Bennett, J.E., Dolin, R., Eds.; Churchill Livingstone: London, UK, 2000; Volume 2.

3. Cornaglia, G.; Courcol, R.; Herrmann, J.-L.; Kahlmeter, G.; Peigue-Lafeuille, H.; Jordi, V. *European Manual of Clinical Microbiology*; European Society for Clinical Microbiology and Infectious Diseases: Basel, Switzerland, 2012; ISBN 978-2-87805-026-4.

4. Finegold, S.M. *Anaerobic Bacteria in Human Disease*; Academic Press: New York, NY, USA, 1977; ISBN 978-0-12-256750-6.

5. Jousimies-Somer, H.; Summanen, P.; Citron, D.M.; Baron, E.J.; Wexler, H.M.; Finegold, S.M. *Wadsworth-KTL Anaerobic Bacteriology Manual*, 6th ed.; Jousimies-Somer, H., Summanen, P., Citron, D.M., Baron, E.J., Wexler, H.M., Finegold, S.M., Eds.; Star Publishing Company: Belmont, CA, USA, 2003.

6. Murray, P.R.; Baron, E.J.; Jorgensen, J.H.; Landry, M.L.; Pfaller, M. *Manual of Clinical Microbiology*, 9th ed.; Murray, P.R., Baron, E.J., Jorgensen, J.H., Landry, M.L., Pfaller, M., Eds.; American Society for Microbiology: Washington, DC, USA, 2007; Volume 1, ISBN 978-1-55581-371-0.

7. Wells, C.L.; Wilkins, T.D. Clostridia: Sporeforming Anaerobic Bacilli. In *Medical Microbiology*; Baron, S., Ed.; University of Texas Medical Branch at Galveston: Galveston, TX, USA, 1996; ISBN 978-0-9631172-1-2.

8. Jenkins, S.G. Infections due to anaerobic bacteria and the role of antimicrobial susceptibility testing of anaerobes. *Rev. Med. Microbiol.* **2001**, *12*, 1–12. [CrossRef]

9. Salonen, J.H.; Eerola, E.; Meurman, O. Clinical significance and outcome of anaerobic bacteremia. *Clin. Infect. Dis.* **1998**, *26*, 1413–1417. [CrossRef] [PubMed]

10. Goldstein, E.J. Anaerobic bacteremia. *Clin. Infect. Dis. Off. Publ. Infect. Dis. Soc. Am.* **1996**, *23* (Suppl. S1), S97–S101. [CrossRef]

11. Hecht, D.W. Anaerobes: Antibiotic resistance, clinical significance and the role of susceptibility testing. *Anaerobe* **2006**, *12*, 115–121. [CrossRef] [PubMed]

12. Lewis, R.P.; Sutter, V.L.; Finegold, S.M. Bone infections involving anaerobic bacteria. *Medicine (Baltimore)* **1978**, *57*, 279–305. [CrossRef] [PubMed]

13. Nolla, J.M.; Murillo, O.; Narvaez, J.; Vaquero, C.G.; Lora-Tamayo, J.; Pedrero, S.; Cabo, J.; Ariza, J. Pyogenic arthritis of native joints due to *Bacteroides fragilis*: Case report and review of the literature. *Medicine (Baltimore)* **2016**, *95*, e3962. [CrossRef] [PubMed]

14. Haggerty, C.L.; Hillier, S.L.; Bass, D.C.; Ness, R.B.; The PID Evaluation and Clinical Health (PEACH). Study Investigators Bacterial Vaginosis and Anaerobic Bacteria Are Associated with Endometritis. *Clin. Infect. Dis.* **2004**, *39*, 990–995. [CrossRef] [PubMed]

15. Saini, S.; Gupta, N.; Aparna; Batra, G.; Arora, D.R. Role of anaerobes in acute pelvic inflammatory disease. *Indian J. Med. Microbiol.* **2003**, *21*, 189–192. [PubMed]

16. Peng, Z.; Jin, D.; Kim, H.B.; Stratton, C.W.; Wu, B.; Tang, Y.-W.; Sun, X. Update on Antimicrobial Resistance in *Clostridium difficile*: Resistance Mechanisms and Antimicrobial Susceptibility Testing. *J. Clin. Microbiol.* **2017**, *55*, 1998–2008. [CrossRef] [PubMed]

17. Khan, F.Y.; Elzouki, A.-N. *Clostridium difficile* infection: A review of the literature. *Asian Pac. J. Trop. Med.* **2014**, *7*, S6–S13. [CrossRef]

18. Janoir, C. Virulence factors of *Clostridium difficile* and their role during infection. *Anaerobe* **2016**, *37*, 13–24. [CrossRef] [PubMed]

19. Terhes, G. Distribution of *Clostridium difficile* PCR ribotypes in regions of Hungary. *J. Med. Microbiol.* **2006**, *55*, 279–282. [CrossRef] [PubMed]

20. La Scola, B.; Fournier, P.E.; Raoult, D. Burden of emerging anaerobes in the MALDI-TOF and 16S rRNA gene sequencing era. *Anaerobe* **2011**, *17*, 106–112. [CrossRef] [PubMed]

21. Riordan, T. Human Infection with *Fusobacterium necrophorum* (Necrobacillosis), with a Focus on Lemierre's Syndrome. *Clin. Microbiol. Rev.* **2007**, *20*, 622–659. [CrossRef] [PubMed]

22. Williams, M.D.; Kerber, C.A.; Tergin, H.F. Unusual Presentation of Lemierre's Syndrome Due to *Fusobacterium nucleatum*. *J. Clin. Microbiol.* **2003**, *41*, 3445–3448. [CrossRef] [PubMed]

23. Brook, I.; Wexler, H.M.; Goldstein, E.J. Antianaerobic antimicrobials: Spectrum and susceptibility testing. *Clin. Microbiol. Rev.* **2013**, *26*, 526–546. [CrossRef] [PubMed]

24. Jousimies-Somer, H.; Summanen, P. Recent taxonomic changes and terminology update of clinically significant anaerobic gram-negative bacteria (excluding spirochetes). *Clin. Infect. Dis.* **2002**, *35*, S17–S21. [CrossRef] [PubMed]

25. Munson, E.; Carroll, K.C. What's in a Name? New Bacterial Species and Changes to Taxonomic Status from 2012 through 2015. *J. Clin. Microbiol.* **2017**, *55*, 24–42. [CrossRef] [PubMed]

26. Murdoch, D.A.; Shah, H.N. Reclassification of *Peptostreptococcus magnus* (Prevot 1933) Holdeman and Moore 1972 as *Finegoldia magna* comb. nov. and *Peptostreptococcus micros* (Prevot 1933) Smith 1957 as *Micromonas micros* comb. nov. *Anaerobe* **1999**, *5*, 555–559. [CrossRef]

27. Lawson, P.A.; Citron, D.M.; Tyrrell, K.L.; Finegold, S.M. Reclassification of *Clostridium difficile* as *Clostridioides difficile* (Hall and O'Toole 1935) Prevot 1938. *Anaerobe* **2016**, *40*, 95–99. [CrossRef] [PubMed]

28. Murdoch, D.A.; Shah, H.N.; Gharbia, S.E.; Rajdendram, D. Proposal to Restrict the Genus *Peptostreptococcus* (Kluyver & van Niel 1936) to *Peptostreptococcus anaerobius*. *Anaerobe* **2000**, *6*, 257–260. [CrossRef]

29. Song, Y.L.; Liu, C.X.; McTeague, M.; Finegold, S.M. 16S ribosomal DNA sequence-based analysis of clinically significant gram-positive anaerobic cocci. *J. Clin. Microbiol.* **2003**, *41*, 1363–1369. [CrossRef] [PubMed]

30. Murdoch, D.A. Gram-positive anaerobic cocci. *Clin. Microbiol. Rev.* **1998**, *11*, 81–120. [PubMed]

31. Murphy, E.C.; Frick, I.M. Gram-positive anaerobic cocci—Commensals and opportunistic pathogens. *FEMS Microbiol. Rev.* **2013**, *37*, 520–553. [CrossRef] [PubMed]

32. Siezen, R.J.; Kleerebezem, M. The human gut microbiome: Are we our enterotypes? *Microb. Biotechnol* **2011**, *4*, 550–553. [CrossRef] [PubMed]

33. Simon, G.L.; Gorbach, S.L. Intestinal flora in health and disease. *Gastroenterology* **1984**, *86*, 174–193. [PubMed]

34. Maier, E.; Anderson, R.C.; Roy, N.C. Understanding how commensal obligate anaerobic bacteria regulate immune functions in the large intestine. *Nutrients* **2014**, *7*, 45–73. [CrossRef] [PubMed]

35. Duranti, S.; Ferrario, C.; van Sinderen, D.; Ventura, M.; Turroni, F. Obesity and microbiota: An example of an intricate relationship. *Genes Nutr.* **2017**, *12*, 18. [CrossRef] [PubMed]

36. Leal-Lopes, C.; Velloso, F.J.; Campopiano, J.C.; Sogayar, M.C.; Correa, R.G. Roles of Commensal Microbiota in Pancreas Homeostasis and Pancreatic Pathologies. *J. Diabetes Res.* **2015**, *2015*, 284680. [CrossRef] [PubMed]

37. Bultman, S.J. Emerging roles of the microbiome in cancer. *Carcinogenesis* **2014**, *35*, 249–255. [CrossRef] [PubMed]

38. Ohtani, N. Microbiome and cancer. *Semin. Immunopathol.* **2015**, *37*, 65–72. [CrossRef] [PubMed]

39. Francescone, R.; Hou, V.; Grivennikov, S.I. Microbiome, inflammation and cancer. *Cancer J.* **2014**, *20*, 181–189. [CrossRef] [PubMed]

40. Shahanavaj, K.; Gil-Bazo, I.; Castiglia, M.; Bronte, G.; Passiglia, F.; Carreca, A.P.; del Pozo, J.L.; Russo, A.; Peeters, M.; Rolfo, C. Cancer and the microbiome: Potential applications as new tumor biomarker. *Expert Rev. Anticancer Ther.* **2015**, *15*, 317–330. [CrossRef] [PubMed]

41. Kelly, J.R.; Kennedy, P.J.; Cryan, J.F.; Dinan, T.G.; Clarke, G.; Hyland, N.P. Breaking down the barriers: The gut microbiome, intestinal permeability and stress-related psychiatric disorders. *Front. Cell. Neurosci.* **2015**, *9*, 392. [CrossRef] [PubMed]

42. Lima-Ojeda, J.M.; Rupprecht, R.; Baghai, T.C. "I Am I and My Bacterial Circumstances": Linking Gut Microbiome, Neurodevelopment and Depression. *Front. Psychiatry* **2017**, *8*, 153. [CrossRef] [PubMed]

43. Zhu, X.; Han, Y.; Du, J.; Liu, R.; Jin, K.; Yi, W. Microbiota-gut-brain axis and the central nervous system. *Oncotarget* **2017**, *8*, 53829–53838. [CrossRef] [PubMed]

44. Aarts, E.; Ederveen, T.H.A.; Naaijen, J.; Zwiers, M.P.; Boekhorst, J.; Timmerman, H.M.; Smeekens, S.P.; Netea, M.G.; Buitelaar, J.K.; Franke, B.; et al. Gut microbiome in ADHD and its relation to neural reward anticipation. *PLoS ONE* **2017**, *12*, e0183509. [CrossRef] [PubMed]

45. Finegold, S.M. State of the art; microbiology in health and disease. Intestinal bacterial flora in autism. *Anaerobe* **2011**, *17*, 367–368. [CrossRef] [PubMed]

46. Shoemaker, N.B.; Vlamakis, H.; Hayes, K.; Salyers, A.A. Evidence for extensive resistance gene transfer among *Bacteroides* spp. and among *Bacteroides* and other genera in the human colon. *Appl. Environ. Microbiol.* **2001**, *67*, 561–568. [CrossRef] [PubMed]

47. Pal, C.; Bengtsson-Palme, J.; Kristiansson, E.; Larsson, D.G.J. The structure and diversity of human, animal and environmental resistomes. *Microbiome* **2016**, *4*, 54. [CrossRef] [PubMed]

48. Loesche, W.J. Oxygen sensitivity of various anaerobic bacteria. *Appl. Microbiol.* **1969**, *18*, 723–727. [PubMed]

49. *Clinical Microbiology Procedures Handbook*, 4th ed.; Leber, A.L. (Ed.) ASM Press: Washington, DC, USA, 2016; ISBN 978-1-55581-880-7.

50. Wexler, H.M. *Bacteroides*: The good, the bad and the nitty-gritty. *Clin. Microbiol. Rev.* **2007**, *20*, 593–621. [CrossRef] [PubMed]

51. Ludwig, R.A. Microaerophilic bacteria transduce energy via oxidative metabolic gearing. *Res. Microbiol.* **2004**, *155*, 61–70. [CrossRef] [PubMed]

52. Morris, R.L.; Schmidt, T.M. Shallow breathing: Bacterial life at low O_2. *Nat. Rev. Microbiol.* **2013**, *11*, 205–212. [CrossRef] [PubMed]

53. Garg, R.; Kaistha, N.; Gupta, V.; Chander, J. Isolation, Identification and Antimicrobial Susceptibility of Anaerobic Bacteria: A Study Re-emphasizing Its Role. *J. Clin. Diagn. Res.* **2014**, *8*, DL01–DL02. [CrossRef] [PubMed]

54. Strobel, H.J. Basic laboratory culture methods for anaerobic bacteria. *Methods Mol. Biol.* **2009**, *581*, 247–261. [CrossRef] [PubMed]

55. Citron, D.M. Specimen collection and transport, anaerobic culture techniques and identification of anaerobes. *Rev. Infect. Dis.* **1984**, *6* (Suppl. S1), S51–S58. [CrossRef] [PubMed]

56. Barreau, M.; Pagnier, I.; La Scola, B. Improving the identification of anaerobes in the clinical microbiology laboratory through MALDI-TOF mass spectrometry. *Anaerobe* **2013**, *22*, 123–125. [CrossRef] [PubMed]

57. Zimbro, M.J.; Power, D.A.; Miller, S.M.; Wilson, G.E.; Johnson, J.A. *Manual of Microbiological Culture Media*, 2nd ed.; BD Diagnostics—Diagnostic Systems: Sparks, MD, USA, 2009; ISBN 978-0-9727207-1-7.

58. Schreckenberger, P.C.; Blazevic, D.J. Rapid methods for biochemical testing of anaerobic bacteria. *Appl. Microbiol.* **1974**, *28*, 759–762. [PubMed]

59. Sondag, J.E.; Ali, M.; Murray, P.R. Rapid presumptive identification of anaerobes in blood cultures by gas-liquid chromatography. *J. Clin. Microbiol.* **1980**, *11*, 274–277. [PubMed]

60. Wust, J.; Smid, I.; Salfinger, M. Experience of gas-liquid chromatography in clinical microbiology. *Ann. Biol. Clin. Paris* **1990**, *48*, 416–419. [PubMed]

61. Lehtonen, L.; Korvenranta, H.; Eerola, E. Intestinal microflora in colicky and noncolicky infants: Bacterial cultures and gas-liquid chromatography. *J. Pediatr. Gastroenterol. Nutr.* **1994**, *19*, 310–314. [CrossRef] [PubMed]

62. Nagy, E.; Becker, S.; Kostrzewa, M.; Barta, N.; Urban, E. The value of MALDI-TOF MS for the identification of clinically relevant anaerobic bacteria in routine laboratories. *J. Med. Microbiol.* **2012**, *61*, 1393–1400. [CrossRef] [PubMed]

63. Nagy, E.; Maier, T.; Urban, E.; Terhes, G.; Kostrzewa, M.; ESCMID Study Group on Antimicrobial Resistance in Anaerobic Bacteria. Species identification of clinical isolates of *Bacteroides* by matrix-assisted laser-desorption/ionization time-of-flight mass spectrometry. *Clin. Microbiol. Infect.* **2009**, *15*, 796–802. [CrossRef] [PubMed]

64. Nagy, E. *MALDI-TOF Mass Spectrometry in Microbiology*; Kostrzewa, M., Schubert, S., Eds.; Caister Academic Press: Norfolk, UK, 2016; ISBN 978-1-910190-41-8.

65. Krishnamurthy, T.; Ross, P.L.; Rajamani, U. Detection of pathogenic and non-pathogenic bacteria by matrix-assisted laser desorption/ionization time-of-flight mass spectrometry. *Rapid Commun. Mass Spectrom.* **1996**, *10*, 883–888. [CrossRef]

66. Croxatto, A.; Prod'hom, G.; Greub, G. Applications of MALDI-TOF mass spectrometry in clinical diagnostic microbiology. *FEMS Microbiol. Rev.* **2012**, *36*, 380–407. [CrossRef] [PubMed]

67. Lin, Y.T.; Vaneechoutte, M.; Huang, A.H.; Teng, L.J.; Chen, H.M.; Su, S.L.; Chang, T.C. Identification of clinically important anaerobic bacteria by an oligonucleotide array. *J. Clin. Microbiol.* **2010**, *48*, 1283–1290. [CrossRef] [PubMed]

68. Jamal, W.Y.; Shahin, M.; Rotimi, V.O. Comparison of two matrix-assisted laser desorption/ionization-time of flight (MALDI-TOF) mass spectrometry methods and API 20AN for identification of clinically relevant anaerobic bacteria. *J. Med. Microbiol.* **2013**, *62*, 540–544. [CrossRef] [PubMed]

69. Veloo, A.C.; Erhard, M.; Welker, M.; Welling, G.W.; Degener, J.E. Identification of Gram-positive anaerobic cocci by MALDI-TOF mass spectrometry. *Syst. Appl. Microbiol.* **2011**, *34*, 58–62. [CrossRef] [PubMed]

70. Veloo, A.C.M.; de Vries, E.D.; Jean-Pierre, H.; Justesen, U.S.; Morris, T.; Urban, E.; Wybo, I.; van Winkelhoff, A.J.; ENRIA Workgroup. The optimization and validation of the Biotyper MALDI-TOF MS database for the identification of Gram-positive anaerobic cocci. *Clin. Microbiol. Infect. Off. Publ. Eur. Soc. Clin. Microbiol. Infect. Dis.* **2016**, *22*, 793–798. [CrossRef] [PubMed]

71. Veloo, A.C.M.; Jean-Pierre, H.; Justesen, U.S.; Morris, T.; Urban, E.; Wybo, I.; Shah, H.N.; Friedrich, A.W.; ENRIA Workgroup; Morris, T.; et al. A multi-center ring trial for the identification of anaerobic bacteria using MALDI-TOF MS. *Anaerobe* **2017**, *48*, 94–97. [CrossRef] [PubMed]

72. Levesque, S.; Dufresne, P.J.; Soualhine, H.; Domingo, M.C.; Bekal, S.; Lefebvre, B.; Tremblay, C. A Side by Side Comparison of Bruker Biotyper and VITEK MS: Utility of MALDI-TOF MS Technology for Microorganism Identification in a Public Health Reference Laboratory. *PLoS ONE* **2015**, *10*, e0144878. [CrossRef] [PubMed]

73. Veloo, A.C.; Knoester, M.; Degener, J.E.; Kuijper, E.J. Comparison of two matrix-assisted laser desorption ionisation-time of flight mass spectrometry methods for the identification of clinically relevant anaerobic bacteria. *Clin. Microbiol. Infect.* **2011**, *17*, 1501–1506. [CrossRef] [PubMed]

74. Hasman, H.; Saputra, D.; Sicheritz-Ponten, T.; Lund, O.; Svendsen, C.A.; Frimodt-Moller, N.; Aarestrup, F.M. Rapid whole-genome sequencing for detection and characterization of microorganisms directly from clinical samples. *J. Clin. Microbiol.* **2014**, *52*, 139–146. [CrossRef] [PubMed]

75. Hardwick, S.A.; Deveson, I.W.; Mercer, T.R. Reference standards for next-generation sequencing. *Nat. Rev. Genet.* **2017**, *18*, 473–484. [CrossRef] [PubMed]

76. Ank, N.; Sydenham, T.V.; Iversen, L.H.; Justesen, U.S.; Wang, M. Characterisation of a multidrug-resistant *Bacteroides fragilis* isolate recovered from blood of a patient in Denmark using whole-genome sequencing. *Int. J. Antimicrob. Agents* **2015**, *46*, 117–120. [CrossRef] [PubMed]

77. Veloo, A.C.M.; de Vries, E.D.; Jean-Pierre, H.; van Winkelhoff, A.J. *Anaerococcus nagyae* sp. nov., isolated from human clinical specimens. *Anaerobe* **2016**, *38*, 111–115. [CrossRef] [PubMed]

78. Haas, K.N.; Blanchard, J.L. *Kineothrix alysoides*, gen. nov., sp. nov., a saccharolytic butyrate-producer within the family Lachnospiraceae. *Int. J. Syst. Evol. Microbiol.* **2017**, *67*, 402–410. [CrossRef] [PubMed]

79. Soki, J.; Hedberg, M.; Patrick, S.; Balint, B.; Herczeg, R.; Nagy, I.; Hecht, D.W.; Nagy, E.; Urban, E. Emergence and evolution of an international cluster of MDR *Bacteroides fragilis* isolates. *J. Antimicrob. Chemother.* **2016**, *71*, 2441–2448. [CrossRef] [PubMed]

80. Salipante, S.J.; Kalapila, A.; Pottinger, P.S.; Hoogestraat, D.R.; Cummings, L.; Duchin, J.S.; Sengupta, D.J.; Pergam, S.A.; Cookson, B.T.; Butler-Wu, S.M. Characterization of a multidrug-resistant, novel *Bacteroides* genomospecies. *Emerg. Infect. Dis.* **2015**, *21*, 95–98. [CrossRef] [PubMed]

81. Rokosz, A.; Meisel-Mikolajczyk, F.; Kot, K.; Zawidzka, E.; Malchar, C.; Nowaczyk, M.; Gorski, A. Toxins of *Bacteroides fragilis* and *Bacteroides thetaiotaomicron* rods as stimulators of adhesion molecule expression on the surface of vascular endothelial cells. *Med. Dosw. Mikrobiol.* **1999**, *51*, 133–142. [PubMed]

82. Sears, C.L. The toxins of *Bacteroides fragilis*. *Toxicon* **2001**, *39*, 1737–1746. [CrossRef]

83. Kasper, D.L. The polysaccharide capsule of *Bacteroides fragilis* subspecies *fragilis*: Immunochemical and morphologic definition. *J. Infect. Dis.* **1976**, *133*, 79–87. [CrossRef] [PubMed]

84. Nguyen, M.H.; Yu, V.L.; Morris, A.J.; McDermott, L.; Wagener, M.W.; Harrell, L.; Snydman, D.R. Antimicrobial resistance and clinical outcome of *Bacteroides* bacteremia: Findings of a multicenter prospective observational trial. *Clin. Infect. Dis.* **2000**, *30*, 870–876. [CrossRef] [PubMed]

85. Merchan, C.; Parajuli, S.; Siegfried, J.; Scipione, M.R.; Dubrovskaya, Y.; Rahimian, J. Multidrug-Resistant *Bacteroides fragilis* Bacteremia in a US Resident: An Emerging Challenge. *Case Rep. Infect. Dis.* **2016**, *2016*, 3607125. [CrossRef] [PubMed]

86. Dunn, D.L.; Barke, R.A.; Ewald, D.C.; Simmons, R.L. Effects of *Escherichia coli* and *Bacteroides fragilis* on peritoneal host defenses. *Infect. Immun.* **1985**, *48*, 287–291. [PubMed]

87. Breitenstein, A.; Wiegel, J.; Haertig, C.; Weiss, N.; Andreesen, J.A.; Lechner, U. Reclassification of *Clostridium hydroybenzoicum* as *Sedimentibacter hydroxibenzoicus* gen. nov., comb. nov. and description of *Sedimentibacter saalensis* sp. nov. *Int. J. Syst. Evol. Microbiol.* **2002**, *52*, 801–807. [CrossRef] [PubMed]

88. Moon, C.D.; Pacheco, D.M.; Kelly, W.J.; Leahy, S.C.; Li, D.; Kopecny, J.; Attwod, G.T. Reclassification of *Clostridium proteoclasticum* as *Butyrivibrio proteoclasticus* comb. nov., a butyrate-producing ruminal bacterium. *Int. J. Syst. Evol. Microbiol.* **2008**, *58*, 2041–2045. [CrossRef] [PubMed]

89. Silva, R.O.; Lobato, F.C. *Clostridium perfringens*: A review of enteric diseases in dogs, cats and wild animals. *Anaerobe* **2015**, *33*, 14–17. [CrossRef] [PubMed]

90. Smith, T.J.; Hill, K.K.; Raphael, B.H. Historical and cultural perspectives on *Clostridium botulinum* diversity. *Res. Microbiol.* **2015**, *166*, 290–302. [CrossRef] [PubMed]

91. Hecht, D.W. Prevalence of antibiotic resistance in anaerobic bacteria: Worrisome developments. *Clin. Infect. Dis.* **2004**, *39*, 92–97. [CrossRef] [PubMed]

92. Goldstein, E.J.C.; Citron, D.M.; Goldman, P.J.; Goldman, R.J. National hospital survey of anaerobic culture and susceptibility methods: III. *Anaerobe* **2008**, *14*, 68–72. [CrossRef] [PubMed]

93. Brook, I. Antimicrobial treatment of anaerobic infections. *Expert Opin. Pharmacother.* **2011**, *12*, 1691–1707. [CrossRef] [PubMed]

94. Tuner, K.; Nord, C.E. Antibiotic susceptibility of anaerobic bacteria in Europe. *Clin. Infect. Dis.* **1993**, *16* (Suppl. S4), S387–S389. [CrossRef] [PubMed]

95. Clinical and Laboratory Standards Institute (CLSI). Available online: https://clsi.org/standards/products/microbiology/ (accessed on 10 September 2017).

96. European Committe for Antimicrobial Susceptibility Testing (EUCAST). Available online: http://eucast.org/ (accessed on 10 September 2017).

97. Brown, D.F.; Wootton, M.; Howe, R.A. Antimicrobial susceptibility testing breakpoints and methods from BSAC to EUCAST. *J. Antimicrob. Chemother.* **2016**, *71*, 3–5. [CrossRef] [PubMed]

98. British Society for Antimicrobial Chemotherapy (BSAC). Available online: http://www.bsac.org.uk/ (accessed on 10 September 2017).

99. Deutsches Institut für Normung (DIN). Available online: https://www.din.de/en (accessed on 10 September 2017).

100. ESCMID Study Group for Anaerobic Infections—ESGAI. Available online: https://www.escmid.org/research_projects/study_groups/anaerobic_infections/ (accessed on 10 September 2017).

101. Anaerobe Society of the Americas. Available online: http://www.anaerobe.org/ (accessed on 10 September 2017).

102. Clinical and Laboratory Standards Institute. *Methods for Antimicrobial Susceptibility Testing of Anaerobic Bacteria*; Approved Standard; CLSI Document M11-A8; CLSI: Wayne, PA, USA, 2012.

103. Justesen, T.; Justesen, U.S. A simple and sensitive quality control method of the anaerobic atmosphere for identification and antimicrobial susceptibility testing of anaerobic bacteria. *Diagn. Microbiol. Infect. Dis.* **2013**, *76*, 138–140. [CrossRef] [PubMed]

104. EUCAST. *The European Committee on Antimicrobial Susceptibility Testing. Breakpoint Tables for Interpretation of MICs and Zone Diameters*, version 7.1; European Committee for Antimicrobial Susceptibility Testing (EUCAST): Växjö, Sweden, 2017.

105. Matuschek, E.; Brown, D.F.; Kahlmeter, G. Development of the EUCAST disk diffusion antimicrobial susceptibility testing method and its implementation in routine microbiology laboratories. *Clin. Microbiol. Infect.* **2014**, *20*, O255–O266. [CrossRef] [PubMed]

106. Wikins, T.D.; Holdeman, L.V.; Abramson, I.J.; Moore, W.E. Standardized single-disc method for antibiotic susceptibility testing of anaerobic bacteria. *Antimicrob. Agents Chemother.* **1972**, *1*, 451–459. [CrossRef] [PubMed]

107. Nagy, E.; Justesen, U.S.; Eitel, Z.; Urban, E.; ESCMID Study Group on Anaerobic Infection. Development of EUCAST disk diffusion method for susceptibility testing of the *Bacteroides fragilis* group isolates. *Anaerobe* **2015**, *31*, 65–71. [CrossRef] [PubMed]

108. Egervarn, M.; Lindmark, H.; Roos, S.; Huys, G.; Lindgren, S. Effects of inoculum size and incubation time on broth microdilution susceptibility testing of lactic acid bacteria. *Antimicrob. Agents Chemother.* **2007**, *51*, 394–396. [CrossRef] [PubMed]

109. El-Halfawy, O.M.; Valvano, M.A. Antimicrobial heteroresistance: An emerging field in need of clarity. *Clin. Microbiol. Rev.* **2015**, *28*, 191–207. [CrossRef] [PubMed]

110. Huang, H.; Weintraub, A.; Fang, H.; Wu, S.; Zhang, Y.; Nord, C.E. Antimicrobial susceptibility and heteroresistance in Chinese *Clostridium difficile* strains. *Anaerobe* **2010**, *16*, 633–635. [CrossRef] [PubMed]

111. Hill, G.B.; Schalkowsky, S. Development and evaluation of the spiral gradient endpoint method for susceptibility testing of anaerobic gram-negative bacilli. *Rev. Infect. Dis.* **1990**, *12* (Suppl. S2), S200–S209. [CrossRef] [PubMed]

112. Pong, R.; Boost, M.V.; O'Donoghue, M.M.; Appelbaum, P.C. Spiral gradient endpoint susceptibility testing: A fresh look at a neglected technique. *J. Antimicrob. Chemother.* **2010**, *65*, 1959–1963. [CrossRef] [PubMed]

113. Wexler, H.M.; Molitoris, E.; Murray, P.R.; Washington, J.; Zabransky, R.J.; Edelstein, P.H.; Finegold, S.M. Comparison of spiral gradient endpoint and agar dilution methods for susceptibility testing of anaerobic bacteria: A multilaboratory collaborative evaluation. *J. Clin. Microbiol.* **1996**, *34*, 170–174. [PubMed]

114. Papanicolas, L.E.; Bell, J.M.; Bastian, I. Performance of phenotypic tests for detection of penicillinase in *Staphylococcus aureus* isolates from Australia. *J. Clin. Microbiol.* **2014**, *52*, 1136–1138. [CrossRef] [PubMed]

115. Pitkala, A.; Salmikivi, L.; Bredbacka, P.; Myllyniemi, A.L.; Koskinen, M.T. Comparison of tests for detection of beta-lactamase-producing staphylococci. *J. Clin. Microbiol.* **2007**, *45*, 2031–2033. [CrossRef] [PubMed]

116. Tierney, D.; Copsey, S.D.; Morris, T.; Perry, J.D. A new chromogenic medium for isolation of *Bacteroides fragilis* suitable for screening for strains with antimicrobial resistance. *Anaerobe* **2016**, *39*, 168–172. [CrossRef] [PubMed]

117. Pumbwe, L.; Curzon, M.; Wexler, H.M. Rapid multiplex PCR assay for simultaneous detection of major antibiotic resistance determinants in clinical isolates of Bacteroides fragilis. *J. Rapid Methods Autom. Microbiol.* **2008**, *16*, 381–393. [CrossRef]

118. Johansson, A.; Nagy, E.; Soki, J. Instant screening and verification of carbapenemase activity in Bacteroides fragilis in positive blood culture, using matrix-assisted laser desorption ionization—Time of flight mass spectrometry. *J. Med. Microbiol.* **2014**, *63*, 1105–1110. [CrossRef] [PubMed]

119. Johansson, A.; Nagy, E.; Soki, J. Esgai Detection of carbapenemase activities of *Bacteroides fragilis* strains with matrix-assisted laser desorption ionization–time of flight mass spectrometry (MALDI-TOF MS). *Anaerobe* **2014**, *26*, 49–52. [CrossRef] [PubMed]

120. Nagy, E.; Becker, S.; Soki, J.; Urban, E.; Kostrzewa, M. Differentiation of division I (cfiA-negative) and division II (cfiA-positive) *Bacteroides fragilis* strains by matrix-assisted laser desorption/ionization time-of-flight mass spectrometry. *J. Med. Microbiol.* **2011**, *60*, 1584–1590. [CrossRef] [PubMed]

121. Sparbler, K.; Schubert, S.; Weller, U.; Boogen, C.; Kostrzewa, M. Matrix-assisted laser desorption ionization-time of flight mass spectrometry-based functional analysis for rapid detection of resistance against beta-lactam antibtiotics. *J. Clin. Microbiol.* **2011**, 927–937. [CrossRef]

122. Hrabák, J.; Chudáčková, E.; Walková, R. Matrix-assisted laser desorption ionization-time of flight (MALDI-TOF) mass spectrometry for detection of antibiotic resistance mechanisms: From research to routine diagnosis. *Clin. Microbiol. Rev.* **2013**, *26*, 103–114. [CrossRef] [PubMed]

123. Hrabák, J.; Walková, R.; Študentová, V.; Chudáčková, E.; Bergerová, T. Carbapenemase activity detection by Matrix-Assisted LaserDesorption Ionization–Time of Flight Mass Spectrometry. *J. Clin. Microbiol.* **2011**, *49*, 3222–3227. [CrossRef] [PubMed]

124. Salipante, S.J.; SenGupta, J.D.; Cummings, L.A.; Land, T.A.; Hoogerstraat, D.R.; Cookson, B.T. Application of Whole-Genome Sequencing for Bacterial Strain Typing in Molecular Epidemiology. *J. Clin. Microbiol.* **2015**, *53*, 1072–1079. [CrossRef] [PubMed]

125. Metcalf, B.J.; Chochua, S.; Gertz, R.E., Jr.; Li, Z.; Walker, H.; Tran, T.; Hawkins, P.A.; Glennen, A.; Lynfield, R.; Li, Y.; et al. Using whole genome sequencing to identify determinants and predict antimicrobial resistance phenotypes for year 2015 invasive pneumococcal disease isolates recovered in the United States. *Clin. Microbiol. Infect.* **2016**, *22*, 1002.e1–1002.e8. [CrossRef] [PubMed]

126. McDermott, P.F.; Tyson, G.H.; Claudine, K.; Chen, Y.; Li, C.; Folster, J.P.; Ayers, S.L.; Lam, C.; Tate, H.P.; Zhao, S. Whole-genome sequencing for detecting antimicrobial resistance in nontyphoidal *Salmonella Antimicrob. Agents Chemother.* **2016**, *60*, 5515–5520. [CrossRef] [PubMed]

127. Köser, C.U.; Ellington, M.J.; Peacock, S.J. Whole-genome sequencing to control antimicrobial resistance. *Trends Genet.* **2014**, *30*, 401–407. [CrossRef] [PubMed]

128. Ellington, M.J.; Ekelund, O.; Aarestrup, F.M.; Canton, R.; Doumith, M.; Giske, C.; Grundman, H.; Hasman, H.; Holden, M.T.; Hopkins, K.L.; et al. The role of whole genome sequencing in antimicrobial susceptibility testing of bacteria: Report from the EUCAST Subcommittee. *Clin. Microbiol. Infect.* **2017**, *23*, 2–22. [CrossRef] [PubMed]

129. Sydenham, T.V.; Soki, J.; Hasman, H.; Wang, M.; Justesen, U.S. Esgai Identification of antimicrobial resistance genes in multidrug-resistant clinical *Bacteroides fragilis* isolates by whole genome shotgun sequencing. *Anaerobe* **2015**, *31*, 59–64. [CrossRef] [PubMed]

130. Owen, J.R.; Noyes, N.; Young, A.E.; Prince, D.J.; Blanchard, P.C.; Lehenbauer, T.W.; Aly, S.S.; Davis, J.H.; O'Rourke, S.M.; Abdo, Z.; et al. Whole-Genome Sequencing and Concordance Between Antimicrobial Susceptibility Genotypes and Phenotypes of Bacterial Isolates Associated with Bovine Respiratory Disease. *G3 Bethesda* **2017**, *7*, 3059–3071. [CrossRef] [PubMed]

131. Hecker, M.T.; Aron, D.C.; Patel, N.P.; Lehmann, M.K.; Donskey, C.J. Unnecessary use of antimicrobials in hospitalized patients: Current patterns of misuse with an emphasis on the antianaerobic spectrum of activity. *Arch. Intern. Med.* **2003**, *163*, 972–978. [CrossRef] [PubMed]

132. Eslami, G.; Fallah, F.; Goudarzi, H.; Navidinia, M. The prevalence of antibiotic resistance in anaerobic bacteria isolated from patients with skin infections. *Gene Ther. Mol. Biol.* **2005**, *9*, 263–268.

133. Hecht, D.W.; Vedantam, G.; Osmolski, J.R. Antibiotic resistance among anaerobes: What does it mean? *Anaerobe* **1999**, *5*, 421–429. [CrossRef]

134. Bach, V.T.; Thadepalli, H. Susceptibility of anaerobic bacteria in vitro to 23 antimicrobial agents. *Chemotherapy* **1980**, *26*, 344–353. [CrossRef] [PubMed]

135. Nagy, E.; Urban, E.; Nord, C.E.; ESCMID Study Group on Antimicrobial Resistance in Anaerobic Bacteria. Antimicrobial susceptibility of *Bacteroides fragilis* group isolates in Europe: 20 years of experience. *Clin. Microbiol. Infect.* **2011**, *17*, 371–379. [CrossRef] [PubMed]

136. Eitel, Z.; Sóki, J.; Urbán, E.; Nagy, E. The prevalence of antibiotic resistance genes in *Bacteroides fragilis* group strains isolated in different European countries. *Anaerobe* **2013**, *21*, 43–49. [CrossRef] [PubMed]

137. Boyanova, L.; Kolarov, R.; Mitov, I. Recent evolution of antibiotic resistance in the anaerobes as compared to previous decades. *Anaerobe* **2015**, *31*, 4–10. [CrossRef] [PubMed]

138. World Health Organisation. *Global Priority List of Antibiotic-Resistant Bacteria to Guide Research, Discovery and Development of New Antibiotics*; WHO: Geneva, Switzerland, 2017; pp. 1–7.

139. Cornick, N.A.; Cuchural, G.J., Jr.; Snydman, D.R.; Jacobus, N.V.; Iannini, P.; Hill, G.; Cleary, T.; O'Keefe, J.P.; Pierson, C.; Finegold, S.M. The antimicrobial susceptibility patterns of the *Bacteroides fragilis* group in the United States, 1987. *J. Antimicrob. Chemother.* **1990**, *25*, 1011–1019. [CrossRef] [PubMed]

140. Snydman, D.R.; Jacobus, N.V.; McDermott, L.A.; Golan, Y.; Goldstein, E.J.; Harrell, L.; Jenkins, S.; Newton, D.; Pierson, C.; Rosenblatt, J.; et al. Update on resistance of *Bacteroides fragilis* group and related species with special attention to carbapenems 2006–2009. *Anaerobe* **2011**, *17*, 147–151. [CrossRef] [PubMed]

141. Snydman, D.R.; Jacobus, N.V.; McDermott, L.A.; Ruthazer, R.; Golan, Y.; Goldstein, E.J.; Finegold, S.M.; Harrell, L.J.; Hecht, D.W.; Jenkins, S.G.; et al. National survey on the susceptibility of *Bacteroides fragilis* group: Report and analysis of trends in the United States from 1997 to 2004. *Antimicrob. Agents Chemother.* **2007**, *51*, 1649–1655. [CrossRef] [PubMed]

142. Snydman, D.R.; Jacobus, N.V.; McDermott, L.A.; Goldstein, E.J.; Harrell, L.; Jenkins, S.G.; Newton, D.; Patel, R.; Hecht, D.W. Trends in antimicrobial resistance among *Bacteroides* species and *Parabacteroides* species in the United States from 2010–2012 with comparison to 2008–2009. *Anaerobe* **2017**, *43*, 21–26. [CrossRef] [PubMed]

143. Snydman, D.R.; McDermott, L.; Cuchural, G.J., Jr.; Hecht, D.W.; Iannini, P.B.; Harrell, L.J.; Jenkins, S.G.; O'Keefe, J.P.; Pierson, C.L.; Rihs, J.D.; et al. Analysis of trends in antimicrobial resistance patterns among clinical isolates of *Bacteroides fragilis* group species from 1990 to 1994. *Clin. Infect. Dis.* **1996**, *23* (Suppl. S1), S54–S65. [CrossRef] [PubMed]

144. Betriu, C.; Culebras, E.; Gomez, M.; Lopez, F.; Rodriguez-Avial, I.; Picazo, J.J. Resistance trends of the *Bacteroides fragilis* group over a 10-year period, 1997 to 2006, in Madrid, Spain. *Antimicrob. Agents Chemother.* **2008**, *52*, 2686–2690. [CrossRef] [PubMed]

145. Hedberg, M.; Nord, C.E.; SCMID Study Group on Antimicrobial Resistance in Anaerobic Bacteria. Antimicrobial susceptibility of *Bacteroides fragilis* group isolates in Europe. *Clin. Microbiol. Infect.* **2003**, *9*, 475–488. [CrossRef] [PubMed]

146. Jeverica, S.; Kolenc, U.; Mueller-Premru, M.; Papst, L. Evaluation of the routine antimicrobial susceptibility testing results of clinically significant anaerobic bacteria in a Slovenian tertiary-care hospital in 2015. *Anaerobe* **2017**, *47*, 64–69. [CrossRef] [PubMed]

147. Nakamura, I.; Aoki, K.; Miura, Y.; Yamaguchi, T.; Matsumoto, T. Fatal sepsis caused by multidrug-resistant *Bacteroides fragilis*, harboring a cfiA gene and an upstream insertion sequence element, in Japan. *Anaerobe* **2017**, *44*, 36–39. [CrossRef] [PubMed]

148. Urban, E.; Horvath, Z.; Soki, J.; Lazar, G. First Hungarian case of an infection caused by multidrug-resistant *Bacteroides fragilis* strain. *Anaerobe* **2015**, *31*, 55–58. [CrossRef] [PubMed]

149. Sadarangani, S.P.; Cunningham, S.A.; Jeraldo, P.R.; Wilson, J.W.; Khare, R.; Patel, R. Metronidazole- and carbapenem-resistant *Bacteroides thetaiotaomicron* isolated in Rochester, Minnesota, in 2014. *Antimicrob. Agents Chemother.* **2015**, *59*, 4157–4161. [CrossRef] [PubMed]

150. Soki, J.; Eitel, Z.; Urban, E.; Nagy, E.; ESCMID Study Group on Anaerobic Infections. Molecular analysis of the carbapenem and metronidazole resistance mechanisms of *Bacteroides* strains reported in a Europe-wide antibiotic resistance survey. *Int. J. Antimicrob. Agents* **2013**, *41*, 122–125. [CrossRef] [PubMed]

151. Soki, J.; Fodor, E.; Hecht, D.W.; Edwards, R.; Rotimi, V.O.; Kerekes, I.; Urban, E.; Nagy, E. Molecular characterization of imipenem-resistant, cfiA-positive *Bacteroides fragilis* isolates from the USA, Hungary and Kuwait. *J. Med. Microbiol.* **2004**, *53*, 413–419. [CrossRef] [PubMed]

152. Nord, C.E. Antimicrobial Resistance Among Anaerobes—The European Experience. *Int. J. Infect. Dis.* **2008**, *12*, E39. [CrossRef]

153. Wareham, D.W.; Wilks, M.; Ahmed, D.; Brazier, J.S.; Millar, M. Anaerobic sepsis due to multidrug-resistant *Bacteroides fragilis*: Microbiological cure and clinical response with linezolid therapy. *Clin. Infect. Dis. Off. Publ. Infect. Dis. Soc. Am.* **2005**, *40*, e67–e68. [CrossRef] [PubMed]

154. Park, J.E.; Park, S.-Y.; Song, D.J.; Huh, H.J.; Ki, C.-S.; Peck, K.R.; Lee, N.Y. A case of *Bacteroides* pyogenes bacteremia secondary to liver abscess. *Anaerobe* **2016**, *42*, 78–80. [CrossRef] [PubMed]

155. Tan, T.Y.; Ng, L.S.Y.; Kwang, L.L.; Rao, S.; Eng, L.C. Clinical characteristics and antimicrobial susceptibilities of anaerobic bacteremia in an acute care hospital. *Anaerobe* **2017**, *43*, 69–74. [CrossRef] [PubMed]

156. Wexler, H.M. Outer-membrane pore-forming proteins in gram-negative anaerobic bacteria. *Clin. Infect. Dis.* **2002**, *35*, S65–S71. [CrossRef] [PubMed]

157. Then, R.L.; Angehrn, P. Low trimethoprim susceptibility of anaerobic bacteria due to insensitive dihydrofolate reductases. *Antimicrob. Agents Chemother.* **1979**, *15*, 1–6. [CrossRef] [PubMed]

158. Bryan, L.E.; Kowand, S.K.; Van Den Elzen, H.M. Mechanism of aminoglycoside antibiotic resistance in anaerobic bacteria: *Clostridium perfringens* and *Bacteroides fragilis*. *Antimicrob. Agents Chemother.* **1979**, *15*, 7–13. [CrossRef] [PubMed]

159. Jimenezdiaz, A.; Reig, M.; Baquero, F.; Ballesta, J.P.G. Antibiotic-Sensitivity of Ribosomes from Wild-Type and Clindamycin Resistant *Bacteroides vulgatus* Strains. *J. Antimicrob. Chemother.* **1992**, *30*, 295–301. [CrossRef]

160. Nikolich, M.P.; Shoemaker, N.B.; Salyers, A.A. A Bacteroides Tetracycline Resistance Gene Represents a New Class of Ribosome Protection Tetracycline Resistance. *Antimicrob. Agents Chemother.* **1992**, *36*, 1005–1012. [CrossRef] [PubMed]

161. Gupta, A.; Vlamakis, H.; Shoemaker, N.; Salyers, A.A. A new *Bacteroides* conjugative transposon that carries an ermB gene. *Appl. Environ. Microbiol.* **2003**, *69*, 6455–6463. [CrossRef] [PubMed]

162. Farrow, K.A.; Lyras, D.; Rood, J.I. Genomic analysis of the erythromycin resistance element Tn5398 from *Clostridium difficile·* Microbiology-Sgm **2001**, *147*, 2717–2728. [CrossRef] [PubMed]

163. Farrow, K.A.; Lyras, D.; Polekhina, G.; Koutsis, K.; Parker, M.W.; Rood, J.I. Identification of essential residues in the Erm(B) rRNA methyltransferase of *Clostridium perfringens*. *Antimicrob. Agents Chemother.* **2002**, *46*, 1253–1261. [CrossRef] [PubMed]

164. Thadepalli, H.; Gorbach, S.L.; Bartlett, J.G. Apparent Failure of Chloramphenicol in Treatment of Anaerobic Infections. *Curr. Ther. Res. Clin. Exp.* **1977**, *22*, 421–426.

165. Balbi, H.J. Chloramphenicol: A review. *Pediatr. Rev.* **2004**, *25*, 284–288. [CrossRef] [PubMed]

166. Golan, Y.; McDermott, L.A.; Jacobus, N.V.; Goldstein, E.J.C.; Finegold, S.; Harrell, L.J.; Hecht, D.W.; Jenkins, S.G.; Pierson, C.; Venezia, R.; et al. Emergence of fluoroquinolone resistance among *Bacteroides* species. *J. Antimicrob. Chemother.* **2003**, *52*, 208–213. [CrossRef] [PubMed]

167. Stein, G.E.; Goldstein, E.J.C. Fluoroquinolones and anaerobes. *Clin. Infect. Dis.* **2006**, *42*, 1598–1607. [CrossRef] [PubMed]

168. Oh, H.; El Amin, N.; Davies, T.; Appelbaum, P.C.; Edlund, C. gyrA Mutations associated with quinolone resistance in *Bacteroides fragilis* group strains. *Antimicrob. Agents Chemother.* **2001**, *45*, 1977–1981. [CrossRef] [PubMed]

169. Dridi, L.; Tankovic, J.; Burghoffer, B.; Barbut, F.; Petit, J.C. gyrA and gyrB mutations are implicated in cross-resistance to ciprofloxacin and moxifloxacin in *Clostridium difficile*. *Antimicrob. Agents Chemother.* **2002**, *46*, 3418–3421. [CrossRef] [PubMed]

170. Brazier, J.S.; Hall, V.; Morris, T.E.; Gal, M.; Duerden, B.I. Antibiotic susceptibilities of Gram-positive anaerobic cocci: Results of a sentinel study in England and Wales. *J. Antimicrob. Chemother.* **2003**, *52*, 224–228. [CrossRef] [PubMed]

171. Podglajen, I.; Breuil, J.; Collatz, E. Insertion of a Novel DNA-Sequence, Is-1186, Upstream of the Silent Carbapenemase Gene Cfia, Promotes Expression of Carbapenem Resistance in Clinical Isolates of *Bacteroides fragilis*. *Mol. Microbiol.* **1994**, *12*, 105–114. [CrossRef] [PubMed]

172. Podglajen, I.; Breuil, J.; Bordon, F.; Gutmann, L.; Collatz, E. A Silent Carbapenemase Gene in Strains of *Bacteroides fragilis* Can Be Expressed after a One-Step Mutation. *Fems Microbiol. Lett.* **1992**, *91*, 21–29. [CrossRef]

173. Appelbaum, P.C.; Spangler, S.K.; Pankuch, G.A.; Philippon, A.; Jacobs, M.R.; Shiman, R.; Goldstein, E.J.C.; Citron, D.M. Characterization of a Beta-Lactamase from *Clostridium clostridioforme*. *J. Antimicrob. Chemother.* **1994**, *33*, 33–40. [CrossRef] [PubMed]

174. Appelbaum, P.C.; Philippon, A.; Jacobs, M.R.; Spangler, S.K.; Gutmann, L. Characterization of Beta-Lactamases from Non-*Bacteroides fragilis* Group *Bacteroides* Spp Belonging to 7 Species and Their Role in Beta-Lactam Resistance. *Antimicrob. Agents Chemother.* **1990**, *34*, 2169–2176. [CrossRef] [PubMed]

175. Cuchural, G.J.; Malamy, M.H.; Tally, F.P. Beta-Lactamase-Mediated Imipenem Resistance in *Bacteroides fragilis*. *Antimicrob. Agents Chemother.* **1986**, *30*, 645–648. [CrossRef] [PubMed]

176. Hurlbut, S.; Cuchural, G.J.; Tally, F.P. Imipenem Resistance in *Bacteroides distasonis* Mediated by a Novel Beta-Lactamase. *Antimicrob. Agents Chemother.* **1990**, *34*, 117–120. [CrossRef] [PubMed]

177. Rasmussen, B.A.; Gluzman, Y.; Tally, F.P. Cloning and Sequencing of the Class-B Beta-Lactamase Gene (Ccra) from *Bacteroides fragilis* Tal3636. *Antimicrob. Agents Chemother.* **1990**, *34*, 1590–1592. [CrossRef] [PubMed]

178. Rogers, M.B.; Parker, A.C.; Smith, C.J. Cloning and Characterization of the Endogenous Cephalosporinase Gene, Cepa, from *Bacteroides fragilis* Reveals a New Subgroup of Ambler Class-a Beta-Lactamases. *Antimicrob. Agents Chemother.* **1993**, *37*, 2391–2400. [CrossRef] [PubMed]

179. Wexler, H.M.; Halebian, S. Alterations to the Penicillin-Binding Proteins in the *Bacteroides fragilis* Group—A Mechanism for Non-Beta-Lactamase Mediated Cefoxitin Resistance. *J. Antimicrob. Chemother.* **1990**, *26*, 7–20. [CrossRef] [PubMed]

180. Edwards, R.; Read, P.N. Expression of the carbapenemase gene (cfiA) in *Bacteroides fragilis*. *J. Antimicrob. Chemother.* **2000**, *46*, 1009–1012. [CrossRef] [PubMed]

181. Gutacker, M.; Valsangiacomo, C.; Piffaretti, J.C. Identification of two genetic groups in *Bacteroides fragilis* by multilocus enzyme electrophoresis: Distribution of antibiotic resistance (cfiA, cepA) and enterotoxin (bft) encoding genes. *Microbiology* **2000**, *146*, 1241–1254. [CrossRef] [PubMed]

182. Mukhopadhya, I.; Hansen, R.; Nicholl, C.E.; Alhaidan, Y.A.; Thomson, J.M.; Berry, S.H.; Pattinson, C.; Stead, D.A.; Russell, R.K.; El-Omar, E.M.; et al. A Comprehensive Evaluation of Colonic Mucosal Isolates of *Sutterella wadsworthensis* from Inflammatory Bowel Disease. *PLoS ONE* **2011**, *6*, e27076. [CrossRef] [PubMed]

183. Wexler, H.M.; Reeves, D.; Summanen, P.H.; Molitoris, E.; McTeague, M.; Duncan, J.; Wilson, K.H.; Finegold, S.M. *Sutterella wadsworthensis* gen. nov., sp. nov., bile-resistant microaerophilic *Campylobacter gracilis*-like clinical isolates. *Int. J. Syst. Bacteriol.* **1996**, *46*, 252–258. [CrossRef] [PubMed]

184. Lewis, K. Platforms for antibiotic discovery. *Nat. Rev. Drug Discov.* **2013**, *12*, 371–387. [CrossRef] [PubMed]

185. Brazier, J.S.; Stubbs, S.L.J.; Duerden, B.I. Metronidazole resistance among clinical isolates belonging to the *Bacteroides fragilis* group: Time to be concerned? *J. Antimicrob. Chemother.* **1999**, *44*, 580–581. [CrossRef] [PubMed]

186. Löfmark, S.; Edlund, C.; Nord, C.E. Metronidazole is still the drug of choice for treatment of anaerobic infections. *Clin. Infect. Dis. Off. Publ. Infect. Dis. Soc. Am.* **2010**, *50* (Suppl. S1), S16–S23. [CrossRef] [PubMed]

187. Presečki Stanko, A.; Sóki, J.; Varda Brkić, D.; Plečko, V. Lactate dehydrogenase activity in *Bacteroides fragilis* group strains with induced resistance to metronidazole. *J. Glob. Antimicrob. Resist.* **2016**, *5*, 11–14. [CrossRef] [PubMed]

188. Soki, J.; Gal, M.; Brazier, J.S.; Rotimi, V.O.; Urban, E.; Nagy, E.; Duerden, B.I. Molecular investigation of genetic elements contributing to metronidazole resistance in *Bacteroides* strains. *J. Antimicrob. Chemother.* **2006**, *57*, 212–220. [CrossRef] [PubMed]

189. Cordero-Laurent, E.; Rodriguez, C.; Rodriguez-Cavallini, E.; Gamboa-Coronado, M.D.; Quesada-Gomez, C. Resistance of *Bacteroides* isolates recovered among clinical samples from a major Costa Rican hospital between 2000 and 2008 to beta-lactams, clindamycin, metronidazole and chloramphenicol. *Rev. Esp. Quimioter.* **2012**, *25*, 261–265. [PubMed]

190. Shilnikova, I.I.; Dmitrieva, N.V. Evaluation of Antibiotic Susceptibility of Gram-Positive Anaerobic Cocci Isolated from Cancer Patients of the N.N. Blokhin Russian Cancer Research Center. *J. Pathog.* **2015**. [CrossRef]

191. Carlier, J.P.; Sellier, N.; Rager, M.N.; Reysset, G. Metabolism of a 5-nitroimidazole in susceptible and resistant isogenic strains of *Bacteroides fragilis*. *Antimicrob. Agents Chemother.* **1997**, *41*, 1495–1499. [PubMed]

192. Trinh, S.; Haggoud, A.; Reysset, G.; Sebald, M. Plasmids Pip419 and Pip421 from *Bacteroides*—5-Nitroimidazole Resistance Genes and Their Upstream Insertion-Sequence Elements. *Microbiology* **1995**, *141*, 927–935. [CrossRef] [PubMed]

193. Theron, M.M.; van Rensburg, M.N.J.; Chalkley, L.J. Nitroimidazole resistance genes (nimB) in anaerobic Gram-positive cocci (previously *Peptostreptococcus* spp.). *J. Antimicrob. Chemother.* **2004**, *54*, 240–242. [CrossRef] [PubMed]

194. Urban, E.; Soki, J.; Brazier, J.S.; Nagy, E.; Duerden, B.I. Prevalence and characterization of nim genes of *Bacteroides* spp. isolated in Hungary. *Anaerobe* **2002**, *8*, 175–179. [CrossRef]

195. Roberts, M.C. Acquired tetracycline and/or macrolide-lincosamides-streptogramin resistance in anaerobes. *Anaerobe* **2003**, *9*, 63–69. [CrossRef]

196. Bartha, N.A.; Soki, J.; Edit, U.; Nagy, E. Investigation of the prevalence of tetQ, tetX and tetX1 genes in *Bacteroides* strains with elevated tigecycline minimum inhibitory concentrations. *Int. J. Antimicrob. Agents* **2011**, *38*, 522–525. [CrossRef] [PubMed]

197. Speer, B.S.; Shoemaker, N.B.; Salyers, A.A. Bacterial resistance to tetracycline: Mechanisms, transfer and clinical significance. *Clin. Microbiol. Rev.* **1992**, *5*, 387–399. [CrossRef] [PubMed]

198. Spengler, G.; Kincses, A.; Gajdacs, M.; Amaral, L. New Roads Leading to Old Destinations: Efflux Pumps as Targets to Reverse Multidrug Resistance in Bacteria. *Molecules* **2017**, *22*. [CrossRef] [PubMed]

199. Pumbwe, L.; Chang, A.; Smith, R.L.; Wexler, H.M. BmeRABC5 is a multidrug efflux system that can confer metronidazole resistance in *Bacteroides fragilis*. *Microb. Drug Resist.* **2007**, *13*, 96–101. [CrossRef] [PubMed]

200. Xu, Z.; Yan, A. Multidrug Efflux Systems in Microaerobic and Anaerobic Bacteria. *Antibiotics (Basel)* **2015**, *4*, 379–396. [CrossRef] [PubMed]

201. Rafii, F.; Park, M. Detection and characterization of an ABC transporter in *Clostridium hathewayi*. *Arch. Microbiol.* **2008**, *190*, 417–426. [CrossRef] [PubMed]

202. Tegos, G.P.; Haynes, M.; Jacob Strouse, J.; Khan, M.T.; Bologa, C.G.; Oprea, T.I.; Sklar, L.A. Microbial Efflux Pump Inhibition: Tactics and Strategies. *Curr. Pharm. Des.* **2011**, *17*, 1291–1302. [CrossRef] [PubMed]

203. Fille, M.; Mango, M.; Lechner, M.; Schaumann, R. *Bacteroides fragilis* group: Trends in resistance. *Curr. Microbiol.* **2006**, *52*, 153–157. [CrossRef] [PubMed]

4

Screening of *E. coli* β-clamp Inhibitors Revealed that Few Inhibit *Helicobacter pylori* more Effectively: Structural and Functional Characterization

Preeti Pandey [1,2], Vijay Verma [3,4], Suman Kumar Dhar [3] and Samudrala Gourinath [1,*]

[1]   School of Life Sciences, Jawaharlal Nehru University, New Delhi 110067, India; preet.satya@gmail.com
[2]   Department of Bioscience and Biotechnology, Banasthali University, Rajasthan 304022, India
[3]   Special Centre for Molecular Medicine, Jawaharlal Nehru University, New Delhi 110067, India;
      vijayscmmjnu@gmail.com (V.V.); skdhar2002@yahoo.co.in (S.K.D.)
[4]   Department of Microbiology, Central University of Rajasthan, Kishangarh 305801, India
*   Correspondence: sgourinath@jnu.ac.in

Abstract: The characteristic of interaction with various enzymes and processivity-promoting nature during DNA replication makes β-clamp an important drug target. *Helicobacter pylori* (*H. pylori*) have several unique features in DNA replication machinery that makes it different from other microorganisms. To find out whether difference in DNA replication proteins behavior accounts for any difference in drug response when compared to *E. coli*, in the present study, we have tested *E. coli* β-clamp inhibitor molecules against *H. pylori* β-clamp. Various approaches were used to test the binding of inhibitors to *H. pylori* β-clamp including docking, surface competition assay, complex structure determination, as well as antimicrobial assay. Out of five shortlisted inhibitor molecules on the basis of docking score, three molecules, 5-chloroisatin, carprofen, and 3,4-difluorobenzamide were co-crystallized with *H. pylori* β-clamp and the structures show that they bind at the protein-protein interaction site as expected. In vivo studies showed only two molecules, 5-chloroisatin, and 3,4-difluorobenzamide inhibited the growth of the pylori with MIC values in micro molar range, which is better than the inhibitory effect of the same drugs on *E. coli*. Therefore, the evaluation of such drugs against *H. pylori* may explore the possibility to use to generate species-specific pharmacophore for development of new drugs against *H. pylori*.

Keywords: DNA replication; surface competition assay; β-clamp; *E. coli* inhibitors; structure; screening

1. Introduction

There are certain pathogens that are affecting the human population worldwide. *Helicobacter pylori* (*H. pylori*) is one of them that infects around 50% of the world's population by causing peptic ulcer, gastritis, and gastric cancer [1]. For the conditions that are associated with *H. pylori*, eradication of infection using antibiotics as well as acid-suppressing medication is highly effective clinical intervention. Current procedure is becoming difficult because of the increasing cases of the antibiotic-resistant strains [2,3]. These resistances are mainly associated with mutation in their target enzyme/protein. Therefore, there is an emergent need to find out promising drug targets that help in eradication of such disastrous pathogen.

The DNA replication machinery offers several important and interesting drug targets [4,5]. Among them one such target is β-clamp. β-clamp, a part of DNA pol III holoenzyme is very crucial protein as it is involved in myriads of steps during DNA replication. It is the key protein that increases the processivity of many important enzymes and complexes by interacting with them. β-clamp prevents the polymerase from dissociating, while polymerase's rapid movement along the DNA molecule. Apart from several DNA polymerases, pol I [6], pol II [7,8], pol IV [9], pol V [10], β-clamp interacts with various proteins such as mismatch repair proteins MutL and MutS [6], DNA ligase [6], and the DnaA-related protein Hda [11].

Biological active form of β-clamp is dimer and each monomeric unit consists of three domains, where the protein-binding site resides in between domain II and III. This interaction site is divided into two subsites and all β-clamp interacting partners bind to these subsites [12–15]. Usually, the proteins that interact with β-clamp in bacteria contain consensus sequence with five or six residues, with the consensus amino acid sequence of "ZXSLF" to bind to the binding pocket of β-clamp [16] where Z represents any amino acid which is hydrophilic in nature while X represents any small hydrophobic residue. This protein-protein interaction site has been target for drug development in different organisms. Recently, we have reported diflunisal a FDA approved drug that binds to this site and can inhibit the growth of *H. pylori* at a micromolar concentration [17]. Many inhibitors and drugs for *E. coli* β-clamp have been identified but regardless of their similar structure, they are not equally effective in other organism [18]. Therefore, drug effective for one organism may not show the same effect on the other. *H. pylori* shows extreme genetic variability and allelic diversity because of intraspecific recombination and mutations [19]. It has been found that many proteins as well as their functions vary in *H. pylori* from that of other bacteria, especially from *E. coli* like helicase and primase strong interaction [20,21], loading of helicase is different from that in *E. coli* [22,23].

In a previous manuscript, we found some differences at DNA binding as well as protein binding regions in native Hpβ-clamp when compared to other β-clamp structures from various organisms [16]. This made us think whether there is any difference in binding pattern of inhibitors or the drugs that are already known to inhibit *E. coli* β-clamp could inhibit *H. pylori* β clamp also. In order to find that, we examined drugs and inhibitors that are known to bind *E. coli* β-clamp, albeit their IC$_{50}$ is in millimolar range [18]. On the basis of docking score, five molecules were selected for in vitro and in vivo studies. All of the five molecules showed competitive binding with ligase and three of them were co-crystallized and determined the complex structure with Hpβ-clamp to show that they bind to the ligase binding site/protein-protein interaction site. Among these three, two molecules 5-chloroisatin and 3,4- difluorobenzamide showed inhibition of *H. pylori* growth with micromolar IC$_{50}$ values.

2. Results and Discussions

2.1. Screening of E. coli β-clamp Drugs/Inhibitors

The structures of *E. coli* β-clamp in complex with some of its inhibitors have already been reported [18,24–26]. In order to check the extent to which these inhibitors would also inhibit Hpβ-clamp, we docked all of them against Hpβ-clamp. Finally, we shortlisted five of these molecules from the PDB depending on their docking scores and availability; these molecules were 5-chloroisatin (C1) (PDB id: 4N95), 6-nitroindazole (C2) (PDB id: 4N96), (S)-carprofen (C3) (PDB id: 4MJR), 5-nitroindole (C4) (PDB id: 4N97), and 3,4-difluorobenzamide (C5) (PDB id: 4N94) (Table S1).

2.2. Competitive Inhibition Using Surface Competition Assay

Due to small size and low molecular weight of the shortlisted molecules we were unable to predict the interaction between them and Hpβ-clamp using the simple SPR binding technique. Therefore, we did a qualitative analysis by choosing an advanced approach of surface competition assay where the sensorgram response decreases with increasing concentration of the analyte molecule. This approach is basically based on competition between two analyte molecules that compete for binding to the same ligand. Here, Hpβ-clamp was used as ligand, HpDNA ligase (a natural binder of β-clamp [16]) was used as analyte 1 and drugs/inhibitor molecules were used as analyte 2, similar to the protocol reported in Pandey et al., 2017. Since mixture of both the analytes, DNA ligase and drugs/inhibitor were passed through the SPR chip, the summation of both analyte contribution was the measured response in this technique. There was an inverse relationship between magnitude of response obtained and amount of small molecule analyte in the sample [27]. Since it was a competition assay so for binding to β-clamp, the drug/inhibitor molecules should compete with ligase. The sensorgram showed a decreased response as we increased the concentration of small molecule (Figure 1), only because now more and more protein binding site is occupied by low molecular weight analyte i.e., drug/inhibitor molecules (which has negligible weight), and thereby blocking the binding of high molecular weight ligase (which was responsible for detectable signals in sensorgram). All five shortlisted molecules showed competitive binding to β-clamp. The inhibitory effect of each of the small molecules is shown by a continuous decrease in the sensorgram response withan increasing small molecule concentration.

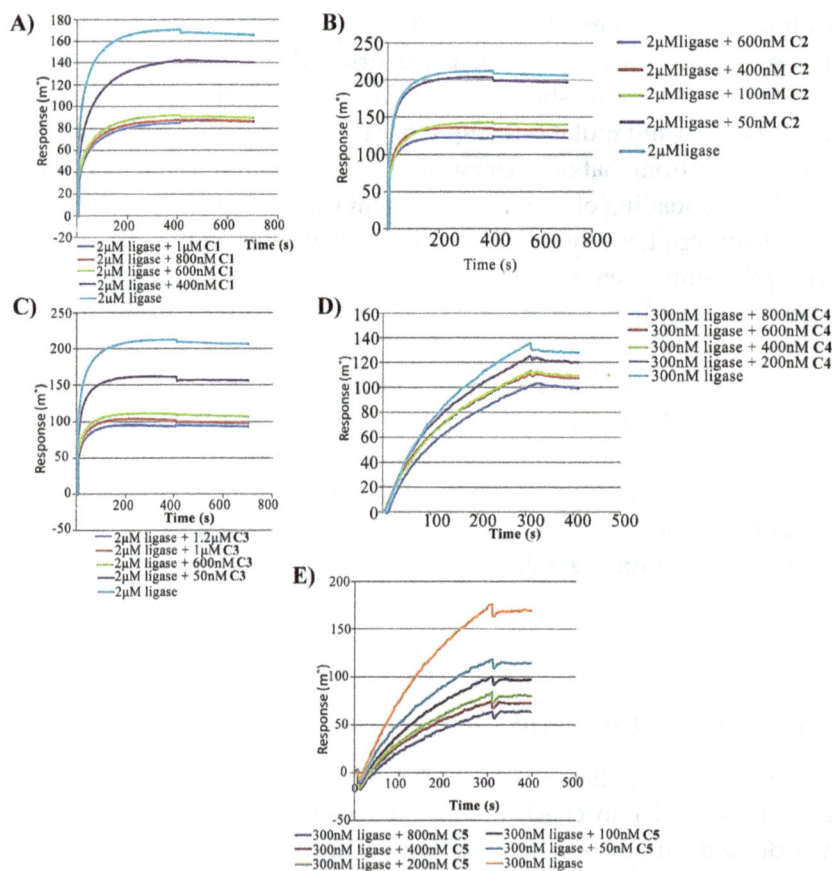

Figure 1. SPR sensorgram. SPR sensorgram showing surface competition assay between HpDNA ligase and the small molecules. A qualitative analysis of the in vitro competition between DNA ligase and small molecules (present in solution) for binding to Hpβ-clamp (immobilized on the chip surface) was carried out. For the small molecules (**A**) 5-chloroisatin (C1); (**B**) 6-nitroindazole (C2) and (**C**) (S)-carprofen (C3), a mass of ~6 ng of Hpβ-clamp gets immobilized on the chip surface while for (**D**) 5-nitroindole (C4) and (**E**) 3,4-difluorobenzamide (C5), a mass of ~4 ng of Hpβ-clamp gets immobilized on the chip surface. The concentration of ligase was kept the same throughout each experiment with a small molecule. As the concentration of the small molecule was increased, the SPR response decreased.

2.3. Binding Pattern Analysis in Complex Crystal Structures

After confirmation of inhibitory activity in surface competition assay, we tried the co-crystallization of those inhibitors with Hpβ-clamp, and three of them were successfully co-crystallized with Hpβ-clamp.

These were 5-chloroisatin (C1) (PDB id: 5G4Q), carprofen (C3) (PDB id: 5FXT) and 3,4-difluorobenzamide (C5) (PDB id: 5FVE) (Figures 2–4). All of these crystals yielded clear electron density for the ligand molecules with good occupancy, except for 5-chloroisatin. The occupancy of 5-chloroisatin was quite low. Moreover, based on data obtained from the soaked crystals, the temperature factor of this inhibitor was high when compared to the average temperature factor of the protein. Some of the following points regarding the binding pattern here were derived from inspection of the co-crystal structures with various inhibitors.

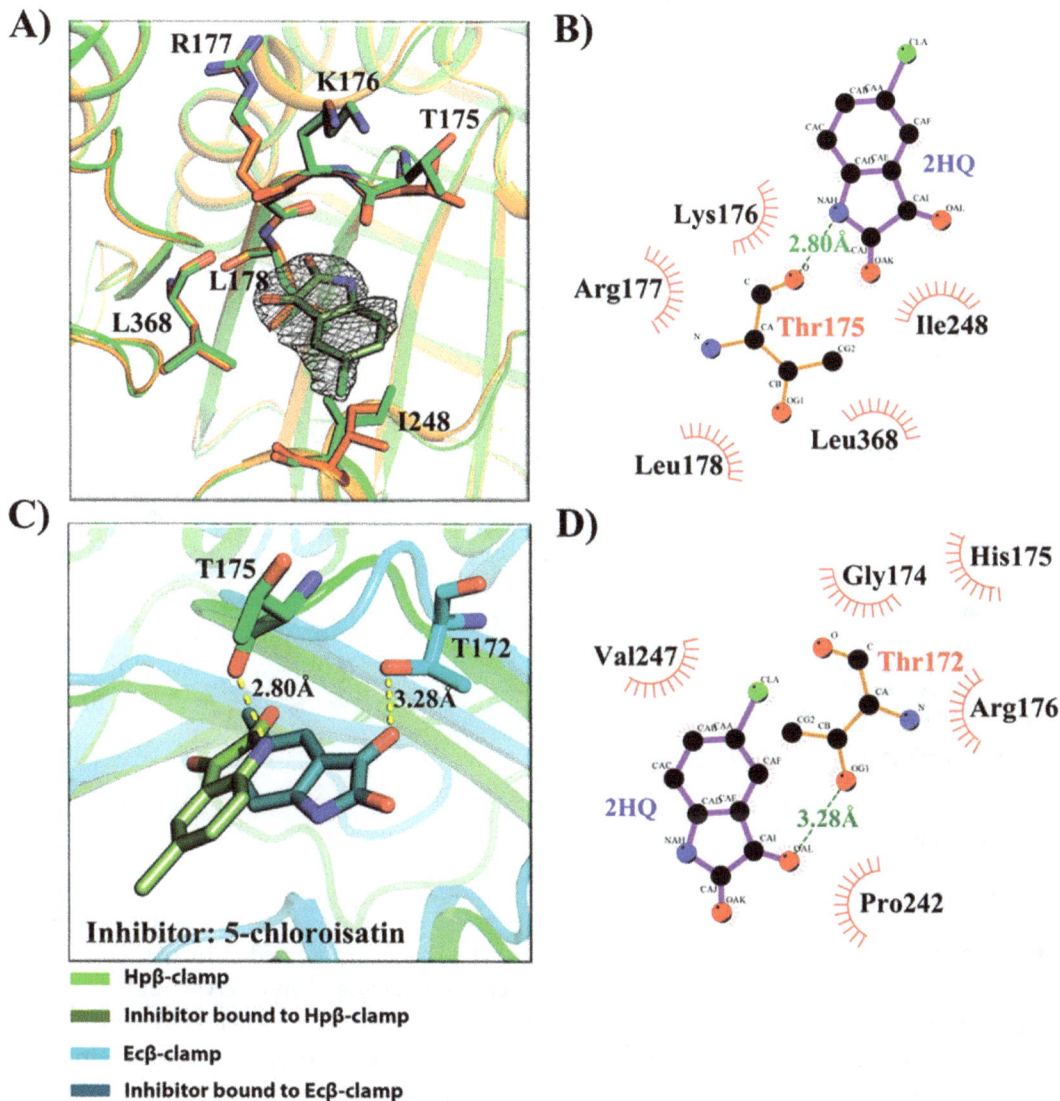

Figure 2. 5-chloroisatin interaction with Hpβ-clamp. (**A**) 2Fo-Fc map, contoured at 1σ, of 5-chloroisatin bound to Hpβ-clamp (PDB ID: 5G4Q). The alignment of the structure of the complex (green) with that of the native (orange) did not yield significant differences in the orientation of interacting residues except for I248; (**B**) Ligplot of the Hpβ-clamp structure near the bound 5-chloroisatin, showing the predominantly hydrophobic interactions between the protein and the inhibitor. T173 of Hpβ-clamp did form an H-bond with the inhibitor molecule; (**C**) Structural alignment of Hpβ-clamp (green) and Ecβ-clamp (cyan) complex with ligand 5-chloroisatin. T172 of Ecβ-clamp makes H-bond with ligand while T175 of Hpβ-clamp makes H-bond with the ligand (PDB ID: 4N95); (**D**) Ligplot of Ecβ-clamp complex with 5-chloroisatin showing the types of interactions between them.

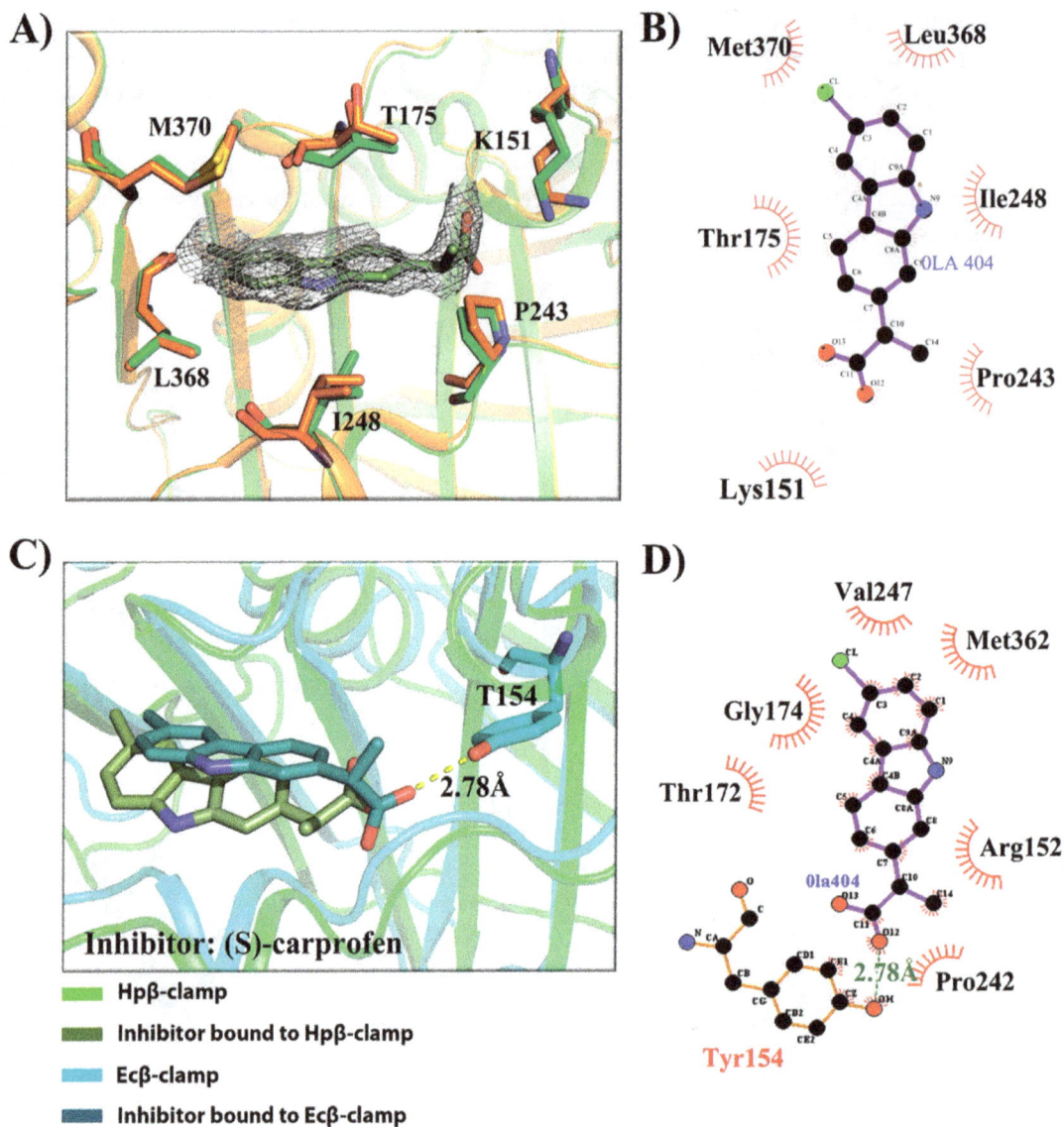

Figure 3. (S)-carprofen interaction with β-clamp. (**A**) 2Fo-Fc map, contoured at 1σ, of (S)-carprofen bound to Hpβ-clamp (PDB ID: 5FXT). The alignment of the structure of the co-crystal of Hpβ-clamp (green) and the inhibitor (olive) with that of the native Hpβ-clamp (orange) showed almost same orientation of interacting molecules in both structures; (**B**) Ligplot of the Hpβ-clamp structure near the bound (S)-carprofen, showing the hydrophobic interactions between the protein and the inhibitor; (**C**) Structural alignment of *H. pylori* (green) and *E. coli* β-clamp (cyan) complex with ligand (S)-carprofen. T154 of Ecβ-clamp makes H-bond with the ligand apart from other hydrophobic interactions while Hpβ-clamp and ligand interactions are dominated by hydrophobic interactions; and, (**D**) Ligplot of Ecβ-clamp with bound ligand showing its various interactions with ligand (PDB ID: 4MJR).

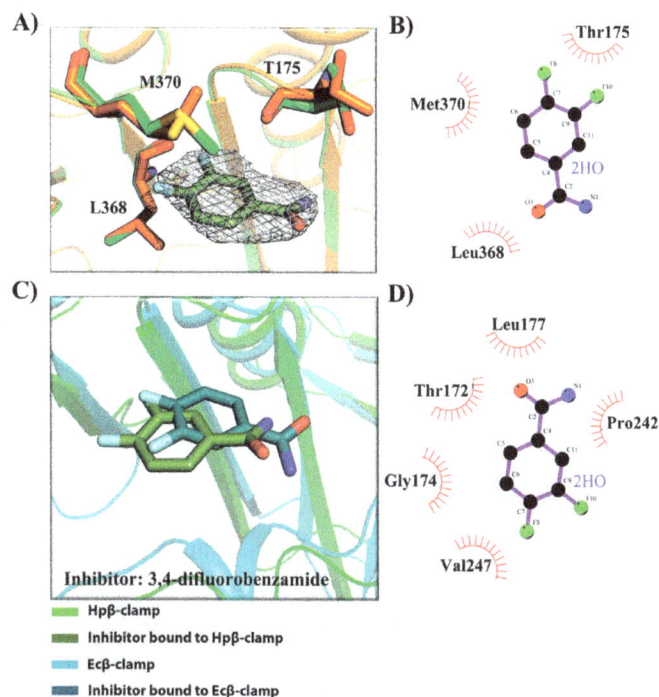

Figure 4. 3,4-difluorobenzamide interaction with β-clamp. (**A**) 2Fo-Fc map, contoured at 1σ, of 3,4-difluorobenzamide in complex with Hpβ-clamp. The alignment of the structure of the co-crystal of Hpβ-clamp (green) and the inhibitor (olive) with that of the native Hpβ-clamp (orange) showed differences in the orientations of residues T175, M370, K176 and I248 between the co-crystal and native structures; (**B**) Ligplot of the Hpβ-clamp structure near the bound 3,4-difluorobenzamide, showing the hydrophobic interactions between the protein and the inhibitor; (**C**) Structural superimposition of Hpβ-clamp (green) and Ecβ-clamp (cyan) complex with ligand 3,4-difluorobenzamide. In both the cases, the contacts are dominated by hydrophobic interactions however the orientation of ligand molecule is differentiated by a rotation of 180 degree; and, (**D**) Ligplot of Ecβ-clamp bound to ligand showing the hydrophobic interactions nearby (PDB ID: 4N94).

(a)   Binding site of β-clamp is conserved in all bacterial species: The ligand-binding site of β-clamp consists of hydrophobic amino acid residues that have been found to be fairly conserved but not identical in the β-clamps of the various species reported so far. As described in introduction, two protein-binding subsites located near each other, subsite I and subsite II, have been identified in β-clamp (Figure S1). All of the proteins and peptides that have been observed to interact with β-clamp in structures that are deposited in the PDB have been shown to bind to the region of β-clamp encompassing subsites I and II as seen in Ecβ-clamp [9,24,28] and in our earlier studies on ligase peptide-bound Hpβ-clamp [17]. Inspection of the crystal structures of the inhibitor-Hpβ-clamp complexes (PDB id: 5g4q, 5FXT, 5FVE) and inhibitor-Ecβ-clamp complexes (PDB id: 4N95, 4MJR, 4N94) revealed the inhibitor-interacting residues of Hpβ-clamp correspond to those of Ecβ-clamp [9,24,28], suggesting the importance of these residues in the protein-binding cleft (Table S2) (Figures 2–4). These residues, especially those corresponding to Thr173, Thr175, Pro243, Ile248, Met370 of subsite I, are quite conserved in β-clamp and are ligand binding residues. Most of these residues also observed to interact with the ligase peptide, clearly indicating that these small molecules will compete with other proteins, like ligase, to bind to β-clamp.

(b)   All of the inhibitors occupy subsite I of the protein interaction site: In the crystal structure of Hpβ-clamp complexed with the FIRSLF peptide from HpDNA ligase (PDB ID: 5FRQ), the peptide was observed to occupy both subsites I and II, like other clamp-interacting proteins/peptides from *E. coli* [16]. Residues Leu360 and Phe361 of this ligase peptide were observed to be buried deep in the Hpβ-clamp cleft and to make hydrophobic contacts with Hpβ-clamp subsite I residues Thr173,

Lys176, Ile248, Pro347, Leu368, and Met370 (PDB ID: 5FRQ). Moreover, all of the inhibitors we crystallized with Hpβ-clamp also bound to subsite I. The ligplots of the Hpβ-clamp residues contacting each inhibitor are shown in Figures 2–4. The inhibitor-interacting residues were found to be the same as those that were observed to interact with HpDNA ligase (Table S2). All of these inhibitors were observed to interact with most of the residues of subsite I that formed contacts with the ligase peptide. A comparison of the ligand-bound Hpβ-clamp structure with the native Hpβ-clamp structure yielded no significant difference in the positions of the ligand-interacting residues (Figures 2–4) except for Lys176 and Met370, which moved a little bit from their native positions to firmly bind the inhibitor. Thr175 of Hpβ-clamp was also observed to make a hydrogen bond with the inhibitor 5-chloroisatin.

(c)   Comparison of co-crystal structures of *H. pylori* and *E. coli* β-clamp: The comparison of co-complex structures of *H. pylori* and *E. coli* with various inhibitors showed some critical differences in the binding pattern. In case of 5-chloroisatin (Figure 2), the Thr175 of Hpβ-clamp makes hydrogen bond with ligand however that in Ecβ-clamp is made by Thr172 in the neighborhood. Out of various hydrophobic contacts between the β-clamp and inhibitor, three of them are common in both *H. pylori* and *E. coli* β-clamp. These residues include Ile248, Lys176, Arg177 in Hpβ-clamp, and Val247, His175, Arg176 in Ecβ-clamp. In case of (S)-carprofen (Figure 3), Thr154 of Ecβ-clamp makes H-bond with the ligand along with other hydrophobic contacts however in *H. pylori* the contact between β-clamp and ligand is favored by only hydrophobic interactions. Five of these interactions are common in both, which includes residues Lys151, Thr175, Pro243, Ile248, Met370 in Hpβ-clamp and Arg152, Gly174, Pro242, Val247, Met362 in Ecβ-clamp. In case of 3,4-difluorobenzamide (Figure 4), the interaction between β-clamp and ligand in both *H. pylori* and *E. coli* is dominated by hydrophobic interactions. Among them, three of these interactions are common in both the clamps, Thr175, Pro243, Ile248 in Hpβ-clamp and Gly174, Pro242, Val247 in Ecβ-clamp, respectively. All of the ligand-interacting residues of Hpβ-clamp as well as Ecβ-clamp are tabulated (Table S2). The structure-based sequence alignment of Hpβ-clamp and Ecβ-clamp is shown in Figure 5 with highlighted ligand-interacting residues, which shows that the mode of interaction between inhibitor/ligand and β-clamp of both organisms are almost same.

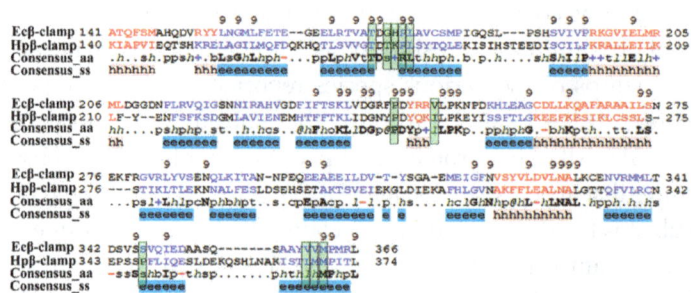

Figure 5. Structure-based sequence alignment. β-clamps of *H. pylori* and *E. coli* were compared using structure based sequence alignment. The ligand-interacting residues are highlighted (in green box). In each block, the first line shows conservation indices for positions with a conservation index above 5. The secondary structure prediction is shown in color red (alpha-helix) and blue (beta-strand). The last two lines show consensus amino acid sequence (consensus_aa) and consensus predicted secondary structures (consensus_ss). Consensus predicted secondary structure symbols: alpha-helix:h; beta-strand:e. Consensus amino acid symbols are: conserved amino acid are in uppercase and bold letter; aliphatic (I,V, L): l; aromatic (YHWF); hydrophobic (W,F,Y,M,L,I,V,A,C,T,H): h; alcohol (S,T):o; polar residues (D,E,H,K,N,Q,R,S,T): p; tiny (A,G,C,S):t; small (A,G,C,S,V,N,D,T,P):s; bulky residues (E,F,I,K,L,M,Q,R,W,Y):b; positively charged (K,R,H):+; negatively charged (D,E): -; charged (D,E,K,R,H):c.

(d) Comparison of the co-crystal Hpβ-clamp structures with docked structure: In all of the docked structures, like in crystal structure, the inhibitors were found to be present in the same pocket (Figure S2). The orientation of the 5-chloroisatin inhibitor in the docked structure did differ from that in the crystal structure (Figure S2), but this difference did not affect much the structure of the binding site. Hpβ-clamp residue Thr173 form hydrogen bond with every docked inhibitor, while residue Lys247 hydrogen bonded the docked inhibitors (S)-carprofen. In contrast, in the actual crystal structure, only 5-chloroisatin was observed to make a hydrogen bond with Thr175 (Figure 2B). In every case, hydrophobic contact dominates the interactions between the protein and inhibitor. Interestingly, all of the docked ligands and ligands in co-crystal structures bound in the same pocket with similar hydrophobic interactions, but the hydrogen bond pattern did not match.

2.4. Antibacterial Activity of Hpβ-clamp Inhibitors

The response of each drug (C1-C5) on *H. pylori* 26695 was evaluated by disk diffusion method [29]. Out of five drugs, C5 (3,4- difluorobenzamide) showed marginal inhibition, while drug C1 (5-chloroisatin) showed significant inhibition zone on BHI agar plate against *H. pylori* (Figure 6A). However, no clear inhibition zones were observed in BHI-agar plates in case of other three drugs (data not shown) suggested that these three drugs have no inhibition on growth of *H. pylori* (data not shown). The results suggested that these two drugs (C1 and C5) might have inhibited the function of Hpβ-clamp thus preventing the *H. pylori* growth in culture. As mentioned in Materials and Methods, the MICs of drugs C1-C5 were measured on BHI-broth culture of *H. pylori*. With an MIC of 18 µM drug C1 (5-chloroisatin) showed significant antimicrobial activity (Figure 6C). In contrast, the drug C5 (3,4-difluorobenzamide) yielded an MIC of 824 µM. These results suggested that drug C5 (3,4-difluorobenzamide) and especially drug C1 (5-chloroisatin) to be effective against *H. pylori*. Although all of the above drugs (C1–C5) bound to Hpβ-clamp and showed their inhibitory effects in surface competition assay, only a few of them showed an inhibition in antimicrobial assay. The drug C1 (5-chloroisatin) showed extra H-bond with Thr173 compared to other complex structures may be responsible for better binding and thus better inhibition. Additionally, differential uptake of drugs into the pathogen could be the other possible reason behind the difference in their inhibition activity.

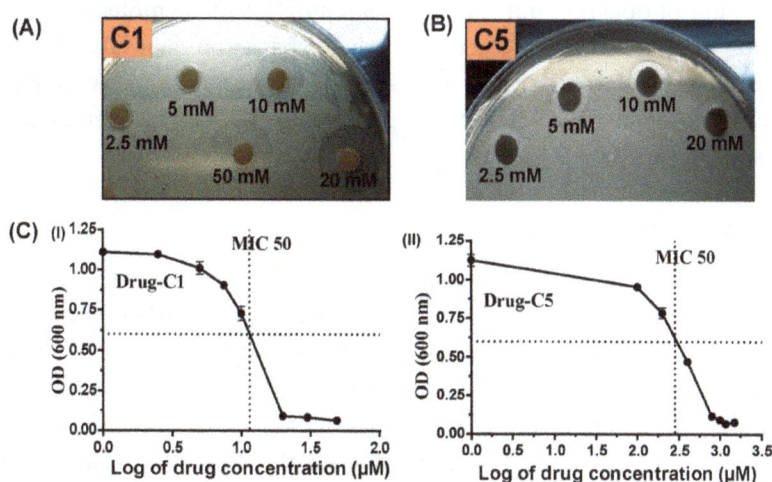

Figure 6. Antimicrobial activities of different drugs against *H. pylori*. (**A**) Anti-*H. pylori* activities of different drugs (**A**) 5-chloroisatin (C1) and (**B**) 3,4-difluorobenzamide (C5) determined by applying the disk diffusion method. Petri dish with drugs containing discs showed inhibition zones for bacterial growth; (**C**) Anti-*H. pylori* activities of drugs determined as minimum inhibitory concentrations (MICs) were obtained via the dilution method. The MIC of drug C1 and C5 are 18 µM and 824 µM, respectively. The experiments were performed in triplicates. Error bars show standard deviation of the mean (Mean ± SD).

3. Material and Methods

3.1. Overexpression and Purification of Hpβ-clamp

As described in our previous work, Hpβ-clamp (Accession id: AJF10096) was cloned, expressed, and purified [16]. The recombinant plasmid of Hpβ-clamp was transformed into *E. coli* BL21 strain. The cells were grown initially at 37 °C till the O.D reaches to 0.6. Induction was given with 0.5 mM IPTG and then cells were incubated at 30 °C in shaker for 6 h. The cells were then harvested at 6000 rpm for 10 min. The cell pellet was suspended in lysis buffer consisting of 10 mM imidazole, 30 mM Tris (pH 7.5), 150 mm NaCl, 0.5% tween20, and 6 mM β-Mercaptoethanol. 0.3% lysozyme. After about 30–45 min of incubation with lysozyme the cells were sonicated and centrifuged at 13,000 rpm for 45 min at 4 °C. The Supernatant was collected and passed through Ni-NTA column, which was pre-equilibrated with buffer having 10 mM imidazole, 30 mM Tris (pH 7.5), 150 mm NaCl, and 6 mM β-Mercaptoethanol. After giving a wash with wash buffer containing 30 mM imidazole, elution was taken with buffer containing 150 mM imidazole, 30 mM Tris (pH 7.5), 150 mM NaCl, 6 mM βMe, and 30 mM arginine. This fraction was then concentrated using a centricon. The concentrated protein was further purified through gel filtration chromatography using Hi-Load G200 16/60 column (GE healthcare). Eluted fraction was checked on a 12% SDS-PAGE gel. The same buffers and procedure was followed to purify HpDNA ligase (Accession id: AJF10437).

3.2. In Silico Screening of Inhibitors

The ligase-binding site on Hpβ-clamp was targeted for screening inhibitors and ligand binding analysis following the protocol, as reported earlier [17]. For grid generation, the site where peptide from ligase was bound [10] (PDB ID: 5FRQ) was used. For docking Maestro was used that includes Schrodinger's Protein Preparation Wizard [30], Schrodinger ligprep wizard, and glide. All known *E. coli* B-clamp inhibitors were chosen from Protein Data Bank (PDB) structures of their complexes with *E. coli* β-clamp with the hope that they would also efficiently inhibit the activity of Hpβ-clamp. Each molecule from *E. coli* β-clamp inhibitor was then prepared using Schrodinger's Ligprep Wizard to generate a maximum of 34 conformations. Finally, docking was carried out using GLIDE [31–33], specifically its extra precision module after preparing the ligand and protein. Initially, we got number of molecules as a result of docking, but we were searching for those molecules, which were easily available. Therefore, we selected five molecules (Table S1) based on their GLIDE rankings as well as their availability. We then tried to co-crystallize these five inhibitor molecules with Hpβ-clamp. To test their inhibitory activities against Hpβ-clamp a biophysical experiment, as well as antimicrobial assay of these molecules, were carried out.

3.3. Surface Competition Assay

We performed a qualitative analysis using a surface competition approach, following the protocol as reported earlier [17]. On SPR sensor surface, β-clamp was immobilized and the analyte, high-molecular-weight DNA ligase was passed over the sensor surface. The DNA ligase was also mixed with low-molecular-weight compounds and was used as competitive analyte. The DNA ligase concentration was kept constant throughout this assay, however the competitive analytes concentration was increased in progressive injections. The sensorgram with different concentrations of analytes are shown in Figure 1. The flow cell 1 was used as a control surface for background subtraction, and in flow cell 2, β-clamp was immobilized. The SPR buffer used consisting of 10 mM HEPES pH 7.4, 150 mM saline-NaCl with 3 mM EDTA (HBS-EP) along with 2% dimethyl sulfoxide (DMSO) and 0.05% surfactant P20. All of the compounds were dissolved in DMSO and diluted in SPR buffer. The concentration of DMSO in buffer was matched with the DMSO amount in the experimental samples to limit bulk refractive index changes. The surface was regenerated between injections using high NaCl (0.5 to 1 M) solution wash.

3.4. Crystallization, Structure Determination and Analysis of the Complex Structures

Hanging drop vapor diffusion method was used to crystalize Hpβ-clamp in complex with the identified *E. coli* β-clamp inhibitors. The protein purified using gel filtration chromatography concentrated up to 6 mg/mL. Crystallization drop was put in 2:2 ratio, where 2 μL of protein was mixed with an equal volume of precipitant solution containing 20% *v/v* PEG MME 550, 0.1 M MOPS/HEPES-Na pH 7.3, 0.2 M ammonium citrate, 6% *w/v* PEG 20,000, 0.01 M $MgCl_2$, and 0.01 M strontium chloride. 2 mM of small molecule (dissolved in DMSO) was added to the crystallization drop and equilibrated against 1 mL of the same precipitant in 24-well plates and incubated at 16 °C. The crystals appeared after about one week. The X-ray diffraction data were collected at DBT-ESRF beamline BM14 to a resolution of 1.9 Å–2.5 Å. To process and integrate the data HKL 2000 [34] was used. Native Hpβ-clamp structure was used as the search model to solve all of the co-crystal structures using the molecular replacement method and using the program Molrep in CCP4 [35]. Further, Refmac5 was used for refinement and COOT [36] was used for fitting the molecular structures into the electron density. Lastly, PROCHECK [37] was used to evaluate the stereochemistry of the model. The refinement statistics are listed in Table 1. The coordinates of complex structure are deposited with PDB IDs: 5G4Q (Hpβ-clamp complex with 5-chloroisatin, C1), 5FXT (Hpβ-clamp complex with carprofen, C3), and 5FVE (Hpβ-clamp complex with 3,4-difluorobenzamide, C5).

Table 1. Crystallographic data and refinement statistics for *H. pylori* β-clamp in complex with various inhibitors.

	Data Collection		
	β-clamp Complexed with 5-chloroisatin	β-clamp Complexed with Carprofen	β-clamp Complexed with 3,4-difluorobenzamide
Space group	P21	C2	C2
Cell dimensions			
a,b,c (Å)	82.1, 65.4, 88.8	89.9, 66.4, 82.8	90.0, 66.3, 82.7
α,β,γ (deg.)	90.0, 115.7, 90.0	90.0, 115.5, 90.0	90.0, 115.4, 90.0
R_{sym} (highest resolution range)	5.0 (43.8)	5.1 (21.6)	5.5 (42.1)
Completeness (highest resolution range)	91.1 (89.0)	98.5 (79.7)	98.8 (90.9)
Mean I/σ	20.2	38.8	33.17
Refinement			
Resolution range (Å)	50.0–2.3	50.0–1.97	50.0–2.07
Rwork/Rfree	22.7/28.5	20.6/24.3	21.3/25.2
Number of atoms			
Protein	5588	3021	2883
Water	57	55	92
R.m.s. deviation			
Bond angles (deg.)	1.78	1.16	1.98
Bond lengths (Å)	0.015	0.005	0.007
Mean B value ($Å^2$)	50.3	50.8	44.5

3.5. Antimicrobial Test

(a) *H. pylori* strain and culture conditions: The *H. pylori* strain and culture conditions were used, as mentioned in our previous work [17]. In brief, Brain heart infusion (BHI) agar/broth medium was used to culture the *H. pylori* strain 26695. The agar/broth medium contains the antibiotics amphotericin B (8 mg/mL), trimethoprim (5 mg/mL), and vancomycin (6 mg/mL), 8% horse blood serum and 0.4% IsoVitaleX. The bacterial plates were incubated under microaerobic conditions (5% O_2, 10% CO_2) at 37 °C for 36 h and the broth cultures were incubated at 37 °C on a shaker operating at 110 rpm under microaerobic conditions (5% O_2, 10% CO_2).

(b) Anti-*H. pylori* susceptibility tests: To screen the susceptibility of *H. pylori* against drugs the Kirby-Bauer disk diffusion susceptibility test was used, as mentioned earlier [17,29]. In brief, 200 μL of the *H. pylori* suspension was spread evenly on 90 mm BHI-agar plates. Because of the slow growth of *H. pylori*, high inoculum was used for the disk diffusion method. Different concentrations of inhibitors (Sigma, St Louis, MI, USA) were inoculated (10 μL of each drug or DMSO as control) on 6 mm disks, which are placed on bacterial lawn surface. The disks were dried and incubated at 37 °C under micro-aerophilic conditions for about 3–5 days.

(c)   Minimum inhibitory concentrations (MICs): The dilution method was applied to determine the MICs of drugs described earlier [17]. In brief, different concentrations of the drugs were used in 2 mL BHI broth that was inoculated with fresh *H. pylori* suspensions (20 μL; 1:100 dilution; initial optical density $OD^{600} < 0.1$). Further, the tubes containing broth and different concentration of drugs were incubated under microaerobic condition for 20 h at 37 °C on a shaker (110 rpm). After 20 h, the OD^{600} were taken and GraphPad software was used for analysis of MICs. OD^{600} measurements were also taken for the *H. pylori* suspension without drugs or with kanamycin (positive control) and with/without bacteria. All of the experiments were done in triplicate.

4. Conclusions

β-clamp is similar to proliferating cell nuclear antigen (PCNA) in higher organisms, including humans. It is required to maintain the fidelity of DNA replication because in prokaryotes, the rate of cell division is very high, and much accuracy of DNA replication and repair is needed. For most of the processes involved in DNA replication and repair, it acts as a protein-protein interaction hub. Therefore, β-clamp is essential for the reproduction as well as the survival of prokaryotes. In spite of having similar function, there is no sequence homology between prokaryotic β-clamp and eukaryotic PCNA. So, the potential drugs that target β-clamp of prokaryotes would be relatively safe for use in humans.

Out of five shortlisted drug molecules 6-Nitroindazole (C2), (S)-Carprofen (C3), and 5-Nitroindole (C4) displayed poor inhibitory activity on the growth of *H. pylori*, which may have been due to their inability to diffuse into the pathogen. Drug 5-chloroisatin (C1) and 3,4-difluorobenzamide (C5) showed significant inhibition in μM range against *H. pylori* in our experimental condition. However, these inhibitors showed inhibition in the mM range on *E. coli* [18]. Interestingly, the sequence comparison of both proteins Hpβ-clamp and Ecβ-clamp showed an identity of 23% with 44% similarity. The inhibitor-binding site is homologous in Hpβ-clamp and Ecβ-clamp, but it is not identical. The binding of 5-chloroisatin differ clearly by one hydrogen bond, in *E. coli* b-clamp Thr172 does form H-bond while equivalent residue Thr173 in *H. pylori* does not form H-bond and interactions are dominated by hydrophobic interactions. Interestingly 3,4-difluorobenzamide interactions are dominated by hydrophobic interactions in both structures, orientation of the molecule and interacting residues are different without any specific notable interaction. When we looked at several physio-chemical properties of these molecules (Table S1), polar surface and relative free binding energy values for 5-chloroisatin (C1) and 3,4-difluorobenzamide (C5) showed contrasting or significantly different values from other molecules, suggesting that these parameters may play an important role in *H. pylori* targeting. Moreover, these molecules may also bind to any other targets in the organism and show better efficiency.

Overall, these results suggest that an inhibitor of a protein in one pathogen may act differently towards the orthologous protein in a different pathogen even if the orthologous proteins share a similar structure. The reason might be due to differential uptake of various drugs/inhibitors in the pathogen. It is, therefore, essential to design and test drugs against the specific pathogen of interest rather than solely relying on drugs that work on other pathogens.

Supplementary Materials: Figure S1: Surface representation of co-crystal structure of Hpβ-clamp monomer with ligase peptide and various inhibitors. Figure S2: Structural alignments of Hpβ-clamp-inhibitor co-complexes with the Hpβ-clamp-inhibitor docking models. Table S1: The list of E. coli β-clamp inhibitors along with their structures, docking scores and binding energy values with Hp β-clamp. Table S2: Table showing residues of Hpβ-clamp that interact with ligase peptide and its inhibitor molecules. Also the corresponding residues of Ecβ-clamp that are involved in binding with inhibitors have been shown.

Acknowledgments: We thank the Advance Instrumentation Research Facility (AIRF) and Jawaharlal Nehru University (JNU) for providing the SPR facility. University for potential excellence II (UPEII) from UGC and JNU, SKD thanks ICMR for financial support. P.P. thanks, D.S.T., V.V. thanks, D.S. Kothari Postdoctoral Fellowship, UGC for fellowship and DST Inspire. We thank ESRF, BM 14 staff, Department of Biotechnology (DBT), Government of India for access to the beamline for data collection. We thank UGC-RNW, DBT-BUILDER, DST-PURSE, DST-FIST for institutional and central instrumentation facility support.

Author Contributions: P.P., S.K.D. and S.G. designed, P.P. and V.V. performed, analyzed experiments; all authors reviewed the results and approved the final version of the manuscript. All work is done under the guidance of S.K.D. and S.G.

References

1. Khatoon, J.; Rai, R.P.; Prasad, K.N. Role of Helicobacter pylori in gastric cancer: Updates. World J. Gastrointest. Oncol. **2016**, 8, 147–158. [CrossRef] [PubMed]

2. Burkitt, M.D.; Duckworth, C.A.; Williams, J.M.; Pritchard, D.M. Helicobacter pylori-induced gastric pathology: Insights from in vivo and ex vivo models. Dis. Model. Mech. **2017**, 10, 89–104. [CrossRef] [PubMed]

3. Rasheed, F.; Campbell, B.J.; Alfizah, H.; Varro, A.; Zahra, R.; Yamaoka, Y.; Pritchard, D.M. Analysis of clinical isolates of Helicobacter pylori in pakistan reveals high degrees of pathogenicity and high frequencies of antibiotic resistance. Helicobacter **2014**, 19, 387–399. [CrossRef] [PubMed]

4. Yin, Z.; Wang, Y.; Whittell, L.R.; Jergic, S.; Liu, M.; Harry, E.; Dixon, N.E.; Kelso, M.J.; Beck, J.L.; Oakley, A.J. DNA replication is the target for the antibacterial effects of nonsteroidal anti-inflammatory drugs. Chem. Biol. **2014**, 21, 481–487. [CrossRef] [PubMed]

5. Guichard, S.M.; Danks, M.K. Topoisomerase enzymes as drug targets. Curr. Opin. Oncol. **1999**, 11, 482–489. [CrossRef] [PubMed]

6. Lopez de Saro, F.J.; O'Donnell, M. Interaction of the beta sliding clamp with muts, ligase, and DNA polymerase I. Proc. Natl. Acad. Sci. USA **2001**, 98, 8376–8380. [CrossRef] [PubMed]

7. Hughes, A.J., Jr.; Bryan, S.K.; Chen, H.; Moses, R.E.; McHenry, C.S. Escherichia coli DNA polymerase II is stimulated by DNA polymerase III holoenzyme auxiliary subunits. J. Biol. Chem. **1991**, 266, 4568–4573. [PubMed]

8. Bonner, C.A.; Stukenberg, P.T.; Rajagopalan, M.; Eritja, R.; O'Donnell, M.; McEntee, K.; Echols, H.; Goodman, M.F. Processive DNA synthesis by DNA polymerase II mediated by DNA polymerase III accessory proteins. J. Biol. Chem. **1992**, 267, 11431–11438. [PubMed]

9. Bunting, K.A.; Roe, S.M.; Pearl, L.H. Structural basis for recruitment of translesion DNA polymerase pol IV/DinB to the beta-clamp. EMBO J. **2003**, 22, 5883–5892. [CrossRef] [PubMed]

10. Patoli, A.A.; Winter, J.A.; Bunting, K.A. The umuc subunit of the E. Coli DNA polymerase V shows a unique interaction with the beta-clamp processivity factor. BMC Struct. Biol. **2013**, 13. [CrossRef] [PubMed]

11. Kurz, M.; Dalrymple, B.; Wijffels, G.; Kongsuwan, K. Interaction of the sliding clamp beta-subunit and Hda, a DnaA-related protein. J. Bacteriol. **2004**, 186, 3508–3515. [CrossRef] [PubMed]

12. Dalrymple, B.P.; Kongsuwan, K.; Wijffels, G.; Dixon, N.E.; Jennings, P.A. A universal protein-protein interaction motif in the eubacterial DNA replication and repair systems. Proc. Natl. Acad. Sci. USA **2001**, 98, 11627–11632. [CrossRef] [PubMed]

13. Lopez de Saro, F.J.; Georgescu, R.E.; O'Donnell, M. A peptide switch regulates DNA polymerase processivity. Proc. Natl. Acad. Sci. USA **2003**, 100, 14689–14694. [CrossRef] [PubMed]

14. Yin, Z.; Kelso, M.J.; Beck, J.L.; Oakley, A.J. Structural and thermodynamic dissection of linear motif recognition by the E. coli sliding clamp. J. Med. Chem. **2013**, 56, 8665–8673. [CrossRef] [PubMed]

15. Wolff, P.; Amal, I.; Olieric, V.; Chaloin, O.; Gygli, G.; Ennifar, E.; Lorber, B.; Guichard, G.; Wagner, J.; Dejaegere, A.; et al. Differential modes of peptide binding onto replicative sliding clamps from various bacterial origins. *J. Med. Chem.* **2014**, *57*, 7565–7576. [CrossRef] [PubMed]

16. Pandey, P.; Tarique, K.F.; Mazumder, M.; Rehman, S.A.A.; kumari, N.; Gourinath, S. Structural insight into β-clamp and its interaction with DNA ligase in *Helicobacter pylori*. *Sci. Rep.* **2016**, *6*, 31181. [CrossRef] [PubMed]

17. Pandey, P.; Verma, V.; Gautam, G.; Kumari, N.; Dhar, S.K.; Gourinath, S. Targeting the beta-clamp in *Helicobacter pylori* with FDA-approved drugs reveals micromolar inhibition by diflunisal. *FEBS Lett.* **2017**, *591*, 2311–2322. [CrossRef] [PubMed]

18. Yin, Z.; Whittell, L.R.; Wang, Y.; Jergic, S.; Liu, M.; Harry, E.J.; Dixon, N.E.; Beck, J.L.; Kelso, M.J.; Oakley, A.J. Discovery of lead compounds targeting the bacterial sliding clamp using a fragment-based approach. *J. Med. Chem.* **2014**, *57*, 2799–2806. [CrossRef] [PubMed]

19. Kawai, M.; Furuta, Y.; Yahara, K.; Tsuru, T.; Oshima, K.; Handa, N.; Takahashi, N.; Yoshida, M.; Azuma, T.; Hattori, M.; et al. Evolution in an oncogenic bacterial species with extreme genome plasticity: *Helicobacter pylori* East Asian genomes. *BMC Microbiol.* **2011**, *11*. [CrossRef] [PubMed]

20. Abdul Rehman, S.A.; Verma, V.; Mazumder, M.; Dhar, S.K.; Gourinath, S. Crystal structure and mode of helicase binding of the C-terminal domain of primase from *Helicobacter pylori*. *J. Bacteriol.* **2013**, *195*, 2826–2838. [CrossRef] [PubMed]

21. Kashav, T.; Nitharwal, R.; Abdulrehman, S.A.; Gabdoulkhakov, A.; Saenger, W.; Dhar, S.K.; Gourinath, S. Three-dimensional structure of N-terminal domain of dnab helicase and helicase-primase interactions in *Helicobacter pylori*. *PLoS ONE* **2009**, *4*, e7515. [CrossRef] [PubMed]

22. Nitharwal, R.G.; Verma, V.; Subbarao, N.; Dasgupta, S.; Choudhury, N.R.; Dhar, S.K. DNA binding activity of *Helicobacter pylori* dnab helicase: The role of the N-terminal domain in modulating DNA binding activities. *FEBS J.* **2012**, *279*, 234–250. [CrossRef] [PubMed]

23. Verma, V.; Kumar, A.; Nitharwal, R.G.; Alam, J.; Mukhopadhyay, A.K.; Dasgupta, S.; Dhar, S.K. Modulation of the enzymatic activities of replicative helicase (DnaB) by interaction with Hp0897: A possible mechanism for helicase loading in *Helicobacter pylori*. *Nucleic Acids Res.* **2016**, *44*, 3288–3303. [CrossRef] [PubMed]

24. Georgescu, R.E.; Yurieva, O.; Kim, S.S.; Kuriyan, J.; Kong, X.P.; O'Donnell, M. Structure of a small-molecule inhibitor of a DNA polymerase sliding clamp. *Proc. Natl. Acad. Sci. USA* **2008**, *105*, 11116–11121. [CrossRef] [PubMed]

25. Wolff, P.; Olieric, V.; Briand, J.P.; Chaloin, O.; Dejaegere, A.; Dumas, P.; Ennifar, E.; Guichard, G.; Wagner, J.; Burnouf, D.Y. Structure-based design of short peptide ligands binding onto the *E. Coli* processivity ring. *J. Med. Chem.* **2011**, *54*, 4627–4637. [CrossRef] [PubMed]

26. Wijffels, G.; Johnson, W.M.; Oakley, A.J.; Turner, K.; Epa, V.C.; Briscoe, S.J.; Polley, M.; Liepa, A.J.; Hofmann, A.; Buchardt, J.; et al. Binding inhibitors of the bacterial sliding clamp by design. *J. Med. Chem.* **2011**, *54*, 4831–4838. [CrossRef] [PubMed]

27. Biacore. *Biacore Concentration Analysis Handbook*; Biacore: Žilina Region, Slovakia, 2001.

28. Jeruzalmi, D.; Yurieva, O.; Zhao, Y.; Young, M.; Stewart, J.; Hingorani, M.; O'Donnell, M.; Kuriyan, J. Mechanism of processivity clamp opening by the delta subunit wrench of the clamp loader complex of *E. coli* DNA polymerase III. *Cell* **2001**, *106*, 417–428. [CrossRef]

29. Nariman, F.; Eftekhar, F.; Habibi, Z.; Falsafi, T. Anti-helicobacter pylori activities of six iranian plants. *Helicobacter* **2004**, *9*, 146–151. [CrossRef] [PubMed]

30. *Schrödinger Release 2016-1: Maestro*, version 10.5; Schrödinger, LLC: New York, NY, USA, 2016.

31. Friesner, R.A.; Murphy, R.B.; Repasky, M.P.; Frye, L.L.; Greenwood, J.R.; Halgren, T.A.; Sanschagrin, P.C.; Mainz, D.T. Extra precision glide: Docking and scoring incorporating a model of hydrophobic enclosure for protein-ligand complexes. *J. Med. Chem.* **2006**, *49*, 6177–6196. [CrossRef] [PubMed]

32. Halgren, T.A.; Murphy, R.B.; Friesner, R.A.; Beard, H.S.; Frye, L.L.; Pollard, W.T.; Banks, J.L. Glide: A new approach for rapid, accurate docking and scoring. 2. Enrichment factors in database screening. *J. Med. Chem.* **2004**, *47*, 1750–1759. [CrossRef] [PubMed]

33. Friesner, R.A.; Banks, J.L.; Murphy, R.B.; Halgren, T.A.; Klicic, J.J.; Mainz, D.T.; Repasky, M.P.; Knoll, E.H.; Shelley, M.; Perry, J.K.; et al. Glide: A new approach for rapid, accurate docking and scoring. 1. Method and assessment of docking accuracy. *J. Med. Chem.* **2004**, *47*, 1739–1749. [CrossRef] [PubMed]

34. Minor, Z.O.A.W. Processing of X-ray diffraction data collected in oscillation mode. *Methods Enzymol.* **1997**, *276*, 307–326.

35. Winn, M.D.; Ballard, C.C.; Cowtan, K.D.; Dodson, E.J.; Emsley, P.; Evans, P.R.; Keegan, R.M.; Krissinel, E.B.; Leslie, A.G.; McCoy, A.; et al. Overview of the CCP4 suite and current developments. *Acta Crystallogr. Sect. D Biol. Crystallogr.* **2011**, *67*, 235–242. [CrossRef] [PubMed]

36. Emsley, P.; Lohkamp, B.; Scott, W.G.; Cowtan, K. Features and development of coot. *Acta Crystallogr. Sect. D Biol. Crystallogr.* **2010**, *66*, 486–501. [CrossRef] [PubMed]

37. Laskowski, R.A.; MacArthur, M.W.; Moss, D.S.; Thornton, J.M. Procheck—A program to check the stereochemical quality of protein structures. *J. Appl. Crystallogr.* **1993**, *26*, 283–291. [CrossRef]

5

Phage-Bacterial Dynamics with Spatial Structure: Self Organization around Phage Sinks can Promote Increased Cell Densities

James J. Bull [1,2,3,*], **Kelly A. Christensen** [4,5], **Carly Scott** [4,6], **Benjamin R. Jack** [7] [iD], **Cameron J. Crandall** [6] and **Stephen M. Krone** [4,5,8,*]

[1]   Department of Integrative Biology, University of Texas, Austin, TX 78712, USA
[2]   The Institute for Cellular and Molecular Biology, University of Texas, Austin, TX 78712, USA
[3]   Center for Computational Biology and Bioinformatics, University of Texas, Austin, TX 78712, USA
[4]   Department of Mathematics, University of Idaho, Moscow, ID 83844, USA;
      chri4898@vandals.uidaho.edu (K.A.C.); scot9278@vandals.uidaho.edu (C.S.)
[5]   Center for Modeling Complex Interactions, University of Idaho, Moscow, ID 83844, USA
[6]   Department of Biological Sciences, University of Idaho, Moscow, ID 83844, USA; cjcrandall91@gmail.com
[7]   The Institute for Cellular and Molecular Biology, University of Texas, Austin, TX 78712, USA;
      benjamin.r.jack@gmail.com
[8]   Institute for Bioinformatics and Evolutionary Studies, University of Idaho, Moscow, ID 83844, USA
*   Correspondence: bull@utexas.edu (J.J.B.); krone@uidaho.edu (S.M.K.)

Abstract: Bacteria growing on surfaces appear to be profoundly more resistant to control by lytic bacteriophages than do the same cells grown in liquid. Here, we use simulation models to investigate whether spatial structure per se can account for this increased cell density in the presence of phages. A measure is derived for comparing cell densities between growth in spatially structured environments versus well mixed environments (known as mass action). Maintenance of sensitive cells requires some form of phage death; we invoke death mechanisms that are spatially fixed, as if produced by cells. Spatially structured phage death provides cells with a means of protection that can boost cell densities an order of magnitude above that attained under mass action, although the effect is sometimes in the opposite direction. Phage and bacteria self organize into separate refuges, and spatial structure operates so that the phage progeny from a single burst do not have independent fates (as they do with mass action). Phage incur a high loss when invading protected areas that have high cell densities, resulting in greater protection for the cells. By the same metric, mass action dynamics either show no sustained bacterial elevation or oscillate between states of low and high cell densities and an elevated average. The elevated cell densities observed in models with spatial structure do not approach the empirically observed increased density of cells in structured environments with phages (which can be many orders of magnitude), so the empirical phenomenon likely requires additional mechanisms than those analyzed here.

Keywords: biofilm; phage therapy; resistance; bacteriophage; models; agent based; mass action

---

1. Introduction

Bacteriophages are ubiquitous predators of bacteria, and they have long been entertained as having possible therapeutic utility in medicine. However, therapeutic utility is typically a matter of controlling the bacterial populations, and population control is not easily inferred from the mere fact that individuals of one species can kill individuals of another species. The difference between killing that achieves population control and killing that has little effect on the population rests on quantitative properties of the killing. Fortunately, phages are easily manipulated in the lab and thus easily studied to address dynamics and the control of bacterial populations.

The history of work on phage-bacterial dynamics has been dominated by liquid cultures in which bacteria are suspended as single cells at uniform density. Such cultures are routinely modeled as ordinary differential equations (ODEs) with assumptions of "mass action." Mass action refers to an environment in which all individuals are "well mixed," as would occur in a chemostat or batch culture, and so collisions occur at random. In such a system (see Equation (7)), interaction terms appear as products of bulk densities and essential parameters are easily estimated. The typical outcome following a lytic phage assault on a dense population of sensitive bacteria in liquid is killing of the bacterial population by many orders of magnitude, followed by a rebound of bacteria genetically resistant to the phage [1,2] with possible long-term coevolutionary arms races [3]. This work has led to many insights about bacterial and bacteriophage biology but has also given rise to a perception that bacterial escape from phages is chiefly through evolution of genetic resistance. However, we now know that many bacteria spend much of their lives in structured environments such as biofilms and aggregates, and bacterial biology in structured environments is fundamentally different than in liquid suspensions [4–6]. Spatially structured bacterial populations are difficult to control—they may persist seemingly indefinitely amid ongoing phage attack (they also survive antibiotic attack), and this persistence does not appear to be from genetic resistance [7–13]. Understanding the nature of this coexistence may be critical to phage therapy. Is it spatial structure itself that allows bacterial escape, or is it an indirect consequence of spatial structure on bacterial habits that allows the escape?

The goal of this study is to use models to understand the maintenance of high densities of sensitive bacteria amid phage attack in spatially structured environments. Our ultimate motivation is to develop phage interventions for controlling bacteria, which requires understanding of how bacteria normally escape. Does spatial structure per se allow for easy persistence, or does escape require cells to behave differently in structured environments than in liquid ones? We use computational models to explore the dynamic nature of the phage-bacterial interaction in spatially structured populations, identifying which mechanisms enable bacterial persistence at high densities. The empirical evidence is that sensitive bacteria easily persist, but identifying a process that may reasonably account for the coexistence is challenging.

2. Empirical Anomalies and Possible Causes

Various observations on bacteria grown under spatial structure suggest that genetically sensitive bacteria can be maintained as the dominant population in the presence of phage, at least in the short term [8,10–12,14]. The environmental contexts in these examples are diverse. The phage typically reduce bacterial numbers 1 or more orders of magnitude, but the remaining population is predominantly sensitive and persists at a much higher density than would occur in liquid. The phage sensitivity of residual populations is sometimes measured directly or is inferred from dynamic principles, such as the continuing high output of phage (which could not grow on genetically resistant cells). In some cases, the surviving bacterial strain is a genetic mutant that is fundamentally sensitive to phage but exhibits reduced adsorption (e.g., mucoidy); the bacteria are merely maintained at higher levels than explicable by basic dynamics principles (e.g., [15]).

As one striking example, Darch et al. [14] grew *Pseudomonas aeruginosa* in a synthetic sputum medium; cell numbers were measured non-destructively with confocal microscopy. The cells grew in aggregates. Addition of phage to an established culture resulted in a less than 1-log drop in bacterial numbers (measured in situ). However, when the bacteria were grown in liquid (albeit in different media), addition of phage resulted in a 7-log drop. In a second example, Lu and Colins [10] grew 24 h *E. coli* biofilms in peg-lid microtiter plates (0.2 mL volumes per well). After media replacement, 24 h treatment with phage T7 led to approximately a 2-log reduction in cell density, but close to 10^5 cells remained (their Fig. 3B). However, treatment with a T7 phage engineered to encode an enzyme that degrades a bacterial matrix component led to another nearly 2-log reduction in cell density. Density of the enzyme-free phage was $\approx 5 \times 10^8$/mL in the surrounding liquid. The fact that the enzyme had such a profound effect indicates that sensitive cells were sequestered from the no-enzyme phage while surrounded with a phage density that should have been more than sufficient to eliminate nearly all of them.

Compared to mass action, the most obvious consequence of spatial structure is local variation in the abundance of bacteria and phage. However, this spatial variation arises, reproduction of phage and bacteria enhances that variation, whereas diffusion diminishes it. Structure leads to expanding concentrations of bacteria (colonies) and to high concentrations of phages near bacterial clusters that have been invaded [16–18]. The spatial variation in abundance will interact with any of several factors that could be contributors to the long-term co-maintenance of sensitive bacteria and lytic phages, as follows.

Resource concentration. Phage growth is known to be reduced on cells that are starved [19,20], a phenomenon easily appreciated from the halting of plaque growth on plates after the bacterial lawn matures. In spatial environments, high concentrations of bacteria will depress resources locally, suppressing phage growth in those zones.

Barriers and gradients. Spatial structure allows the local buildup of substances exuded from cells, such as expolysaccharides (EPS), ions, signalling molecules, and outer membrane vesicles [1,8,21]. These agents may trap phages, drive phages away with electrostatic forces, or alter the concentration of factors necessary for phage adsorption.

Phage-adsorbing debris. The remnants of cells lysed by phages may continue to adsorb phage perhaps irreversibly and thereby reduce the number of phage encountering live cells. Spatial structure will facilitate the buildup of debris around clusters of cells.

Co-infection and superinfection. Phage growth with spatial structure will often concentrate phages around cells, which for many phages will lead to high numbers of phages infecting the same cell [18]. This property will reduce the effective number of phage progeny and may allow cells to reach higher densities than in liquid.

Altered gene expression. Cells may vary gene expression specifically in response to surface attachment or signals received from adjacent cells (e.g., [22]). Changes in gene expression are not necessarily effects of spatially structured dynamics per se, but gene expression changes may themselves enable phage-bacterial co-existence. As an example, non-genetic variation in receptor abundance on cells can lead to high levels of the survival of genetically sensitive bacteria challenged with phages [23–26]. If bacterial growth with spatial structure amplifies variation in gene expression, that variation could enable bacterial escape and subsequent growth, more than in liquid.

3. Perspective: Does Spatial Structure Increase Bacterial Density?

The question addressed here is whether phage and cell dynamics that are spatial in nature allow cells to attain a higher density than if everything is well mixed. As our approach uses mathematical and computational models, this question requires understanding the difference between spatial structure and well-mixed conditions. Phage dynamics have traditionally been modeled under the assumptions of mass action, which assumes cells and phages are fully mixed and that interactions occur at rates determined by population averages. Mass action means that cells and phage have no assigned locations; they just exist. This mathematical convenience allows the process to be studied with ordinary differential equations [1,27–29]. With spatial structure, the locations of cells and phages are tracked over time, and interactions are location dependent. Typically, phages move through diffusion and cells remain in fixed locations (adjacent to parent cells). Thus, high densities of cells or phages can build up in parts of the environment while other parts have few or no individuals. Phage killing is local to the areas of high phage density.

Extensive computational analyses of spatially structured phage-bacterial dynamics have been undertaken in a few previous studies [16–18]. This pioneering work described many properties of dynamics unique to spatial structure, such as strong spatial co-localization of bacteria and phage, as well as spatial structure enabling coexistence over a wider range of parameter values than does mass action (due to greater oscillations with mass action).

Our study uses that foundation to ask a specific question: does spatially structured phage dynamics per se maintain a greater cell density than under mass action? The fact that spatial structure more easily allows coexistence [17] might suggest that spatial structure also increases bacterial density, but the effect of spatial structure was reported to stem from reduced global oscillations rather than an increase in (mean) bacterial density. Reduced oscillations could lead to greater coexistence without affecting mean density.

The reason for using models to study these processes is to develop understanding that cannot feasibly be obtained from empirical studies alone. The models allow control of variables so that effects of single variables can be isolated. From there, one may proceed to empirical studies to test specific processes.

4. Setting the Stage for Evaluating the Effect of Spatial Structure: Biological Consequences of Mass Action Are Well Studied

We use a variety of computational approaches to understand phage-bacterial dynamics in spatially structured environments. Whereas the outcomes of simulations are easy to interpret, understanding the causal parameters can be challenging because of the many environmental details that must simultaneously be specified to model dynamics in space. To help understand simulation results, and especially to motivate the types of analyses done with simulations, we offer a brief review of specific mass action results from previous studies using ordinary differential equations.

1. Mass action does not preclude high cell density. Although the typical pattern of phage-bacterial dynamics under mass action is one in which phages decimate the bacterial populations, there are mass action conditions in which high densities of sensitive bacteria can be maintained, typically with a low adsorption rate [28].
2. Maintenance of phages and bacteria requires some form of phage death. The ODE models typically assume a constant rate of phage death or clearance from the system.
3. Numerical solutions to the equations often exhibit undamped and even accelerating oscillations [17,28,29]. The oscillations complicate comparisons of cell density across systems (see below).

5. Formal Spatial Structure

We use computational simulations to consider the formal dynamics of phage and bacteria with spatial structure. Our simulations were based on a two-dimensional 'grid' of sites and included a mix of stochastic (random) and deterministic processes. In these models, every cell, phage or other agent has a location on the grid; at each time step, infection, reproduction and movement may occur (explained in Methods). These models have many components similar to those in mass action models, but with explicit spatial structure and rates that are locally determined. We are primarily interested in whether and how spatial structure affects the cell density maintained in the presence of phages. The grid models include versions that enforce spatial structure as well as mass action versions, although nearly all trials assumed spatial structure. In the mass action versions of the grid models, each individual gets relocated every time step.

Biologically, there are two general types of bacterial avoidance of phages that may be entertained. One is that bacteria are protected from phages, whether by reduced adsorption rate or by surrounding themselves with anti-phage protection. The second is that cells either produce or associate with phage-killing products but are otherwise intrinsically susceptible when phages encounter them. We focus on the latter here, chiefly because it is non-trivial. It is otherwise clear that fully protected bacteria will be able to grow to the limits permitted by the environment—as is well known from ODE models allowing evolution of genetically resistant bacteria. If spatially structured cell growth combined with phage death does not intrinsically promote higher bacterial densities by several orders of magnitude, then protection of individual bacteria becomes plausible as the main driver.

A challenge in switching from mass action to spatial structure lies in accommodating attachment of phage to bacteria. With mass action models, an adsorption rate coefficient (k) subsumes both the chance encounter of a bacteria with phage and the rate at which the phage sticks to the bacterium given an encounter [1]. With spatial structure, we are forced to separate encounter from attachment because the two processes are operating at different scales in different parts of the environment [16].

Although some types of physiological protection of cells may be imposed by the environment (e.g., temperature, metal ions that affect adsorption, pH), of interest here is how the bacteria can potentially influence the local environment to enact protection by blocking encounter with phages. Excretion of extracellular polysaccharides and other substances may directly slow or block phage access altogether, and some of the extracellular matrix may effectively kill phages by binding them irreversibly. Dead cells and outer membrane vesicles may act as decoys that bind phages and cause them to eject their genomes.

6. Results

The maintenance of sensitive cells amid phage attack depends fundamentally on phage density and thus on phage death mechanisms. In a closed environment with cells and phages, such as a flask, the absence of phage death (or other form of permanent loss/sequestration) will ensure that phage ultimately eliminate all sensitive cells. Once cells are abundant, even phages with poor adsorption rates will ultimately increase to such densities that cells are rapidly eliminated. In the absence of cells being completely protected from phage, some form of phage death is required to prevent the ultimate buildup of phage to the point that all cells are killed. While it is obvious that fully protected cells can grow with impunity in the presence of phages, it is less obvious how the interplay between phage growth and death will collaborate to allow coexistence of sensitive cells and phage. The latter is our focus here—how phage death mechanisms influence the density of cells maintained.

6.1. The Nature of Phage Death Used Here: EPS and Cellular Debris

We will model two phage death mechanisms: adsorption to exopolysaccharides (EPS) and adsorption to dead cells (debris). The main difference in implementation of these two mechanisms is that EPS is treated as a spatially static and permanent mechanism of phage death; debris is also assumed to be spatially static, but its creation waxes and wanes as phage kill more or fewer cells, and it is not permanent, instead having an intrinsic decay rate. The association of debris with phage abundance may lead to substantially different outcomes than with a static phage sink. EPS will be the mechanism employed in all but the last set of studies presented here (for reasons explained below).

We accept that the empirical evidence from liquid cultures does not support a major role of debris in causing phage death (e.g., phage titers in lysed cultures are often stable for months—even when the lysate is not filtered or cleared of bacterial debris—J.J. Bull personal observations). The implementation of death by debris is offered in the spirit of any mechanism that rises and falls with phage attack on cells. Furthermore, if debris is short-lived, it may have an impact but the mechanism be difficult to detect empirically. We note that our mechanisms of phage death do not necessarily obey any empirically established process, mostly for lack of effort to detect such processes. Nonetheless, our assumed processes are seemingly more realistic than the usual assumption of a constant, intrinsic phage death rate, and they fall within the broad realm of mechanisms that cells can use to potentially kill off phages (e.g., outer membrane vesicles). It will be shown that our assumption of a fixed level of permanent EPS is equivalent to a constant phage death rate in mass action models.

Spatial structure will alter the dynamics in several ways [16–18], and indeed, it is likely that different models of spatial structure will do so differently. Most fundamentally, a lack of uniform densities will often result, allowing cells to amplify in zones that are temporarily phage-free. As regards phage death, phage reproduction from individual cells will have progeny phage spatially clustered at least temporarily and thus subject to a common fate. In addition, cells may find refuge and amplify behind materials that bind phage and act as phage sinks.

6.2. A Formal Measure of Whether Cell Density Is Elevated

If spatial structure leads to an elevated cell density above that with complete mixing (mass action), it might seem sufficient to merely observe cell density alone. However, any comparison of cell densities between spatial structure and mass action is not straightforward, in part because there is no single cell density expected under mass action—the cell density, even at equilibrium, depends on many parameters, such as phage burst size, adsorption rate, and death rate, to mention a few. Complicating matters further, mass action processes can themselves lead to a high cell density at equilibrium. Thus, cell density alone cannot tell us whether spatial structure elevates cell density. The effect of spatial structure must be measured via some comparison to cell density in the absence of spatial structure, a comparison that otherwise avoids confounding the many differences between the two types of models.

One such approach is to directly compare cell density when spatial structure is present to that when it is absent in the simulation; abolishing spatial structure can be done by increasing the diffusion rates of phage and cells [16,17]. This approach is free of alternative interpretations, but it has the drawback that bacterial and phage numbers often oscillate with mass action [16,17,28]. Given the limited dynamical range of cell densities afforded by the simulations, bacteria may often go extinct in the simulations even when the equilibrium density is well above extinction (see below).

We adopt a related approach, one that takes advantage of a universal property of equilibrium under mass action, at which phage and bacterial densities are unchanging. Our approach identifies a reproduction number constant that will be used to scale bacterial densities, with a similar use in [29]. Every successful phage infection of a cell will, on average, lead to one new successful infection. This dynamical property of populations in reproductive equilibrium is commonly used in ecology [30]. In the context of phage-bacterial dynamics under mass action, it means that the following equality holds:

$$\frac{\text{rate of productive phage infection}}{\text{all sources of phage loss from the free state}} \times \text{phage fecundity per infection} = 1. \tag{1}$$

The ratio on the LHS (left hand side) is merely the fraction of all rates leading to phage loss that result in phage reproduction. Since only one phage offspring from an infected cell will go to establish a new successful infection, the product equals unity on average. We denote the ratio on the LHS of Equation (1) as α. Phage fecundity per infection, known as burst size, is represented here as b. We have analytically confirmed that $\alpha b = 1$ at equilibrium in various mass action models (e.g., those in [27,28,31]) and not found any that violate the equality.

For the specific sources of phage loss in the spatial models, we propose

$$\alpha = \frac{k_C C}{k_C C + k_I I + k_D D + k_E E} \tag{2}$$

where C, I, D, E represent the densities of uninfected cells, infected cells, debris, and EPS, and k with appropriate subscripts denotes the various attachment/infection probabilities. The time-variable quantities in Equation (2) are C, I, and D, but not all models here allow infection of I and D; moreover, α is an increasing function of C and a decreasing function of I and D.

In this implementation, α is calculated with the parameters used and values observed in the simulations of spatial structure, but the value of α is otherwise interpreted as that which would obtain if the population obeyed mass action. In particular, the quantities in Equation (2) are calculated globally, ignoring the spatial structure that played a role in their generation. The extent to which αb exceeds 1 then measures the effect of spatial structure in conspiring to allow a higher density of cells than would accrue without spatial structure. It indicates, in effect, the added degree of protection experienced by cells in a spatial setting. If, for example, the current value is $\alpha b = 5$ in a spatial simulation, this should be interpreted to mean that if the system suddenly transformed to mass action dynamics, the phage progeny from a burst would infect an average of five uninfected cells. (Of course, this excess of infections would be sustained only briefly.) We have qualitatively confirmed this behavior with spatial simulations that had equilibrated by suddenly (in the middle of the simulation run) increasing phage diffusion and allowing cells to move as an approximation to mass action. Finally, in any trial, the maximum possible value of αb is b, but arbitrarily large values of b can be tested for compatibility with cell maintenance.

The observed αb in spatially structured trials is not a measure of cell density directly. However, in the absence of debris attachment ($k_D = 0$) and superinfection of infected cells ($k_I = 0$), it may be used to calculate the equilibrium cell density expected under mass action. From Equation (2), the cell density satisfying $\alpha b = 1$ is

$$\hat{C} = \frac{k_E E}{k_C(b-1)}. \tag{3}$$

$\hat{C}$ provides a constant baseline against which the observed cell density (C_o) may be compared under the above assumptions. The amplification of cell density due to spatial structure (what we will denote as A_g, for the grid model, in anticipation of defining an A for a second model) is thus the ratio of observed cell density to $\hat{C}$:

$$A_g = \frac{C_o}{\hat{C}}. \tag{4}$$

A_g is dimensionless, thus does not depend on cell density units. For convenience, and to emancipate the results from specific values of grid size, cell densities will be measured as the fraction of patches in the grid occupied by cells.

It is evident from inspection of (4) that A_g must have an upper bound ($A_{ub,g}$) whenever cell density has an upper bound. In our model, the upper bound does not arise from grid size, rather it stems from the maximum ratio of cells to EPS:

$$A_{ub,g} = \frac{1}{\hat{C}} = \frac{k_C(b-1)}{k_E E}, \tag{5}$$

where E is measured as the fraction of the grid occupied by EPS and the 1 in $1/\hat{C}$ is for a grid filled with cells.

The foregoing applies only if the causes of phage death are unchanging. When superinfection occurs or debris traps phages,

$$\hat{C} = \frac{k_I I + k_D D + k_E E}{k_C(b-1)}. \tag{6}$$

As I and D are dynamic variables, their values will not generally be the same at the mass action equilibrium as at equilibrium with spatial structure. The calculation of $\hat{C}$ when superinfection and/or debris are admitted, and thus requires some means of determining those values; it may be possible to put bounds on them, however.

6.3. Simulations

6.3.1. Increased Cell Densities Especially with Large Burst Sizes

Any effect of spatial structure on cell density, even relative density, is likely to depend on details of phage and cell biology. To look for generalities that transcend specifics, simulations were studied for each of a variety of EPS levels, burst sizes, diffusion rates, and cell growth rates (Figure 1). There are in fact general trends, especially that spatial structure often leads to higher cell densities than mass action, but only under some conditions, especially large phage burst sizes.

In each trial, our measure of relative cell density, A_g, as well as αb and cell density were averaged over the last 3000 steps of runs lasting 10,000 steps, so that the system should have been approaching its equilibrium behavior and any fluctuations would be averaged out. These trials disallowed superinfection of infected cells and attachment to debris: as explained above, this allows calculation of the cell density expected under mass action ($\hat{C}$). An otherwise equivalent set of trials was run allowing superinfection; the αb values were largely unaffected by superinfection, nearly always differing in the first or second decimal place.

Figure 1 shows averages of A_g from 15 trials with different random number seeds and three initial conditions (the averages shown exclude extinctions). These A_g averages sometimes exceeded 1 by more than an order of magnitude, but were also less than 1 for some parameter combinations (as Figure 1 rounds to the nearest integer, values between 0.5 and 1 are not evident). Not all parameter combinations led to sustained coexistence of bacteria and phage, and parameter combinations leading to extinctions for all 15 trials are omitted from the figure. The largest effects on A_g were from changes in EPS and burst size, but changes in the other parameters also had detectable effects. Some of the effects are easily appreciated; for example, it is expected and observed that higher diffusion rates will shift A_g toward 1, as the system gets closer to mass action—if cells and phage in fact coexist.

As expected from previous work [16,17], these systems did not always go to a static equilibrium. The trials recorded distributions of αb and A_g values for the last 3000 time steps; the distributions were narrow for many parameter combinations but were large for some others. There was no suggestion that high αb or A_g was due to large (or small) oscillations, a point that will become reinforced when considering spatially clustered EPS (below). For example, for trials in the upper right corner of Figure 1C (the highest A_g averages observed), 80% of the αb values from the run were usually contained in a range spanning 1.0 around the average. In general, there was wider variance in αb with larger bursts and small EPS values. Within the same figure panel (the same cell reproduction and diffusion rates), there was wider variance the closer the burst size and EPS values approached the extinction zone in the upper left quadrant, although trials with burst sizes of 2 and 6 typically did not show a wide variance.

All trials in Figure 1 used the same attachment probabilities, k_C and k_E. To see if the patterns generalize, additional trials considered different combinations of attachment rates for three burst sizes and two EPS values (Table 1); diffusion and cell reproduction rates were those of Figure 1C, and superinfection was again precluded. There is overlap in A_g values between burst sizes of 2 and 10 and between 10 and 60. Within an EPS level, the smaller A_g value is associated with the smaller burst (with one exception). However, there does not appear to be any single variable strongly determining A_g value across all variables. It is also clear that both large and small A_g values are not limited to the attachment rates used in Figure 1.

To address the possibility that the observed A_g values are bounded artificially by the model, Table 1 includes the upper-bound A_g value for each set of parameters, $A_{ub,g}$. In some cases, the observed A_g is indeed near its upper bound, raising the possibility that the observed value would be higher with a model structure allowing a higher limit. However, not all high A_g values appear to be constrained in this way. This argument will be addressed further when the model is modified to cluster EPS.

The table includes a parallel set of trials and corresponding A_g values for mass action in the grid model; the ratio of A_g for spatial structure over that for mass action is explicitly the ratio of average cell densities maintained under the two conditions, an empirical comparison that bypasses any use of $\hat{C}$.

The major difference between mass action and spatial structure is extinction of the former. For the mass action trials that avoided extinction, none of the spatially structured counterparts had A_g averages as high as 2.0.

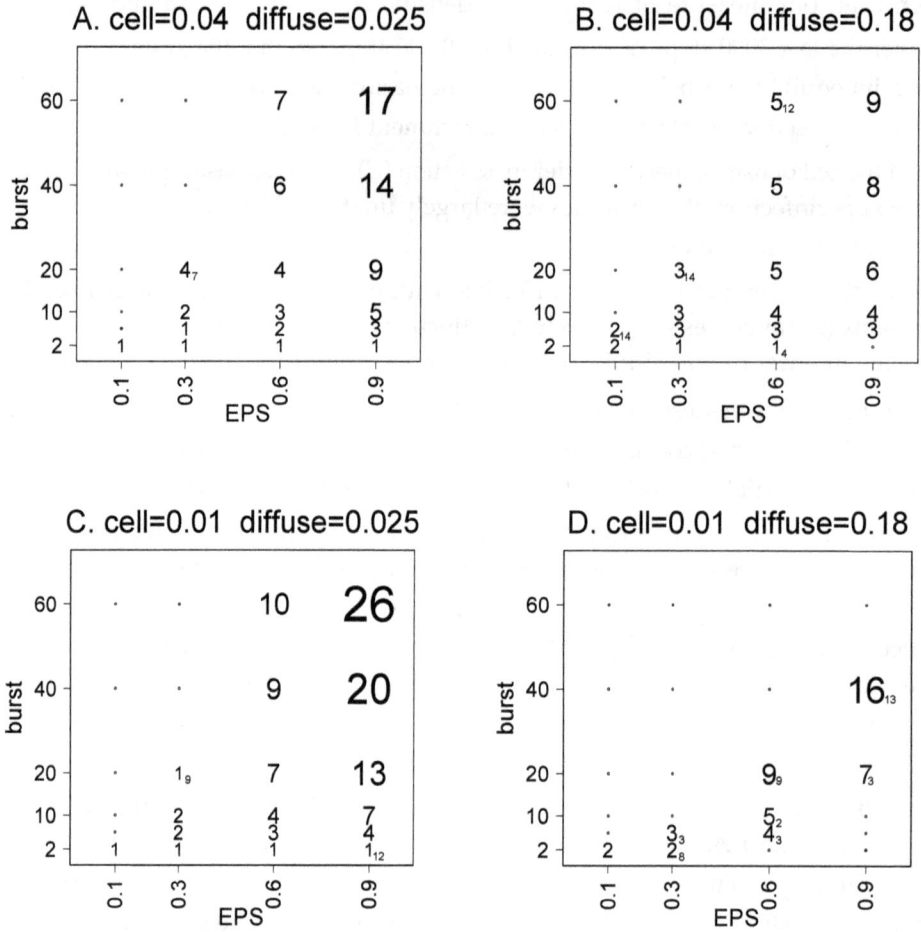

Figure 1. The density of cells maintained in the presence of phage is often increased by spatial structure. Shown in each panel are the A_g values, giving the fold increase in cell density over that with mass action. A_g values are greatly influenced by EPS levels and burst sizes, exceeding 10 only in the upper right quadrant, with large bursts and high EPS densities, and then only for some values of diffusion and cell reproduction rate. Values within each panel give average A_g values from 15 trials each using the same burst and EPS levels, with rate of cell reproduction and phage diffusion rate given at the top of each panel; trials leading to extinction of phage or cells are not included in the averages. EPS was assigned randomly to each patch at the start and remained in the patch for the life of the run; superinfection of infected cells was not allowed ($k_I = 0$), nor was debris attachment ($k_D = 0$). Each trial ran 10,000 time steps, and A was averaged over the last 3000 steps; values are rounded to the nearest integer (values rounded to 1 were often less than 1). A black subscript denotes the number of trials with bacterial and/or phage extinction; a dot indicates that all 15 trials led to extinction. The 'cell=' value given above each panel is the probability that an uninfected cell reproduced at each time step; the 'diffuse=' value is the fraction of phage that left the patch in each time step. In all trials, the adsorption probability to uninfected cells was $k_C = 0.25$, and that to EPS was $k_E = 0.35$.

Table 1. Effect of attachment probabilities on cell density in grid models.

				Spatial		Mass Action		
Burst	EPS	k_C	k_E	A_g	ext	A_g	ext	$A_{ub,g}$
2	0.3	0.05	0.05	1.2	-	1.4	-	3.3
2	0.3	0.05	0.15	0.5	-	1.0	-	1.1
2	0.3	0.05	0.25	0.3	-	-	10	0.7
2	0.3	0.15	0.05	3.1	-	-	10	10.0
2	0.3	0.15	0.15	1.3	-	-	10	3.3
2	0.3	0.15	0.25	0.8	-	1.1	1	2.0
2	0.3	0.25	0.05	5.1	-	-	10	16.7
2	0.3	0.25	0.15	2.2	-	-	10	5.6
2	0.3	0.25	0.25	1.4	-	-	10	3.3
2	0.9	0.05	0.05	—	10	1.0	-	1.1
2	0.9	0.05	0.25	0.2	9	-	10	0.2
2	0.9	0.15	0.05	3.3	8	-	10	3.3
2	0.9	0.15	0.15	1.1	7	1.0	8	1.1
2	0.9	0.15	0.25	0.7	7	-	10	0.7
2	0.9	0.25	0.05	5.5	6	-	10	5.6
2	0.9	0.25	0.15	1.8	7	-	10	1.9
2	0.9	0.25	0.25	1.1	9	-	10	1.1
10	0.3	0.05	0.15	0.8	-	-	10	10.0
10	0.3	0.05	0.25	0.7	-	-	10	6.0
10	0.3	0.15	0.15	1.8	2	-	10	30.0
10	0.3	0.15	0.25	1.3	-	-	10	18.0
10	0.3	0.25	0.15	0.9	4	-	10	50.0
10	0.3	0.25	0.25	2.0	-	-	10	30.0
10	0.9	0.05	0.05	4.4	-	-	10	10.0
10	0.9	0.05	0.15	2.9	-	-	10	3.3
10	0.9	0.05	0.25	1.9	-	1.1	4	2.0
10	0.9	0.15	0.05	9.7	-	-	10	30.0
10	0.9	0.15	0.15	7.7	-	-	10	10.0
10	0.9	0.15	0.25	5.5	-	-	10	6.0
10	0.9	0.25	0.05	14.4	-	-	10	50.0
10	0.9	0.25	0.15	12.2	-	-	10	16.7
10	0.9	0.25	0.25	9.2	-	-	10	10.0
60	0.9	0.05	0.15	8.8	-	-	10	21.9
60	0.9	0.05	0.25	8.2	-	-	10	13.1
60	0.9	0.15	0.15	17.3	-	-	10	65.6
60	0.9	0.15	0.25	18.0	-	-	10	39.3
60	0.9	0.25	0.15	31.4	1	-	10	109.3
60	0.9	0.25	0.25	25.0	-	-	10	65.6

Average amplification of cell density (A_g) due to spatial structure compared to the amplification under mass action across a range of EPS values, burst sizes, and attachment probabilities (k_C, k_E). Columns 5 and 6 are for spatial structure, 7 and 8 for mass action. For each combination, the A_g shown in the row is the mean of 10 runs differing in the random seed and spanning 2 different initial concentrations of phage and bacteria (extinctions were excluded from the averages, and superinfection was not allowed). Both EPS values (0.3, 0.9) were tested at each burst size (2, 10, 60) for each possible combination of k_C and k_E in (0.5, 0.15, 0.25); rows are omitted when all 10 trials resulted in extinction for both mass action and spatial structure (17 cases, including all nine trials with a burst of 60 and EPS value of 0.3); numbers of extinctions are otherwise given when more than 0. A_g modestly exceeds 1.0 due to oscillations in density being asymmetric around 1.0. The mass action assumptions were applied in the grid model, so the model parameters are directly comparable except that cells and phage were randomly assigned to locations each generation.

6.3.2. Understanding the Puzzle of Why Larger Phage Burst Sizes Lead to Higher Cell Densities

The results show clearly that some sets of parameter values lead to large elevations of cell density. The next step is to understand how this elevation happens. In particular, some patterns seem to defy intuition, such as why our relative cell density measures (A_g and αb) increase with b when holding other parameters constant. It is clear that increasing burst size will affect whether cells and phage are both maintained indefinitely, but the fact that αb changes with b indicates that some properties of the infection do not scale proportionally with burst. (ab is more easily addressed in this respect than is A_g.) Changing EPS abundance is also expected to affect coexistence, but the reason for its affect on ab is not clear. Understanding this absence of proportionality is potentially critical to understanding the effect of spatial structure on cell density, and is addressed next.

To understand how spatial structure enables A_g (and thus ab) to exceed 1 and why A_g varies with b, additional statistics were calculated for the parameter combinations used in Figure 1C (Table 2). The statistics included (i) losses of phage to EPS, (ii) the spatial association of cells and phage with EPS (probability that an uninfected cell or free phage was found in a patch with EPS), and (iii) the proportion of infections that happened in patches with EPS. As true of Figure 1, (i) all statistics were averaged over the last 3000 time steps of 10,000 step runs, and (ii) all statistics were averaged over all runs that led to coexistence.

One striking observation is that, holding all other parameters constant, increases in burst size led to directly corresponding increases in phage lost to EPS, while the losses to uninfected cells were only slightly affected. Thus, as burst size increased, the fraction of phage lost to EPS increased disproportionately. Proportionality is expected unless the association of phage or cells with EPS is changing.

Table 2. Spatial grid model outcomes with random placement of EPS, no superinfection or debris.

Burst	EPS	A_g	$A_{ub,g}$	ab	P→E	C:E	P:E	I:E
2	0.1	0.9	7.1	0.9	1.0	0.2	0.01	0.10
2	0.3	1.0	2.4	1.0	1.0	0.5	0.02	0.19
2	0.6	1.1	1.2	1.0	1.0	0.6	0.03	0.25
2	0.9	0.8	0.8	0.9	1.0	0.9	0.04	0.27
6	0.3	1.9	11.9	1.6	5.0	0.5	0.02	0.34
6	0.6	2.9	6.0	2.2	5.0	0.8	0.06	0.51
6	0.9	3.9	4.0	2.6	5.0	0.9	0.09	0.59
10	0.3	1.9	21.4	1.8	9.0	0.4	0.02	0.37
10	0.6	4.3	10.7	3.2	9.0	0.8	0.07	0.58
10	0.9	6.9	7.1	4.3	9.0	0.9	0.12	0.69
20	0.3	0.5	45.2	0.5	18.6	0.4	0.02	0.39
20	0.6	6.8	22.6	5.2	19.0	0.8	0.08	0.65
20	0.9	13.2	15.1	8.2	19.0	0.9	0.17	0.79
40	0.6	9.5	46.4	7.8	39.0	0.7	0.08	0.68
40	0.9	20.4	31.0	13.7	39.0	1.0	0.24	0.87
60	0.6	10.1	70.2	8.8	59.0	0.7	0.08	0.67
60	0.9	26.1	46.8	18.4	59.0	1.0	0.28	0.90

For these numerical trials, parameter values and initial conditions were as in Figure 1C. For each combination of burst size and EPS, the output values shown in the row are the means of 15 runs differing in the random seed and spanning three different initial concentrations of phage and bacteria. All four EPS values (0.1, 0.3, 0.6, 0.9) were tested at each burst size (2, 6, 10, 20, 40, 60); values are not shown when all 15 trials resulted in extinction. The numbers of extinctions for the data shown are given in Figure 1. Burst is phage burst size. EPS is the fraction of grid sites containing EPS, assigned randomly. A_g is the magnitude to which total grid cell density is increased above that expected with mass action. P→E is the average number of phage per burst lost to EPS. C:E is the fraction of uninfected cells found in patches with EPS. P:E is the fraction of free phage found in patches with EPS. I:E is the fraction of infections occurring in patches with EPS.

A second observation is that uninfected cells are somewhat associated with EPS (the association is often only modestly greater than the fraction of patches with EPS), whereas free phage are strongly associated with an absence of EPS. These latter observations suggest that spatial structure favors the retention of cells and phage into separate refuges where they are differentially protected from loss.

There are also apparent trends that, as burst size increases, (i) an increasing proportion of all infections happen on patches with EPS, and (ii) phage are increasingly associated with EPS. As burst size increases, the phage appears to be spreading to less protected areas and incurring greater loss.

6.3.3. Reasons for Higher Cell Densities Become Clearer When EPS Is Clumped: Cells Have More Protection from Spatial Structure

The patterns seen in Tables 1 and 2 are somewhat noisy. Those trials assigned EPS randomly to patches across the grid. Although random assignment may be realistic, it may also complicate understanding. Random assignment gives rise to varied and inconsistent boundaries between EPS-containing and EPS-free regions, possibly complicating inferences about associations of phage and cells with EPS. A clustering of EPS into a single area can overcome those difficulties by ensuring that all trials have the same boundaries around EPS. Trials were conducted so that EPS was laid down contiguously within the grid (adjacent rows were filled until the total EPS allotment was reached). This design resulted in a band of EPS on the grid. One straightforward effect of deterministic clustering is that the size of the boundary between EPS and EPS-free zones is now unaffected by the overall level of EPS. Table 3 provides values from a set of runs corresponding to those in Table 2.

Table 3. Spatial grid model outcomes with deterministically clustered EPS, no superinfection or debris.

Burst	EPS	A_g	$A_{ub,g}$	αb	P$\rightarrow$E	C:E	P:E	I:E
2	0.1	0.7	7.1	0.8	1.0	1.0	0.00	0.274
2	0.3	0.7	2.4	0.8	1.0	1.0	0.00	0.273
2	0.6	0.7	1.2	0.8	1.0	1.0	0.00	0.276
2	0.9	0.7	0.8	0.8	1.0	1.0	0.00	0.272
6	0.1	3.3	35.7	2.4	4.9	1.0	0.00	0.594
6	0.3	3.5	11.9	2.5	4.9	1.0	0.00	0.593
6	0.6	3.5	6.0	2.5	4.9	1.0	0.00	0.594
6	0.9	3.5	4.0	2.5	5.0	1.0	0.01	0.600
10	0.1	5.8	64.3	3.9	8.9	1.0	0.00	0.699
10	0.3	6.2	21.4	4.1	8.9	1.0	0.00	0.698
10	0.6	6.3	10.7	4.1	8.9	1.0	0.00	0.697
10	0.9	6.3	7.1	4.1	9.0	1.0	0.01	0.703
20	0.1	11.7	135.7	7.6	19.0	1.0	0.00	0.805
20	0.3	12.9	45.2	8.1	19.0	1.0	0.00	0.805
20	0.6	13.2	22.6	8.2	19.0	1.0	0.00	0.805
20	0.9	13.4	15.1	8.3	19.0	1.0	0.01	0.804
40	0.1	22.4	278.6	14.6	39.2	1.0	0.00	0.889
40	0.3	26.0	92.9	16.0	39.2	1.0	0.00	0.889
40	0.6	26.9	46.4	16.3	39.2	1.0	0.00	0.890
40	0.9	27.2	31.0	16.4	39.0	1.0	0.02	0.887
60	0.1	30.5	421.4	20.5	59.4	1.0	0.00	0.935
60	0.3	38.0	140.5	23.5	59.3	1.0	0.00	0.943
60	0.6	40.1	70.2	24.3	59.3	1.0	0.01	0.942
60	0.9	40.8	46.8	24.5	59.0	1.0	0.04	0.939

For these numerical trials, parameter values were as in Figure 1C, except that EPS was laid down deterministically in a single cluster. For each combination of EPS and burst size, the output values shown in the row are the means of 15 trials differing in the random seed, spanning three different initial abundances of phage and cells. The range of values as a percent of the mean obtained from the 15 trials never exceeded 11%, except for P:E (the range reaching as high as 110% of the mean, which was invariably tiny). No extinctions occurred. Notation is as in Table 2.

Patterns are clearer than with random EPS assignment and support intuition about the effect of spatial structure in enabling high cell densities over those with mass action:

1. A_g (αb) is now moderately constant across different EPS levels within the same burst size. The constancy is stronger at smaller burst sizes. This suggests that the width of the EPS zone itself is unimportant to the properties being measured until bursts get large.
2. The span of A_g (αb) values across the table is higher than with random EPS, not profoundly so, and some A_g (αb) are consistently less than 1, even when $A_{ub,g}$ cannot have imposed the low value. Spatial structure does not invariably increase cell density over mass action.

3. Phage and cells coexist over a wider range of parameter values with clustered EPS than with random EPS. There were no extinctions, in contrast to the many extinctions when EPS was placed randomly.
4. The association of cells with EPS and phage avoidance of EPS is more extreme than with random placement of EPS.
5. There is now a consistent trend that increasing burst size increases the fraction of infections occurring in patches with EPS.
6. Within a burst size, the value A_g is far more stable than is the $A_{ub,g}$, suggesting that the observed A_g is not often constrained by the upper bound.

An intuitive interpretation of these results is that free phage and uninfected cells tend to occupy different patches (phages live in EPS-free patches, cells live in patches with EPS: Figure 2). At low burst sizes, phage are lost to EPS at a high enough rate relative to burst that they virtually only persist in patches without EPS, and they amplify when cells migrate into those patches. This pattern can be argued from the fraction of infections that occur in EPS-free patches. As burst size increases, phages increasingly diffuse into zones with EPS, where they encounter otherwise protected cells. However, these successful infections also result in high rates of phage lost to EPS.

Burst sizes measured from infected cells grown in rich media are often much larger than those evaluated here [1]. However, it should first be appreciated that our simulations of spatial structure are two-dimensional, and a smaller burst size will operate in two dimensions than in three. Since our 2D model characterizes the horizontal spread of phage, it is appropriate to think of only a fraction of the full 3D burst contributing to horizontal spread. Since the volume of a thin slice (say of thickness equal to a tenth of the radius) that intersects the center of a sphere of radius r is less than 10% of the volume of the sphere, a full 3D burst B should correspond to an analogous 2D burst of size $b < B/10$. For example, a burst of 60 in two dimensions corresponds to a burst of over 600 in three dimensions.

Nonetheless, trials with burst sizes of 100 and 300 were evaluated for the same EPS levels and adsorption rates as in Table 3. Analyses of these large bursts were reserved for the clumped EPS model because of the repeatability of outcomes provided by this model. The largest A_g values were observed for the EPS levels of 0.9: 48 for a burst of 100 and 66 for a burst of 300. Thus, increasing burst sizes several-fold led to only modest increases in A_g values. As in Table 3, nearly all phage per burst were lost to EPS. All trials with EPS of 0.1 and a burst of 300 went extinct, revealing that phage can indeed overwhelm cells if the EPS is clustered in small enough patches (no extinctions were observed for the smaller bursts in Table 3). Furthermore, strong oscillations were typical of all trials, again suggesting that, with the larger burst sizes, phages are invading deeper into the EPS-protected refuges. These dynamical effects of large burst sizes on extinction and dynamics would likely disappear with sufficiently large grid sizes (much larger than 10,000 patches) because the zones of EPS protection would be larger and thus require phages to traverse greater distances before reaching the centers of the EPS zones. From the perspective of how spatial structure contributes to an elevated density of cells, larger bursts increase the elevation, but much less than proportionally.

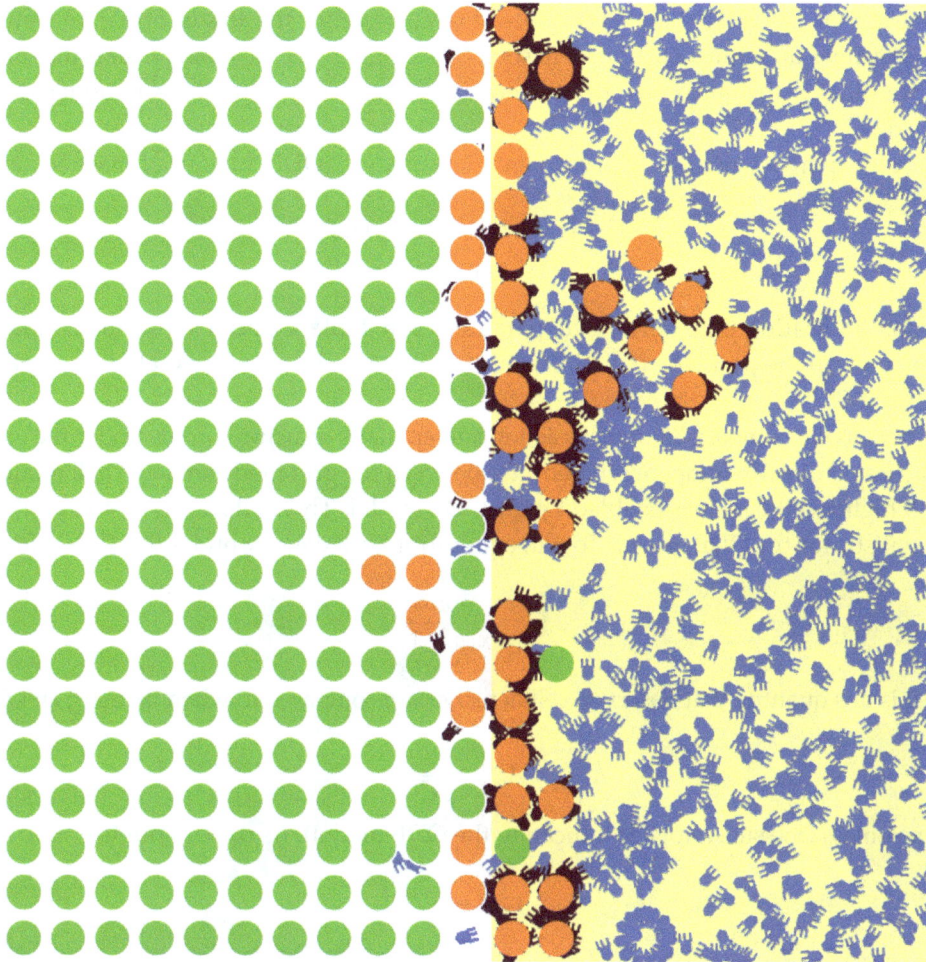

Figure 2. Illustration of self-organization of phages and cells with clumped EPS. White background indicates EPS, yellow is absence of EPS. A green (orange) circle is an uninfected (infected) cell. A blue or black legged icon is a phage (blue is free, black is attached to a cell). Phages are mostly confined to the EPS-free zone and the first row of EPS. Figure was generated from a NetLogo trial with a grid size of 21×21, a burst of 20, diffusion step size of 0.45 and attachment probabilities as in Figure 1C. There were 32 phage (partially obscured by cells) in the first three rows of EPS; αb for the entire grid was 7.26.

6.3.4. Average Densities under Differential Equation Mass Action Are Also Sometimes Elevated but Not as Much and for a Different Reason

The analysis so far has compared simulated cell densities under spatial structure to densities expected for mass action equilibrium, except for a few trials in Table 1. It is well known that models of mass action dynamics do not obey equilibrium for wide parameter ranges, instead exhibiting either stable oscillations or accelerating oscillations [29]. It is thus possible that average cell densities under mass action will themselves systematically differ from the expected equilibrium. That is, A-values for mass action may not equal 1, as has been implied above.

Two efforts were undertaken to calculate A-values for mass action: a simulated version of mass action based on adding 'mixing' to the spatial grid model, and a version based on an ODE model. The first mass action model merely modified the simulation code of spatial structure so that phage and cells were each assigned grid positions randomly every time step. However, the comparison of A-values for spatial structure and mass action is most informative when the A-values for spatial structure are well above 1, as those are the only cases in which there appears to be a meaningful effect of spatial structure on cell density. As was shown in Table 1, cell-phage coexistence under mass action was obtained only with parameter values for which the spatial structure A_g values were

1–2. (Increasing the grid size 9-fold did not lead to coexistence for any informative combinations either.) The A-values under mass action were sometimes higher, but the main result is that mass action extinction was always the outcome for parameter combinations leading to even moderate A_g under spatial structure.

In contrast to the comparison of mass action and spatially structured trials under the grid model, it is not practical to directly compare cell densities between the grid model and an ODE model because of the much higher cell densities enabled by the ODE model. This realization motivates the use of a parallel A statistic for the ODE model. To wit, equilibrium cell density under this ODE model is

The second approach used ordinary differential equation (ODE) models of mass action:

$$\dot{C} = rC(1 - C/K) - \kappa CP,$$
$$\dot{P} = b\kappa C_L P_L - \kappa CP - \delta P, \tag{7}$$

with the "dot" indicating time derivative, parameters in Table 4, and a subscript L indicating the value L time units in the past. The $(1 - C/K)$ term slows bacterial growth as cell density nears K, the carrying capacity.

In contrast to the comparison of mass action and spatially structured trials under the grid model, it is not practical to directly compare cell densities between the grid model and an ODE model because of the much higher cell densities enabled by the ODE model. This realization motivates the use of a parallel A statistic for the ODE model. To wit, equilibrium cell density under this ODE model is

$$\bar{C} = \frac{\delta}{\kappa(b-1)}$$

and hence it is this quantity that observed cell densities are compared to when defining an ODE-based A value:

$$A_{ode} = \frac{C}{\bar{C}}$$

also dimensionless (the subscript ode indicating the ODE model). Its upper limit is

$$A_{ub,ode} = K/\bar{C}. \tag{8}$$

Table 4. Model variables and parameters.

Notation	Description	Units
Variables		
C	density of uninfected bacteria	/mL
P	density of phage	/mL
Parameters		
κ	adsorption rate of phage to cells	mL/min
δ	loss rate of phage to EPS	/min
b	burst size of phage	
L	lysis time	min
K	carrying capacity of environment	/mL

Using ODEs presents the additional challenge establishing a correspondence between attachment probabilities in the grid model to attachment rates in the ODE model. To develop such a correspondence, we used the fact that, over a single unit of time (1 min in ODE corresponds to 1 time step in grid-based model), a phage avoids EPS in the grid-based model with probability $1 - k_E E$ and in the ODE model with probability $e^{-\delta}$. Thus, $\delta = -\ln(1 - k_E E)$ is an approximate equivalence. For $k_E = 0.35$ and $E \in 0.1, 0.3, 0.6, 0.9$, this gives a range for δ of $(0.04, 0.38)$, but the range goes down to 0.005 for the lowest k_E and E values used in Table 1. A similar basis was used to obtain equivalence between k_C and κ; in contrast to the equivalence for EPS, however, cell density is not fixed, so it is necessary to choose a density for the equivalence. Here, that density was the maximum for the system (K for the ODE versus 1 in the grid model). For those cell densities and the k_C values used in Table 1, κ was in the range $(5 \times 10^{-11}, 3 \times 10^{-10})$. For an ODE model scaled per-minute, these are reasonable values [28], although on the low end for some phages [26]. An exact correspondence between mass action and spatial models is not required, of course, because we are interested in whether any realistic mass action process can give high A-values; the conversions derived above merely suggest that the ODE model equivalence lies in established regions of parameter space for phages grown in liquid culture.

ODE numerical trials were run for 50,000 time steps using appropriate parameters (Table 5). Many parameter combinations led to expanding oscillations and premature termination of the run (effective extinction). Coexistence of cells and phage was obtained for many runs as well, typically with stable oscillations. For those, average A_{ode} values ranged from slightly above 1 to 10. The average exceeds 1.0 because of the asymmetry in the range of values: A_{ode} periodically goes up to the limit ($A_{ub,ode}$) but can go no lower than 0 (reflecting an asymmetry in the range of bacterial densities).

The highest A_{ode} averages were associated with the highest oscillations in cell densities (up to 18 orders of magnitude for the trial with an average A_{ode} of 10). No attempt was made to evaluate parameter space comprehensively, as our goal was merely to discover whether sustained oscillations resulted in a deviation of A_{ode} from 1.0. In the absence of oscillations, A_{ode} was 1.0, as expected (one example shown).

Summary of ODE model versus spatial grid model. For the differential equation model, an average A_{ode} above 1 is due entirely to sustained oscillations, whereas for the spatial grid model, an elevated A_g is not from oscillations but is intrinsic to the dynamics. Thus, the mechanism of high A-values are completely different for spatial structure and mass action; in the former, they are intrinsic to the environment and are approximately constant. In the latter, they arise because of oscillations in cell density and the asymmetry of limits on A.

Table 5. A_{ode} values for the ODE mass action model.

A_{ode}	$A_{ub,ode}$	Burst	δ	κ	L	r
3.9–4.1	9.0	10	0.1	1×10^{-10}	20	0.03
1.7	4.5	10	0.1	5×10^{-11}	20	0.03
5.8	18.0	10	0.05	1×10^{-10}	20	0.03
1.1	3.0	10	0.3	1×10^{-10}	20	0.03
4.2–4.4	9.0	10	0.1	1×10^{-10}	25	0.03
1.0	1.9	20	0.3	3×10^{-11}	20	0.03
1.2	3.3	20	0.4	7×10^{-11}	20	0.03
5.0	9.5	20	0.2	1×10^{-10}	20	0.03
5.6–5.8	9.8	60	0.3	5×10^{-11}	25	0.04
3.8	7.4	60	0.4	5×10^{-11}	20	0.03
10.1–10.2	39.3	60	0.045	3×10^{-11}	21	0.03

A_{ode} values for a small sample of numerical trials of Equation (7) in which bacteria-phage coexistence was observed for the full 50,000 time units. Parameter combinations leading to extinctions are not shown and often resulted with small changes in a single parameter from a parameter set in which coexistence was otherwise observed. A_{ode} was calculated as the arithmetic mean of cell density divided by $\delta / (\kappa(b-1))$; averages were calculated every 10,000 time units spanning time 10,000 to 50,000, and when the four values differed, the range is given. Parameters used in the trial are defined in Table 4. Carrying capacity K was 10^9 for all trials.

6.3.5. Debris: Adding Greater Reality Does Not Change the Trends

The preceding results from the grid model exclude all mechanisms of phage death except irreversible attachment to EPS, and EPS locations and levels were fixed. Other cell-based mechanisms of phage death are plausible and likely temporary. To consider whether our results continue to hold when other phage death mechanisms are present, we expanded the spatial grid model in include cellular debris—remnants of lysed cells that cause phage to bind irreversibly or inject their genomes non-productively. In mass action (liquid culture), this effect appears to be negligible empirically, as phage concentrations are often stable over months ([1], and personal observations). It is unknown whether debris may constitute a greater element of phage death in biofilms and other structured habitats, but we entertain it as an example of a possibly general phenomenon of local phage death resulting from the lysis of cells. Furthermore, the killing effect of debris may be short-lived, thus difficult to detect empirically, but such effects can be studied in the models.

Following [16,31,32], debris was introduced as infected cells that persisted after death (after lysing). In our trials, they were assigned a fixed lifespan, during which they could act as a phage sink in the same capacity as an infected (but unlysed) cell; α is correspondingly recalculated to include this new loss term, and, because of its inclusion, we can no longer use (3) to calculate an expected cell density under mass action. Our presentation is thus of αb instead of A, but αb is a suitable proxy. Additionally, superinfection of infected cells was allowed in these trials. The main effect of this debris model is that the dead cell is present after burst and thus is an additional source of death in the patch when phage densities are highest. Even limiting debris longevity to a mere two time steps had a huge effect on shifting the source of phage loss from EPS to debris but had only a modest effect on αb (as well as on coexistence) (Table 6, columns were added to indicate phage lost to debris and infected cells). Coexistence of phage and cells was typically not observed when debris was present and EPS was absent (not shown), but this outcome is necessarily sensitive to debris longevity (our trials assumed a moderately short life for debris).

Table 6. Random EPS with debris lasting two steps, superinfection allowed.

EPS	Burst	αb	P→C	P→I	P→E	P→D	C:E	P:E	I:E
0.1	6	2.2	1.08	0.71	1.58	2.58	0.17	0.01	0.097
0.3	6	2.4	1.07	0.60	1.83	2.50	0.49	0.02	0.218
0.6	6	2.8	1.11	0.74	1.69	2.46	0.68	0.04	0.257
0.9	6	2.7	1.14	0.83	1.61	2.46	0.90	0.05	0.255
0.1	10	0.3	1.13	1.22	3.51	4.28	0.14	0.00	0.100
0.3	10	3.1	1.13	0.92	3.85	4.10	0.48	0.02	0.272
0.6	10	3.9	1.17	1.04	3.80	3.99	0.76	0.05	0.356
0.9	10	4.4	1.25	1.35	3.44	3.96	0.90	0.07	0.343
0.3	20	3.9	1.24	1.62	9.06	8.09	0.43	0.02	0.297
0.6	20	6.4	1.26	1.42	9.60	7.72	0.77	0.07	0.451
0.9	20	8.7	1.40	1.86	9.16	7.59	0.91	0.11	0.461
0.3	40	4.2	1.47	2.97	19.71	16.12	0.36	0.02	0.272
0.6	40	10.4	1.38	1.88	21.62	15.13	0.76	0.08	0.501
0.9	40	16.4	1.56	2.16	21.62	14.67	0.93	0.17	0.558
0.6	60	13.5	1.47	2.30	33.67	22.55	0.75	0.08	0.510
0.9	60	22.4:	1.63	2.23	34.45	21.69	0.95	0.20	0.616

αb values and other properties of dynamics when debris is included and superinfection of infected cells is allowed. Dead cells persisted for two time steps after cell lysis and acted as a phage sink during this time (adsorption to debris was the same as to live cells, 0.25). Parameter values were otherwise as in Figure 1C. For each combination of EPS and burst size, the output values shown in the row are the means of 15 trials differing in the random seed and using three different initial densities of cells and phage. All four EPS values were tested at each burst size; values are not shown when all 15 trials resulted in extinction. For those rows shown, 10 extinctions occurred for (EPS = 0.9, burst =6), 13 extinctions for (0.1, 10), and two extinctions each for (0.9, 10) and (0.3, 40). Ranges of the 15 values as a per cent of the mean were mostly less than 20% and never exceeded 42%, except that the range of αb values was almost as large as the mean for (0.3, 40); some of those trials experienced large variation in αb values with occasional low numbers of cells. Notation as in Table 2, with $P \rightarrow I$ indicating the approximate number of phage per burst lost to infected cells and $P \rightarrow D$ indicating the loss to debris. In contrast to Tables 1–3, A_g is not provided because the baseline calculation of equilibrium cell density for mass action includes terms that depend on dynamics.

7. Discussion

Phage and their hosts exist in a predator–prey relationship, the dynamics of which have been modeled for over half a century. These models have assumed population structures of well-mixed environments (mass action), both for mathematical convenience and because laboratory studies of phage have used conditions that represent mass action—flasks in shakers and chemostats. However, it is increasingly evident that bacteria grown in biofilms and other spatial contexts are able to persist at much higher densities than apparent from the models, and it is not clear why. This study used a computational approach to investigate the simple question of whether and how spatially structured cell and phage growth might allow higher equilibrium cell densities than with the well mixed conditions of mass action. This question is motivated by empirical observations suggesting that genetically sensitive cells are often profoundly more protected from phage when grown with structure (e.g., biofilms or aggregates) than when grown in liquid. By uncovering the mechanisms behind these high densities, it may be possible to improve the prospects for phage therapy.

Our main findings are:

1. Spatial structure sometimes, but not always, led to cell densities above those maintained at equilibrium under mass action. However, average cell densities under mass action were also often greater than expected at equilibrium. Any effect of spatial structure in elevating cell densities thus appears to be less than an order of magnitude.

2. The mechanisms of 'elevated' cell densities are different between spatial structure and mass action. The effect of spatial structure appears to stem from phage and cells dynamically sorting to occupy different patches in the environment, with cells in patches that otherwise kill phage, and phage occupying patches that did not kill them but were largely free of cells. The elevation under mass action arises from sustained oscillations, due to a large dynamic range for $A > 1$ but A being bounded to lie above 0.

3. Under spatial structure, increasing burst size was usually observed to increase the relative cell density—to increase the effect of spatial structure in raising cell density—holding other parameters constant. However, a high abundance of environmental protection (EPS) contributed to relative cell density; phage diffusion rates, cell reproduction rates and attachment rates also had influences.

4. The burst size effect was shown to result from a curious effect of the spatial segregation between phages and cells. At higher burst sizes, phages increasingly invaded refuges occupied by cells and suffered proportionally greater losses. Thus, the per capita phage loss to EPS was higher with higher burst sizes, thus accounting for their poorer efficacy in suppressing cell density.

7.1. Back to Nature: Do Our Spatial Models Explain What We Observe?

Our efforts were primarily to look for mechanisms that might promote high cell densities as observed in nature. Having found possible mechanisms, the question then turns whether those mechanisms do indeed operate in nature. The latter question is empirical and is a far greater challenge than merely identifying possible mechanisms. Understanding of the empirical side of phage-bacterial dynamics with spatial structure is rudimentary, and our discussion of it is correspondingly speculative. It is premature to suggest that the mechanisms promoting high cell density in our models are empirically important, but they at least suggest directions of inquiry. Indeed, a recent study accounts for bacterial colony survival amid phage attack merely by considering the rate of colony growth versus the rate of phage penetration; when the colony reaches a certain size before phage encounter, it grows faster than the rate at which phage can penetrate—due in no small part to the large number of phages infecting the same cell in the close confines of the bacterial colony [33]. In their model, therefore, cells persist in spatial structure because phages are slow to invade the structure and because many different phage infect the same cell—an effect we intentionally excluded in most of our trials.

The largest effect of spatial structure on cell density observed in our trials is well short of the apparent effects of spatial structure observed in some empirical systems. Furthermore, mass action models were also observed to maintain average cell densities above the expected equilibrium, albeit that this elevated average arises from oscillations. In some natural systems, cells are maintained at densities several orders of magnitude above those in liquid systems. It could be that the cell density increase under spatial structure observed in a numerical trial is artificially bounded by the construct of the model, hence that a more realistic model would exhibit a far higher equilibrium cell density. While a larger grid size or allowing multiple cells per site could increase the dynamic range of A, we speculate that a fully 3D system would better capture the large cell densities seen in biofilms that are subjected to phage attack. Imagining our clustered EPS zone as a 2D slice of a biofilm, a 3D version would have a two-dimensional (surface) interface between the protected and unprotected regions. This surface would be more permeable to phage incursions, but the potential gain in cell density in the EPS zone when going from a 2D to a 3D model could vastly increase the dynamic range of A.

An alternative interpretation is that empirically high cell densities arise with spatial structure mostly from mechanisms other than those considered here. At one extreme, cells grown with structure may be resistant to infection. This resistance need not even be genetic [23–26]. Resistance could stem from changes in gene expression that arise when cells are attached to surfaces. Such gene expression changes could lower phage receptor densities or could lead to the secretion of protective layers.

Alternatively, cell protection with spatial structure could be an automatic consequence of limited diffusion and not even involve changes in gene expression. Thus, if cells normally secrete diffusible substances that can form gradients or protective boundaries, spatial structure would allow those gradients to form and protect cells from all sides, whereas liquid culture would not. In contrast, our models allowed protection purely from phage death: cells could escape phage merely because phage were killed before they could attack cells. That phage death was spatially structured, allowing cells to associate with refuges within that structure. Spatial structure offers many possible mechanisms of cellular escape from phages, and our models point a direction toward more biologically comprehensive processes. Empirical progress in understanding bacterial escape will obviously be useful in directing further modeling efforts.

7.2. Our Models in Context

Whereas it is straightforward to measure an average cell density with spatial structure any time cells and phage are maintained, it is difficult to use the same approach to determine the cell density that would obtain under the same conditions if phage and cells were fully mixed: the dynamic ranges of cell and phage densities are limited in the simulations, and the oscillations that typically accompany mass action dynamics lead to extinctions in finite populations, even when the average densities are well above the extinction threshold. We thus developed a metric for calculating the equilibrium cell density expected under mass action that could be compared to the cell densities observed in many of the simulations.

For cells to persist amid phages, the cells must either be fully protected from infection (i.e., some form of resistance, genetic or otherwise), or phages must die often enough to keep from overwhelming the cells. We explored the latter process here. Many of our observations as regards dynamics with spatial structure are similar to those of [17], but we took the analysis one step farther by making a comparison of the effect of spatial structure versus mass action on cell density. Another difference is that we did not impose an intrinsic phage death rate, instead allowing phages to die either from sticking to spatially static substances that could in principle be produced by cells (exopolysaccharide, or EPS), or from infection of 'debris,' represented here as short-lived parts of dead cells that persist after lysis (inspired by [31,32]). EPS, which is fixed spatially in our model, and thereby allows cells and phages to differentially organize around them, is similar to the fixed refuge model in [17], the main difference being that we have a specific mechanism for inhibiting phage growth. In our model, superinfection results in phage loss; results in our Figure 1 and Tables 1–3 specifically precluded superinfection, but parallel trials that allowed superinfection yielded similar outcomes. In [16], superinfection is beneficial to phage since it is assumed to inhibit lysis with a resultant increase in burst size; in [17], there is no superinfection.

Our chief interest in this study was to evaluate the effect of spatial structure on long-term or equilibrium cell density, comparing it to the density expected under mass action. For the purpose of evaluating the effect of spatial structure on phage-bacterial coexistence, Heilman et al. [17] provided a direct comparison of coexistence under the the two conditions. However, oscillations in cell and phage densities under mass action often led to extinction in the grid-based simulations of mass action we attempted, except in cases for which spatial structure appeared to have a small or no elevating effect on cell density. To evaluate the effect of mass action on cell density for cases of interest, we used an ordinary differential equation model, with parameters chosen to correspond to those of the spatial structure model.

To evaluate the effect of spatial structure on cell density, compared to mass action, we used the well-known principle that, in populations at reproductive equilibrium, each individual merely replaces itself, on average—each offspring has one successful offspring during its lifetime (in asexual populations). For a phage with burst size b, this means that for each infection of a cell that survives to burst, only one of those b progeny will itself establish a surviving infection. We defined α as the ratio of successful infections divided by all sources of free phage loss, hence this equilibrium condition is $\alpha b = 1$. Under some conditions easily implemented in numerical trials, this equilibrium condition can be used to calculate an equilibrium cell density for mass action. The dimensionless statistic A was then used as the ratio of observed cell density over the equilibrium cell density under mass action—the 'amplification' effect of spatial structure. This statistic could be derived for the grid model (with or without spatial structure) and for the ODE model of mass action, allowing easy comparisons of the effect of different structures.

Across different parameter combinations in the model of spatial structure, grid-based A_g values ranged from slightly less than 1 to nearly 30. Thus, spatial structure sometimes conspired to reduce cell density below that maintained with mass action, but also commonly led to an elevation of cell density—depending on parameter values. However, a similar elevation of average density was also observed under mass action whenever the dynamics exhibited sustained oscillations.

A large effect on A was from burst size (b). It was not immediately clear why increasing burst size should increase the effect of spatial structure on cell density, so various metrics of phage dynamics were analyzed, and a simple explanation was found. The environmental structure allows cells to reside in protected areas (those with EPS) and phages to exist in death-free areas (those without EPS). This is a type of self organization due to the different causes of death for cells (phage kill them) and phage (EPS kills them). When this organization is established, infections result from cells growing into unprotected areas and/or phage diffusing into zones in which they are rapidly killed but where cells reside. The balance between these two processes shifts as burst size is increased—a larger burst means that phages diffuse further into protected-cell zones, but at a cost that more phage progeny are killed. It is also clear that large burst sizes result in the EPS-free zone being essentially devoid of bacteria; this is reflected in a large fraction of infections being limited to the EPS zone. In contrast, with low burst sizes, cells are growing into unprotected zones, where they are killed by phages and where phages do not die (as in Figure 2). In the case of no superinfection or debris attachment, it is also clear that the denominator in A decreases as a function of b.

7.3. Caveats

One potentially important omission from our models is local variation in cell growth rate (as might be mediated by variation in resource concentration). Bacterial growth is known to be important to phage growth (e.g., [1]), with starved cells reducing burst sizes and increasing times to lysis [34]; a change in susceptibility of cell populations at high density requires non-standard models and leads to alternative stable states of the bacterial system even with mass action [35]. Biofilms are thought to be highly structured for resources and consequent cell growth rates [9,36]. To what extent starvation of cells or delayed spread of phages contributes to high cell densities is not addressed by our model but is certainly a worthy avenue of further analysis. Also excluded are temperate phages, whereby infection can lead to a viable cell carrying the phage genome (a lysogen); dynamics of temperate phages with spatial structure presents a fundamentally different set of challenges [37].

The theory advanced here motivates the empirical search for phage death mechanisms, especially those that operate with spatial structure. We yet know little of how rapidly phage are inactivated by exopolysaccharides, outer membrane vesicles, or other materials produced in situ. Such measurements will be difficult when phages are actively growing on live cells in structured environments, but it should be possible to inactivate cells while leaving the structure intact, then measuring the effect on phages.

8. Methods: Simulation Model Basics

Three computer programs were used to model spatial dynamics: a program written in C, a program written in Python, and a program written in NetLogo. Due to its superior runtime and versatility, the C program was used for all results presented; the Python program was written to verify the C program results. The Netlogo program was used early in the study to visualize spatial dynamics and develop intuition about the processes. All three models are broadly similar to those in [16,17].

The C code was also adapted to model mass-action dynamics in a grid model. This version of mass action allows an "apples-to-apples" comparison of mass action and spatial dynamics on the same computational platform—including finite population size and identical parameters. With finite population size, the grid based mass action model is stochastic and thus differs somewhat from an ODE-based mass action model. (The randomness actually disappears in the limit as population size goes to infinity.) Aside from the randomness and heightened probability of extinction due to finite population size in simulations of grid-based mass action, they produce similar behavior to numerical solutions of ODE-based mass action.

C program for spatial grid model. The spatial C program was typically run with a 100×100 grid of patches with no boundary effects (migration on a torus). Figure 1 and Tables 1–3 were generated using this program. All phage, infected cells, dead cells, and EPS were assigned to a patch, and all interactions of phage within a patch occurred with other entities in that patch. A patch could harbor at most one cell (infected or uninfected), but in runs allowing debris (dead cells), a dead cell could occur in a patch with an infected or uninfected cell. Independent phage infection probabilities were assigned to the entities of EPS, cells, infected cells, and dead cells, such that a phage could remain uninfected or infect only one of the other entities. Once infected, cells had a finite lifespan (20 steps).

Within a time step, phage migration from a patch was limited to its eight neighbors, with probabilities according to a truncated symmetric, bivariate normal distribution centered on the patch and with a single variance parameter, as follows. Writing

$$f(x,y) = \frac{1}{2\pi\sigma^2} e^{-\frac{(x^2+y^2)}{2\sigma^2}},$$ (9)

if $F(z) = P(Z \leq z)$ denotes the cumulative distribution of the standard (1-dimensional) normal, we have the following probabilities for phage diffusion to the eight patches (of side length 1) in the basic neighborhood:

center patch: A^2 (no diffusion),
each "orthogonal" neighboring patch: AB,
each diagonal patch: B^2,
where $A = 2F(0.5/\sigma) - 1$ and $B = F(1.5/\sigma) - F(0.5/\sigma)$.
These values were normalized by dividing each by $C = A^2 + 4AB + 4B^2$ to give the fractions of phage diffusing and remaining in the central patch.

In our trials, most of the probability was to remain on the central patch (no diffusion), so a phage was unlikely to move to a neighboring patch in a single time step. Phage diffusion was calculated deterministically (assigning appropriate fractions of the phage in a patch to that patch and the eight neighboring patches), but the overall net effect of migration on the patch was converted to an integral value by assigning any decimal fraction to 0 or 1 with a random draw in proportion to its magnitude.

Cell reproduction was permitted in every time step, each cell's reproductive fate chosen randomly according to a fixed probability, and independently of other cells' fates. Cells could reproduce only if one or more of their eight neighboring patches were unoccupied by a live cell (infected or uninfected), and preference was given that a daughter cell move into an orthogonal (off-diagonal) patch. All runs began with cells distributed randomly to 30% of patches and phage distributed randomly to 30% of patches (a patch getting phage received a burst size of phage).

C program for mass action grid model. For mass action, the C program was altered in three ways: (i) after burst and before new infections were allowed, all individuals in the entire population of phage were randomly assigned to patches in the grid; (ii) localized phage diffusion was turned off; and (iii) after cell reproduction, the entire population of infected and uninfected cells was reassigned to new patches, with at most one cell (infected or not) per patch. All other aspects of the mass-action C code are identical to those in the spatial C code, allowing us to assess the effects of spatial structure using the same computational platform. There was no simulation of mass-action dynamics in the case of spatially clumped EPS since only the amount of EPS makes a difference in this case.

Python program for spatial grid model. The second spatial simulation, written in Python, assumed a 20×20 grid of patches without boundary effects. This simulation served as a prototype for the C simulation, and operates similarly with some exceptions. During each time step in the simulation, following a randomized order, each patch executed cell lysis (if applicable), cell reproduction, infection, and phage diffusion. Then, the simulation repeated the same steps in the next randomly-selected patch until all patches were updated for that time step. Contrast this process with the C simulation, where a single event (e.g., lysis) executed across all patches before the next type of event (e.g., reproduction) executed. In the Python simulation, phage and cells only diffused to orthogonal patches. Allowing for diagonal diffusion did not qualitatively impact the simulation results, as long as both phage and cells followed similar diffusion rules. Early simulations in which cells were allowed to diffuse diagonally (but phage were not) decreased the proportion of infections (I:E) that occurred in EPS under deterministic EPS clustering, and also made I:E sensitive to EPS abundance. Such disparity in diffusion capabilities of phage and cells was determined to be unrealistic, so in the C version of the program, both cells and phage were allowed to diffuse both orthogonally and diagonally. In summary, the differences between the Python and C simulations are minor, and both simulations produced comparable output.

NetLogo program for spatial grid model. The third spatial simulation, written in the agent-based platform NetLogo, assumed a 51×51 grid of patches without boundary effects. This discrete-time simulation updates all patches simultaneously according to probabilities that are based on the current configuration. It is similar to the C simulation except for the following: (a) individual phage diffuse randomly and independently by taking steps in random directions with a prescribed step size; (b) nutrient-dependent cell growth and lysis, where an initial allocation of nutrient was provided and then replenished periodically by pulsing in fresh nutrient across the grid (though the simulations used here had nutrient pulsing every time step to match the nutrient-independent dynamics of the other two simulations); (c) the offspring of a reproducing cell is placed at one of the eight neighboring patches as long as there is space available. Reproduction is suppressed whenever all these local patches are at their carrying capacity; and (d) an approximation to mean-field dynamics is simulated by using large phage step size and random placement of cell offspring (but no subsequent cellular diffusion). Trends observed with the NetLogo program were similar to those with the other two programs.

The choices of a 20×20 grid size for the Python simulation, a 51×51 grid size for the NetLogo simulation, and a 100×100 grid size for the C simulation were made because of computational constraints but are arbitrary. An increase in grid size moderately increased αb in some conditions and decreased it in others. However, the magnitude of these changes was small, and the larger grid size simulations showed smaller variances in αb than in smaller grid size simulations. For example, in one set of simulations with the C program (EPS = 0.9, burst = 60, random placement of EPS), αb was 18.19, 17.98, 17.96 at grid sizes of 30×30, 100×100, and 300×300, respectively. Thus, the choice of grid size does not affect the overall trends in αb described here.

Numerical ODE trials were carried out with Mathematica 11.1.0 (Wolfram Research Inc., Champaign, IL, USA) using NDSolve.

9. Conclusions

Phages are predators of bacteria. Their predator-prey dynamics have been studied for decades in the ideal conditions of liquid culture, where a reasonable agreement has been obtained between models and observations. More recent studies of phages and bacteria grown on surfaces and other 'structured' environments suggest that bacterial densities are often much higher than expected from liquid culture results.

Our study focused on the simple question of how spatial structure alone might allow densities of sensitive cells to be maintained at higher levels than in liquid. Our approach relied on computational models in which bacteria could escape phage only by residing adjacent to environmental phage traps, such as exopolysaccharide or cellular debris that irreversibly binds phage. We found that these types of environments could enable an elevation of cell density in which phage and cells self-organized into different regions of the environment: cells persisted in protected areas, phages persisted in areas that lacked phage-killing agents. However, the magnitude to which cell densities were elevated was always less than 2 orders of magnitude, often less than one order—and less than reported in empirical contexts. Other mechanisms are thus needed to account for bacterial survival amid phage attack in structured environments.

Acknowledgments: We thank Benji Oswald for assistance with the IBEST computer cluster. We are pleased to acknowledge the following grant support for this work: to B.R.J. and J.J.B.: National Institutes of Health Grants R01 GM 088344 and GM 122079; to K.C. and C.S.: National Science Foundation UBM (DMS-1029485); to S.M.K.: Center for Modeling Complex Interactions at the University of Idaho (NIH grant P20GM104420), and the IBEST Computational Resources Core (NIH grant UL1 TR000423).

Author Contributions: J.J.B. and S.M.K. conceived of the problem, the general approach and were responsible for all analytical work. All authors contributed to one or more simulation codes and carried out trials. The manuscript was written by J.J.B. and S.M.K.

References

1.   Adams, M.H. *Bacteriophages*; Interscience Publishers: New York, NY, USA, 1959.
2.   Bohannan, B.J.M.; Lenski, R.E. Linking genetic change to community evolution: Insights from studies of bacteria and bacteriophage. *Ecol. Lett.* **2000**, *3*, 362–377.
3.   Weitz, J.S.; Hartman, H.; Levin, S.A. Coevolutionary arms races between bacteria and bacteriophage. *Proc. Natl. Acad. Sci. USA* **2005**, *102*, 9535–9540.
4.   Donlan, R.M.; Costerton, J.W. Biofilms: Survival mechanisms of clinically relevant microorganisms. *Clin. Microbiol. Rev.* **2002**, *15*, 167–193.
5.   Briandet, R.; Lacroix-Gueu, P.; Renault, M.; Lecart, S.; Meylheuc, T.; Bidnenko, E.; Steenkeste, K.; Bellon-Fontaine, M.N.; Fontaine-Aupart, M.P. Fluorescence correlation spectroscopy to study diffusion and reaction of bacteriophages inside biofilms. *Appl. Environ. Microbiol.* **2008**, *74*, 2135–2143.
6.   Alhede, M.; Kragh, K.N.; Qvortrup, K.; Allesen-Holm, M.; van Gennip, M.; Christensen, L.D.; Jensen, P.O.; Nielsen, A.K.; Parsek, M.; Wozniak, D.; et al. Phenotypes of Non-Attached Pseudomonas aeruginosa Aggregates Resemble Surface Attached Biofilm. *PLoS ONE* **2011**, *6*, e27943.
7.   Hanlon, G.W.; Denyer, S.P.; Olliff, C.J.; Ibrahim, L.J. Reduction in exopolysaccharide viscosity as an aid to bacteriophage penetration through Pseudomonas aeruginosa biofilms. *Appl. Environ. Microbiol.* **2001**, *67*, 2746–2753.
8.   Sutherland, I.W.; Hughes, K.A.; Skillman, L.C.; Tait, K. The interaction of phage and biofilms. *FEMS Microbiol. Lett.* **2004**, *232*, 1–6.
9.   Xavier, J.B.; Foster, K.R. Cooperation and conflict in microbial biofilms. *Proc. Natl. Acad. Sci. USA* **2007**, *104*, 876–881.

10. Lu, T.K.; Collins, J.J. Dispersing biofilms with engineered enzymatic bacteriophage. *Proc. Natl. Acad. Sci. USA* **2007**, *104*, 11197–11202.

11. Cornelissen, A.; Ceyssens, P.J.; T'Syen, J.; Van Praet, H.; Noben, J.P.; Shaburova, O.V.; Krylov, V.N.; Volckaert, G.; Lavigne, R. The T7-related Pseudomonas putida phage phi-15 displays virion-associated biofilm degradation properties. *PLoS ONE* **2011**, *6*, e18597.

12. Hosseinidoust, Z.; Tufenkji, N.; van de Ven, T.G.M. Formation of biofilms under phage predation: Considerations concerning a biofilm increase. *Biofouling* **2013**, *29*, 457–468.

13. Soothill, J. Use of bacteriophages in the treatment of *Pseudomonas aeruginosa* infections. *Expert Rev. Anti-Infect. Ther.* **2013**, *11*, 909–915.

14. Darch, S.E.; Kragh, K.N.; Abbott, E.A.; Bjarnsholt, T.; Bull, J.J.; Whiteley, M. Phage Inhibit Pathogen Dissemination by Targeting Bacterial Migrants in a Chronic Infection Model. *mBio* **2017**, *8*, doi:10.1128/mBio.00240-17.

15. Schmerer, M.; Molineux, I.J.; Bull, J.J. Synergy as a rationale for phage therapy using phage cocktails. *PeerJ* **2014**, *2*, e590.

16. Heilmann, S.; Sneppen, K.; Krishna, S. Sustainability of virulence in a phage-bacterial ecosystem. *J. Virol.* **2010**, *84*, 3016–3022.

17. Heilmann, S.; Sneppen, K.; Krishna, S. Coexistence of phage and bacteria on the boundary of self-organized refuges. *Proc. Natl. Acad. Sci. USA* **2012**, *109*, 12828–12833.

18. Taylor, B.P.; Penington, C.J.; Weitz, J.S. Emergence of increased frequency and severity of multiple infections by viruses due to spatial clustering of hosts. *Phys. Biol.* **2016**, *13*, 066014.

19. Robb, S.M.; Woods, D.R.; Robb, F.T. Phage growth characteristics on stationary phase Achromobacter cells. *J. Gen. Virol.* **1978**, *41*, 265–272.

20. Los, M.; Golec, P.; Łoś, J.M.; Weglewska-Jurkiewicz, A.; Czyz, A.; Wegrzyn, A.; Wegrzyn, G.; Neubauer, P. Effective inhibition of lytic development of bacteriophages lambda, P1 and T4 by starvation of their host, Escherichia coli. *BMC Biotechnol.* **2007**, *7*, doi:10.1186/1472-6750-7-13.

21. Manning, A.J.; Kuehn, M.J. Contribution of bacterial outer membrane vesicles to innate bacterial defense. *BMC Microbiol.* **2011**, *11*, 258.

22. Erez, Z.; Steinberger-Levy, I.; Shamir, M.; Doron, S.; Stokar-Avihail, A.; Peleg, Y.; Melamed, S.; Leavitt, A.; Savidor, A.; Albeck, S.; et al. Communication between viruses guides lysis-lysogeny decisions. *Nature* **2017**, *541*, 488–493.

23. Lenski, R.E. Dynamics of interactions between bacteria and virulent bacteriophage. *Adv. Microb.Ecol.* **1988**, *10*, 1–44.

24. Chapman-McQuiston, E.; Wu, X.L. Stochastic receptor expression allows sensitive bacteria to evade phage attack. Part I: Experiments. *Biophys. J.* **2008**, *94*, 4525–4536.

25. Chapman-McQuiston, E.; Wu, X.L. Stochastic receptor expression allows sensitive bacteria to evade phage attack. Part II: Theoretical analyses. *Biophys. J.* **2008**, *94*, 4537–4548.

26. Bull, J.J.; Vegge, C.S.; Schmerer, M.; Chaudhry, W.N.; Levin, B.R. Phenotypic resistance and the dynamics of bacterial escape from phage control. *PLoS ONE* **2014**, *9*, e94690.

27. Campbell, A. Conditions for the existence of bacteriophage. *Evolution* **1961**, *15*, 143–165.

28. Levin, B.R.; Stewart, F.M.; Chao, L. Resource—Limited growth, competition, and predation: A model and experimental studies with bacteria and bacteriophage. *Am. Nat.* **1977**, *977*, 3–24.

29. Weitz, J.S. *Quantitative Viral Ecology: Dynamics of Viruses and Their Microbial Hosts*; Princeton University Press: Oxford, UK, 2015.

30. Charnov, E.L. *Life History Invariants: Some Explorations of Symmetry in Evolutionary Ecology*; Oxford University Press: Oxford, UK, 1993.

31. Aviram, I.; Rabinovitch, A. Dynamical types of bacteria and bacteriophages interaction: Shielding by debris. *J. Theor. Biol.* **2008**, *251*, 121–136.

32. Rabinovitch, A.; Aviram, I.; Zaritsky, A. Bacterial debris-an ecological mechanism for coexistence of bacteria and their viruses. *J. Theor. Biol.* **2003**, *224*, 377–383.

33. Eriksen, R.S.; Svenningsen, S.L.; Sneppen, K.; Mitarai, N. A growing microcolony can survive and support persistent propagation of virulent phages. *Proc. Natl. Acad. Sci. USA* **2018**, *115*, 337–342.

34. Bryan, D.; El-Shibiny, A.; Hobbs, Z.; Porter, J.; Kutter, E.M. Bacteriophage T4 Infection of Stationary Phase *E. coli*: Life after Log from a Phage Perspective. *Front. Microbiol.* **2016**, *7*, 1391.

35. Weitz, J.S.; Dushoff, J. Alternative stable states in host-phage dynamics. *Theor. Ecol.* **2008**, *1*, doi:10.1007/s12080-007-0001-1.

36. Nadell, C.D.; Drescher, K.; Foster, K.R. Spatial structure, cooperation and competition in biofilms. *Nat. Rev. Microbiol.* **2016**, *14*, 589–600.

37. Mitarai, N.; Brown, S.; Sneppen, K. Population dynamics of phage and bacteria in spatially structured habitats using phage λ and *Escherichia coli*. *J. Bacteriol.* **2016**, *198*, 1783–1793.

6

Diversification of Secondary Metabolite Biosynthetic Gene Clusters Coincides with Lineage Divergence in *Streptomyces*

Mallory J. Choudoir ⓘ, Charles Pepe-Ranney and Daniel H. Buckley *

School of Integrative Plant Science, Bradfield Hall 705, Cornell University, Ithaca, NY 14853, USA;
mjchoudoir@gmail.com (M.J.C.); chuck.peperanney@gmail.com (C.P.-R.)
* Correspondence: dbuckley@cornell.edu

Abstract: We have identified *Streptomyces* sister-taxa which share a recent common ancestor and nearly identical small subunit (SSU) rRNA gene sequences, but inhabit distinct geographic ranges demarcated by latitude and have sufficient genomic divergence to represent distinct species. Here, we explore the evolutionary dynamics of secondary metabolite biosynthetic gene clusters (SMGCs) following lineage divergence of these sister-taxa. These sister-taxa strains contained 310 distinct SMGCs belonging to 22 different gene cluster classes. While there was broad conservation of these 22 gene cluster classes among the genomes analyzed, each individual genome harbored a different number of gene clusters within each class. A total of nine SMGCs were conserved across nearly all strains, but the majority (57%) of SMGCs were strain-specific. We show that while each individual genome has a unique combination of SMGCs, this diversity displays lineage-level modularity. Overall, the northern-derived (NDR) clade had more SMGCs than the southern-derived (SDR) clade (40.7 ± 3.9 and 33.8 ± 3.9, mean and S.D., respectively). This difference in SMGC content corresponded with differences in the number of predicted open reading frames (ORFs) per genome (7775 ± 196 and 7093 ± 205, mean and S.D., respectively) such that the ratio of SMGC:ORF did not differ between sister-taxa genomes. We show that changes in SMGC diversity between the sister-taxa were driven primarily by gene acquisition and deletion events, and these changes were associated with an overall change in genome size which accompanied lineage divergence.

Keywords: *Streptomyces*; biogeography; comparative genomics; diversification; secondary metabolite biosynthetic gene clusters; SMGC; natural products

1. Introduction

Microbial secondary metabolism encapsulates a remarkable diversity of natural products with an extensive range of biological activities. Secondary metabolites differ from primary metabolites in that they are not involved in essential catabolic and anabolic activities required for normal growth and reproduction, but may contribute significantly to an individual's fitness [1]. While primary metabolic pathways are often conserved deeply within a phylogeny, secondary metabolic pathways are more divergent, often being species or strain-specific, with conservation sometimes observed among closely related species and genera [2]. This phylogenetic pattern suggests an adaptive role for secondary metabolites, and if secondary metabolism pathways provide adaptive benefits, their evolution might drive or reinforce evolutionary processes that result in microbial diversification and speciation [3].

The values of natural products to humanity are widely recognized, yet because most research has focused on their discovery and human-centric relevance, we are still far from understanding their biological role in natural systems. The discovery and application of antibiotics revolutionized medicine in the 1940's, sparking the "golden age" of antibiotics between 1950 and 1960, during which time approximately half of the microbial-derived drugs we use today were discovered [4]. Presently, thousands of bioactive compounds with antibacterial, antifungal, and antitumor activities are cataloged [5,6], and yet these represent only a fraction of actual natural product diversity [7]. In addition, microbial populations in situ are exposed to natural products at concentrations far below the lethal clinical dose, and hence these compounds may serve different functions in the environment from those observed during therapeutic application. We know that secondary metabolites can mediate diverse biotic interactions including mutualistic interactions, competition for nutrients, metal scavenging, and plant-microbe and insect-microbe symbioses [8–10], which can all have profound impacts on microbial fitness. It is clear that natural products must have considerable impacts on microbial ecology and evolution and that understanding the biology and evolutionary history of natural products will enhance our ability to use these agents therapeutically.

Soil-dwelling actinomycetes are the predominant source of microbial-derived therapeutic natural products, and the majority of described bioactive compounds originate from the genus *Streptomyces* [6,7]. The *Streptomyces* life cycle resembles that of many fungi, consisting of filamentous growth, formation of mycelia, and production of aerial hyphae and spores. Indeed, *Streptomyces* were thought to be an intermediary between bacteria and fungi until as recently as the 1950's [11]. However, *Streptomyces* are Gram-positive *Actinobacteria* with long linear chromosomes that have a high G+C content [12]. Traditionally, *Streptomyces* species are often known to produce several secondary metabolites when grown in culture. Genome sequencing, however, reveals that *Streptomyces* contain an enormous reservoir of "cryptic secondary metabolites" which are not expressed under standard laboratory conditions [13]. For instance, while *Streptomyces coelicolor* A3(2) was known to produce several well characterized secondary metabolites, genome sequencing discovered that it actually contained >20 biosynthetic gene clusters not expressed when grown in culture [14]. Genes within secondary metabolite biosynthetic gene clusters (SMGCs) are co-localized as operons within discrete genomic regions. SMGCs have recognizable functional domains, so SMGCs are readily predicted using bioinformatics [15]. Phylogenetic conservation of SMGCs between closely related microbes suggests that these secondary metabolites may have ecological roles which facilitate microbial diversification [16–18].

The evolutionary and ecological processes that govern SMGC diversity remain largely unexplored. The richness of SMGCs within soils is linked to both edaphic and biotic factors [19,20]. For example, the production of antibiotics by *Streptomyces* isolated from prairie soils is highly variable between strains and correlates poorly with 16S rRNA gene phylogeny, suggesting a role of selection acting at small spatial scales [21,22]. Conversely, at larger spatial scales, *Streptomyces* SMGC composition varies in relation to both spatial distance and environmental dissimilarity [23]. Furthermore, evidence within *Streptomyces* for endemism at inter-continental and regional geographic scales [16,24,25] suggests limits to dispersal at large spatial scales. These data indicate that both adaptive and neutral processes contribute to patterns of SMGC biogeography.

Microbial biogeography is readily explored with geographically explicit microbial culture collections (reviewed in [26]), and the genus *Streptomyces* is an ideal model system to evaluate the influence of SMGC dynamics on patterns of diversification. We previously assembled a culture collection of *Streptomyces* from sites spanning the United States, and we observed evidence for dispersal limitation, as well as a latitudinal gradient of species riches and intraspecific nucleotide diversity [27,28]. From this culture collection, we have identified *Streptomyces* sister-taxa that have geographic ranges delimited by latitude and have patterns of gene flow and genomic diversity consistent with their diversification from a recent common ancestor [28,29]. Here, we evaluate changes in SMGC diversity between these *Streptomyces* sister-taxa to explore SMGC evolutionary dynamics during the divergence of *Streptomyces* species.

2. Results and Discussion

2.1. Genomic Divergence between Streptomyces Sister-Taxa

We used comparative genomics to analyze patterns of genomic diversity and SMGC content in 24 *Streptomyces* representing sister-taxa and related strains. These strains were identified through a phylogenetic analysis of a *Streptomyces* culture collection [28] generated from soils of ecologically similar grassland sites spanning 6000 km across the continental United States (Figure 1, Table S1). The sister-taxa, which we have designated the northern-derived (NDR) and southern-derived (SDR) clades, were defined by their geographic range and genomic similarity (Figure 1). Each clade contains ten isolates, and an additional four genomes represent intermediate (INT) taxa.

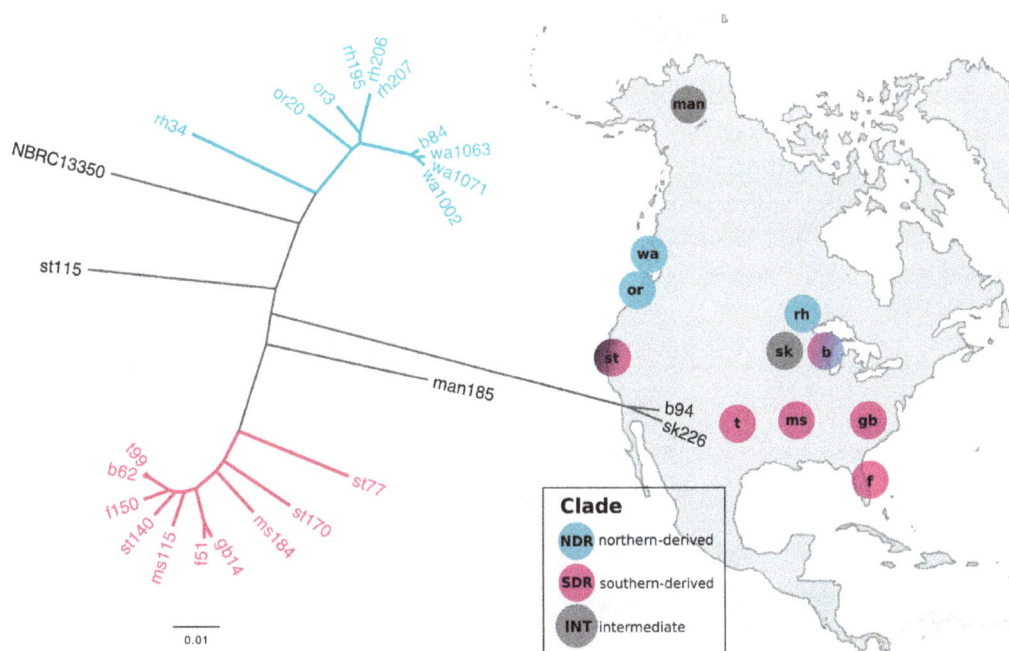

Figure 1. The northern-derived (NDR) and southern-derived (SDR) clades are closely related sister-taxa and yet were isolated from soils of different latitude. The un-rooted tree was constructed from multiple whole genome alignments with maximum likelihood and a GTRGAMMA model of evolution. Scale bar represents nucleotide substitutions per site. Colored branches depict the northern-derived (NDR) and southern-derived (SDR) clades. Strain names reflect the sample site they were isolated from (Table S1). Genome NBRC 13350 is the publically available type strain *Streptomyces griseus* subsp. *griseus* NBRC 13350. Sample locations are shown in the right panel and labeled with the site code. Circles are colored to reflect the geographic distribution of clades. (Figure modified from [29]).

Assembled genomes are 7.5–9.1 Mb with a G+C content of 71.4–72.5% and 6776–8078 predicted open reading frames (ORFs) (Table S2). The core gene content across all 24 strains is comprised of 3234 orthologous genes (representing 2778 single-copy genes), with a total of 22,054 genes in the overall pan-genome. All isolates affiliate taxonomically with the *Streptomyces griseus* species cluster [30] and share >90% average nucleotide identity (ANI) with the type strain *Streptomyces griseus* subsp. *griseus* NBRC 13350 (Figure 1).

The NDR core genome is comprised of 4234 genes, and the SDR core genome is comprised of 4400 genes. The NDR and SDR clades share a recent phylogenetic ancestor and have nearly identical 16S rRNA genes (inter-lineage nucleotide dissimilarity of 0–0.21% between strains). Strains within each clade have a whole genome ANI value ranging from 95.6% to 99.9%, while the ANI between strains of NDR and SDR range from 92.6% to 93.3% (Figure 1). Distinct microbial species are typically distinguished by ANI in the range of 95–96% [31]. Comparative population genomics reveals signatures of genomic differentiation and gene flow limitation between NDR and SDR consistent with expectations of allopatric diversification [29]. Collectively, these results indicate that NDR and SDR clades represent distinct microbial species which have recently diverged from a common ancestor.

2.2. Secondary Metabolite Biosynthetic Gene Cluster (SMGC) Identification and Classification

We used antiSMASH [32] to identify SMGCs in the genomes of our *Streptomyces* sister-taxa. To assess the novelty of these SMGCs, we utilized antiSMASH's downstream annotation pipeline, which annotates SMGCs based on similarity to genes and pathways present within the Minimum Information about a Biosynthetic Gene cluster (MIBiG) database. The antiSMASH pipeline annotated 120 SMGCs across the 24 strains (Table S3). Each genome had between 28 and 47 SMGCs which ranged in size from 1 to 137 Kb (20.9 ± 15.7 Kb, mean $\pm$ S.D., respectively) (Figure 2). This range in SMGC content is consistent with the results obtained from previous genomic surveys of *Streptomyces* [14,33–36]. The NDR clade has a greater number of SMGCs per genome than the SDR clade (40.7 ± 3.9, 33.8 ± 3.9, mean $\pm$ S.D., respectively; t-test, $p < 0.001$; Figure 2a). The NDR clade also has a greater number of ORFs per genome than the SDR clade (7775 ± 196 and 7093 ± 205, mean and S.D., respectively; t-test, $p < 0.001$; Table S2). Correspondingly, NDR strains also have larger genomes than SDR strains (8.7 ± 0.25 Mb and 7.9 ± 0.21 Mb, mean $\pm$ S.D., respectively; t-test, $p < 0.001$; Table S2). We observed a strong positive correlation between genome size and number of SMGCs across all genomes examined (Pearson's $r = 0.66$, $p < 0.001$).

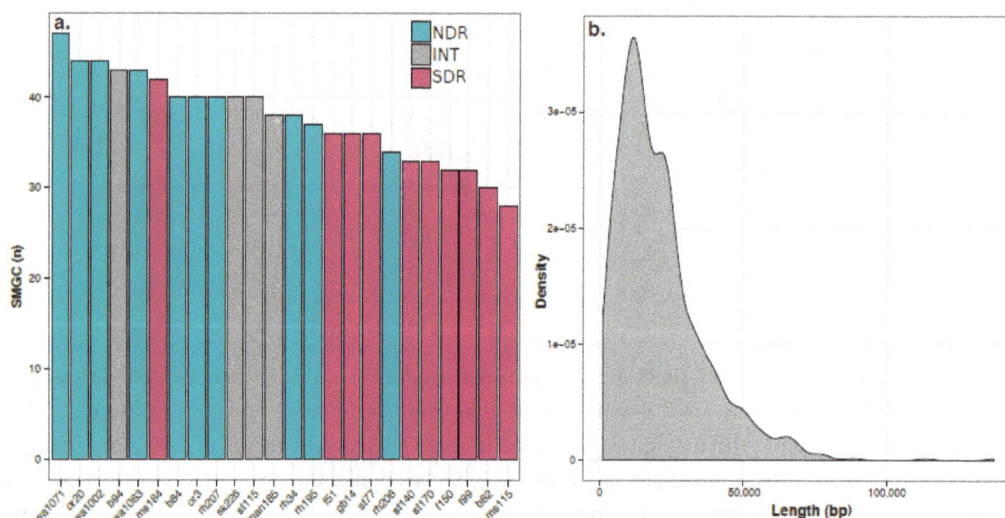

Figure 2. NDR strains have more secondary metabolite biosynthetic gene clusters (SMGCs) than SDR strains (t-test, $p < 0.001$). (**a**). Bars indicate the number of SMGCs identified in each genome and are colored according to clade affiliation, and genome names reflect the site of isolation as identified in Table S1; (**b**). Kernal density plot shows the distribution of SMGC length (bp).

Only 21% ($n = 25$) of the MIBiG-annotated SMGCs represent well-characterized biosynthetic gene clusters (in which $\geq 70\%$ of the genes in a SMGC show similarity to genes within the most similar known cluster from the MIBiG database) (Table S3). In addition, each genome harbors five to 25 potentially novel SMGCs with low similarity to biosynthetic pathways within the MIBiG database. These findings indicate that the diversity of *Streptomyces* SMGCs found within public databases remains low and that a vast reservoir of *Streptomyces* SMGC diversity remains to be characterized within natural populations.

The SMGCs predicted by antiSMASH within our *Streptomyces* sister-taxa encompass 22 classes of natural products. Most of these classes, including bacteriocin, butyrolactones, ectoine, lantipeptide, melanin, non-ribosomal peptide synthases (NRPS), siderophore, polyketide synthases (PKS), and terpene gene clusters, are widely conserved at the genus level [2]. The most abundant SMGC classes in our genomes are NRPS and terpene clusters (Figure 3, Table S3). Many of the predicted gene clusters are NRPS-PKS hybrids (Table S3). Given the similar structure and activity between NRPS and PKS [37], it is unsurprising that hybrid NRPS-PKS clusters are commonly detected in *Streptomyces* genomes [38,39]. Most SMGC classes are present in both NDR and SDR clades, but the relative abundance of each class differs between genomes, as well as between clades (Figure 3). We observe the significant enrichment of melanin and ladderane gene clusters in NDR compared to SDR (t-test with Bonferrori correction, $p < 0.002$). Additionally, NDR genomes harbor linaridin gene clusters, which are entirely absent from SDR genomes (Figure 3) but are found in the type strain *Streptomyces griseus* NBRC subsp. *griseus* 13350 [40]. Interestingly, antiSMASH did not identify aminoglycoside biosynthetic clusters in our *Streptomyces* isolates, and all of these genomes presumably lack genes for streptomycin biosynthesis (Figure 3). Schatz and Waksman reported the isolation of streptomycin from *Streptomyces griseus* in 1944, and this was the first antibiotic used to successfully combat tuberculosis [41]. However, not all *Streptomyces griseus* isolates produce streptomycin [42,43].

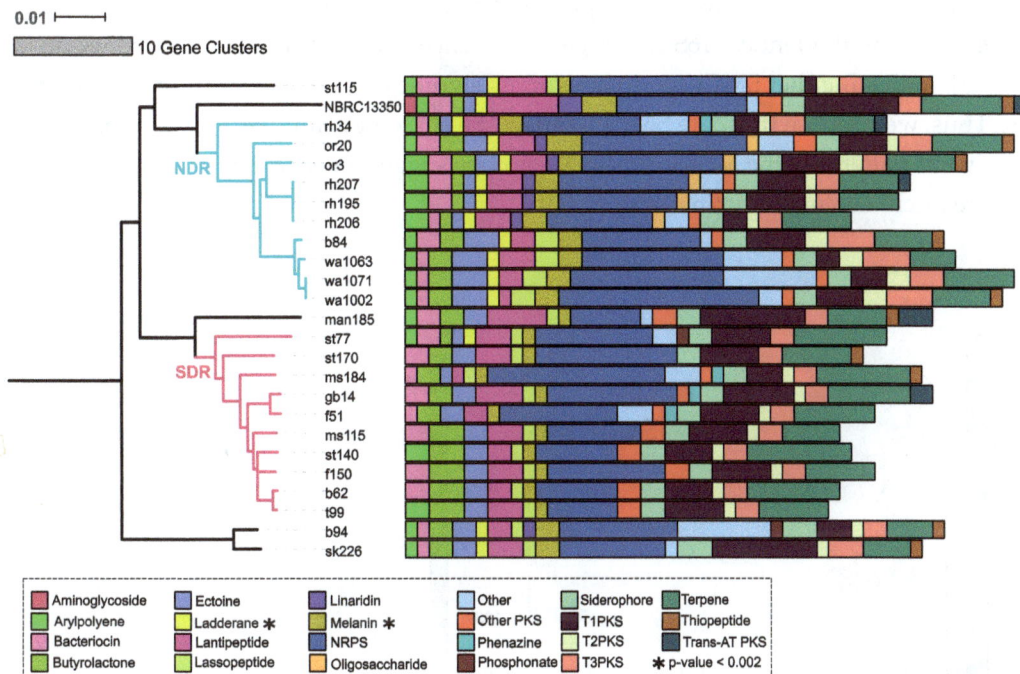

Figure 3. A total of 22 SMGC classes were observed in NDR and SDR genomes by antiSMASH [32]. The tree reflects phylogenetic relationships between *Streptomyces* sister-taxa genomes and was constructed from multiple whole genome alignments (see Figure 1). Scale bar represents nucleotide substitutions per site. Tree branches are colored according to clade affiliation. Bars depict the number of gene clusters belonging to each class for each genome. Colors illustrate gene cluster class as provided by the legend. Asterisks note gene cluster classes that are significantly enriched between clades (t-test and Bonferonni correction for multiple comparisons, $p < 0.002$).

2.3. Core and Accessory SMGCs of Streptomyces Sister-Taxa

Comparative population genomics and pan-genome analyses can offer powerful insights into the processes underlying species divergence [44,45]. Given that many of our SMGCs have low similarity to biosynthetic pathways in public databases, we determined shared orthologous SMGCs within our genomes using an annotation-independent approach that compares SMGCs based on similarity in nucleotide composition and gene content (see Materials and Methods). This approach identified 310 non-redundant SMGCs within the pan-genome of all 24 strains (Figures 4 and 5); this number is greater than the number of MIBiG-annotated SMGCs because it classified both known and unknown pathways into distinct non-redundant gene clusters. Only two SMGCs are conserved in all 24 genomes, an ectoine gene cluster and the siderophore desferrioxamine B (Figure 6). Desferrioxamine siderophores are commonly observed in other species of *Streptomyces* and acintomycetes [46,47].

We observed that core SMGC content increased with phylogenetic similarity, but that more than half of the SMGCs were strain-specific (Figures 4 and 5). NDR and SDR shared nine core SMGCs (present in ≥80% of genomes), while NDR strains shared 11 core SMGCs (nine in the conserved core and two in the NDR-specific core), and SDR strains shared 15 core SMGCs (nine in the conserved core and six in the SDR-specific core) (Figure 6). In addition, there were 158 accessory SMGCs (present in <80% genomes) in NDR and 114 accessory SMGCs in SDR (Figure 4). Most SMGCs were observed at low to intermediate frequencies (Figures 4 and 5), and 177 SMGCs were strain-specific, with each *Streptomyces* genome harboring one to 19 exclusive SMGCs. These estimates are generally consistent with previous observations that indicate each different *Streptomyces* species will harbor a distinct repertoire of natural product pathways [17]. For example, Seipke [36] estimated 18 core SMGCs for six *Streptomyces albus* isolates. However, despite the phylogenetic conservation of core SMGC content, even *Streptomyces* with identical 16S rRNA gene sequences can have distinct secondary metabolite profiles [48], indicating that SMGC content exhibits significant strain to strain variability within a species. Thus, we propose that core SMGCs reflect the shared evolutionary history of *Streptomyces* genomes, while patterns of the accessory SMGC carriage suggest lineage and strain-specific processes across more recent evolutionary time scales.

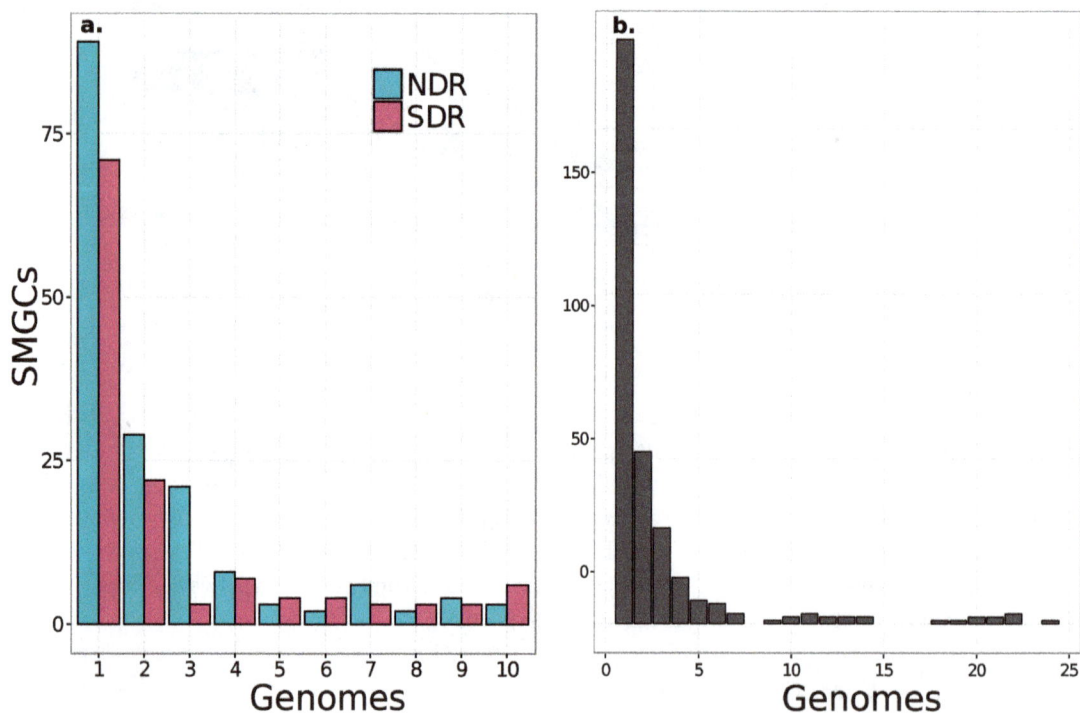

Figure 4. The frequency distribution of SMGCs across strains shows that most SMGCs are strain-specific and fewer are species-specific. Results are shown both for NDR and SDR. (**a**) and for all 24 genomes; (**b**). Non-redundant orthologous SMGCs were defined using our annotation-independent approach (see Materials and Methods).

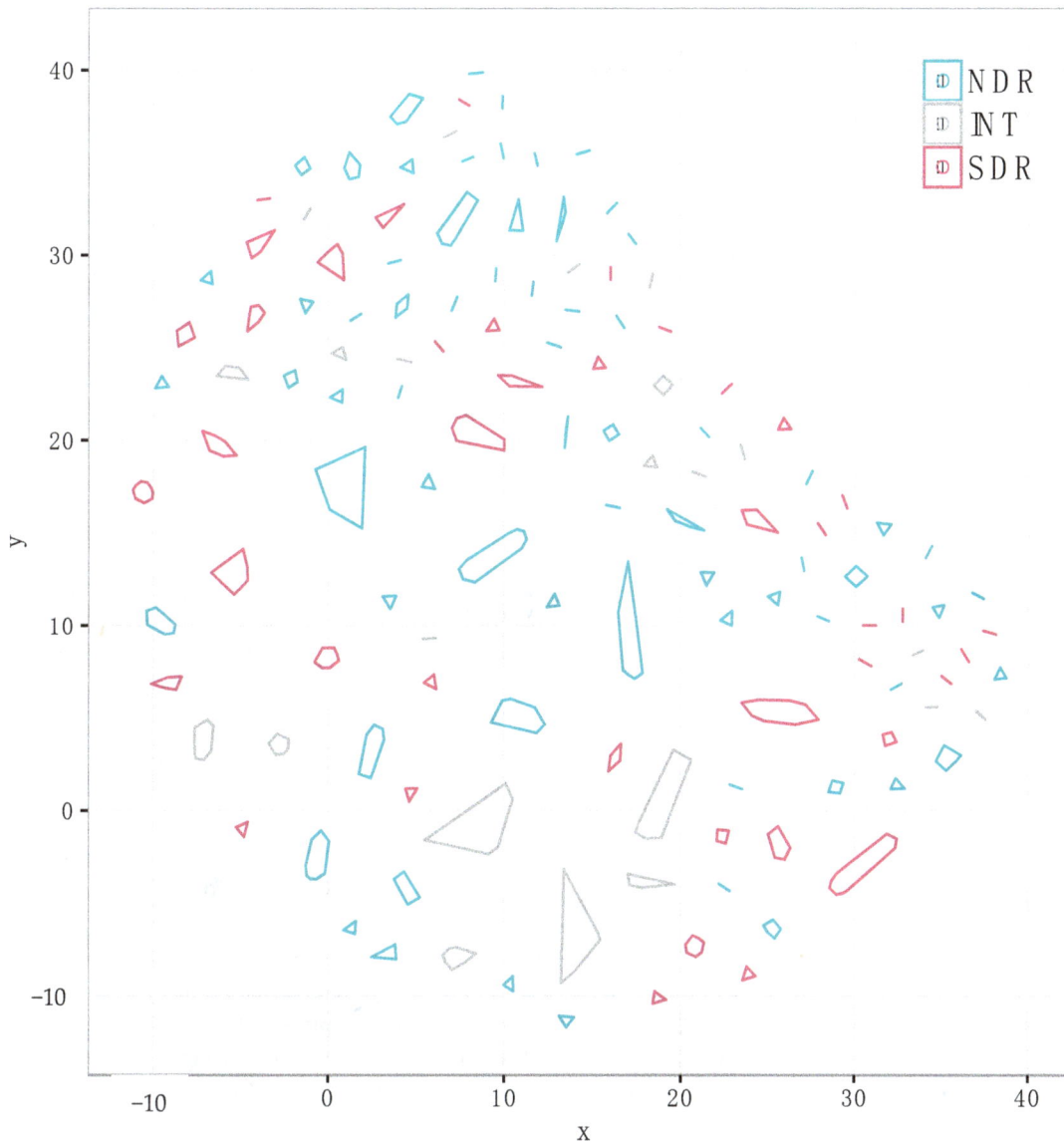

Figure 5. We identified 310 non-redundant distinct SMGCs using our annotation-independent gene clustering approach (see Materials and Methods). Each point represents a unique SMGC from a single genome, and colors correspond to clade affiliation. SMGCs with a similar gene composition are clustered spatially, and cluster membership is depicted with polygons. The same data is presented in a different network diagram in Figure S1.

2.4. Evolutionary Dynamics of Core and Accessory SMGCs

To address potential lineage-specific mechanisms of divergence, we next evaluated the evolutionary dynamics of SMGCs. Most shared SMGCs occur within rather than between clades (Figures 5 and S1). A total of 78 SMGCs are shared among two or more NDR genomes, and 55 are shared among SDR genomes, but only 37 SMGCs are shared across clade boundaries (i.e., found in both NDR and SDR genomes). Furthermore, network analysis reveals unique patterns of SMGC sharing that manifests as nodes of connectivity within clades (Figure S1). This network indicates that there is a core set of SMGC content which links NDR and SRD and which must be ancestral, that there is a clade-specific core set of SMGCs which link the strains of each clade together based on shared SMGC content, and that there are a large number of strain-specific SMGCs (Figures 5 and S1).

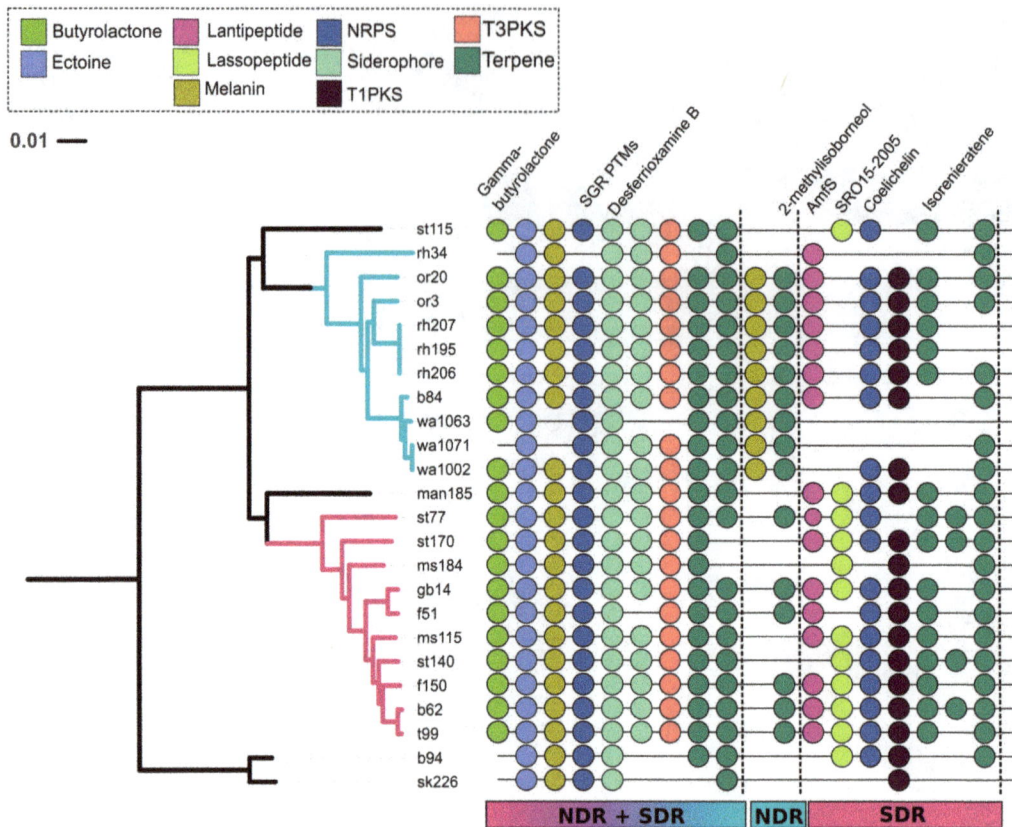

Figure 6. A total of nine core (i.e., conserved in ≥80% of genomes) SMGCs were found in both NDR and SDR. The NDR clade had 11 core SMGCs and the SDR clade had 15 core SMGCs. The tree reflects phylogenetic relationships between *Streptomyces* sister-taxa genomes and was constructed from multiple whole genome alignments (see Figure 1). Scale bar represents nucleotide substitutions per site. Tree branches are colored according to clade affiliation. Core orthologous SMGCs (depicted by colored circles) were determined using the antiSMASH [32] MIBiG annotation pipeline or were defined using our annotation-independent approach (see Materials and Method). Colors correspond to SMGC class (see legend), and natural product annotations are labeled if available.

Differences in gene content between closely related microbes ultimately result from gene gain and loss events [49–51]. Although deletion bias is strong in bacterial genomes [52], gene acquisitions can drive rapid genome innovation and evolution [53]. Gene clusters are often acquired through horizontal gene transfer leading to the formation of new operons in bacterial genomes [54], and many SMGCs in actinomycetes are believed to be the result of horizontal gene transfer [16,18,33,55]. Parsimony predicts that low frequency and strain-specific genes are likely the result of a recent acquisition, while high frequency "near core" genes are the likely result of recent deletion events [56]. Hence, we are able to infer SMGC gain and loss dynamics in our *Streptomyces* sister-taxa from SMGC frequency distributions (Figure 4).

The majority of SMGCs observed within the sister-clades occurred in only one or a few strains, and this suggests that gene acquisition is a major force that drives the diversity of SMGC pathways in *Streptomyces*. However, each clade has a distinct set of core and accessory SMGCs (Figures 3, 5, 6 and S1), and this suggests that SMGC composition (Figure 7) may underlie ecological traits that promote or reinforce lineage divergence. For example, nearly all genomes within the NDR clade (with the exception of rh34) harbor a melanin gene cluster which is absent from both the intermediate (INT) and SDR genomes, suggesting that horizontal gene transfer of the melanin gene cluster into the immediate ancestor of NDR accompanied lineage divergence (Figures 6 and 7). Overall, NDR has more low frequency SMGCs (present in one to three strains) than SDR (139 and 96, respectively) (Figure 4). This result suggests a greater rate of gene acquisition in NDR than in SDR and is consistent with the observation that NDR has more SMGCs (Figure 2) and larger genomes overall than SDR. While this difference in gene content is potentially adaptive, it could also be explained as a consequence of neutral demographic processes such as genome surfing (reviewed in [57]). However, the distribution of SMGC frequencies does not differ significantly between clades (Kolmogorov-Smirnov test, $p = 0.4$). Hence, while it seems clear that gene acquisition is a major driver of SMGC biodiversity, the role of gene acquisition in driving lineage divergence remains unclear.

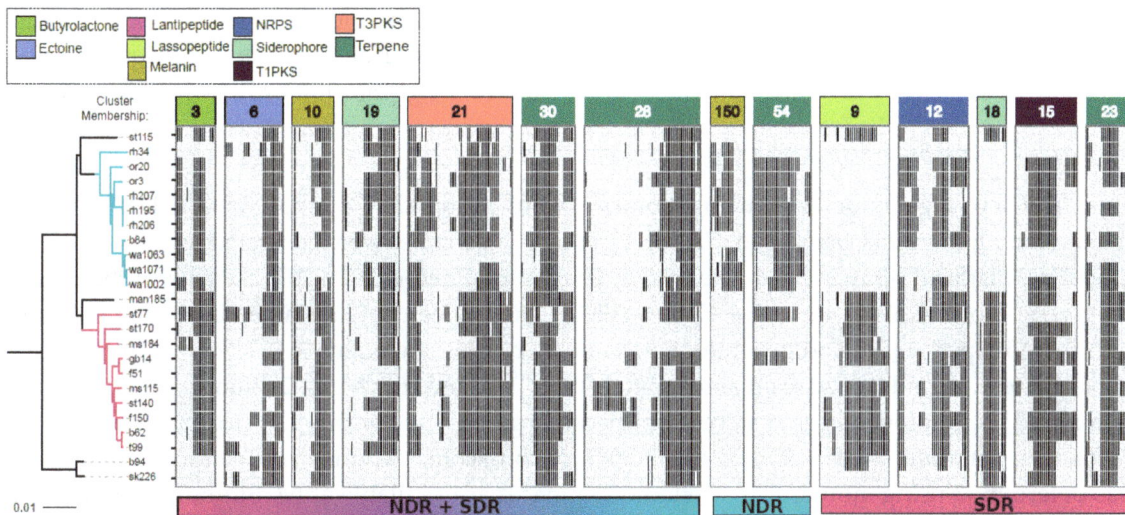

Figure 7. Gene content of core SMGCs vary within and between clades as a result of gene acquisition and deletion events. Panels depict the gene content (i.e., genetic architecture) of core SMGCs (i.e., conserved in ≥80% of genomes), the NDR-specific SMGC core, and the SDR-specific SMGC core. Black bars within the panels represent orthologous genes. The tree reflects phylogenetic relationships between *Streptomyces* sister-taxa genomes and was constructed from multiple whole genome alignments (see Figure 1). Scale bar represents nucleotide substitutions per site. Panel colors correspond to SMGC class (see legend). Panels are labeled with the SMGC cluster membership (see Table S3) defined using our annotation-independent approach (see Materials and Methods).

We also see evidence that NDR has undergone the deletion of SMGC-associated genes inherited from the common ancestor of NRD and SDR. For example, the SRO15-2005 lassopeptide gene cluster is conserved in SDR and found in INT but absent from NDR, suggesting that deletion of this lassopeptide accompanied NDR divergence (Figures 6 and 7). We also find that core SMGC gene loss is more common in NDR than SDR (strain-level deletions occur in six out of nine core gene clusters within NDR and two out of nine core gene clusters in SDR) (Figure 6). Similarly, we can observe SDR species-specific core gene clusters (AmfS, coelichelin, a T1PKS, and a terpene) that are found in only 70% (i.e., near core) of NDR strains (Figure 6). This pattern suggests that these SMGCs were present in the common ancestor of the two clades and subsequently deleted from NDR isolates. In addition, the butyrolactone operon (cluster 3) is comprised of more genes in SDR than in NDR, and this likely indicates active gene loss within this pathway for NDR strains (Figure 7).

Taken together, these results suggest that the sister-clades are under different evolutionary pressures which drive dissimilarity in SMGC composition. NDR genomes have increased in size relative to their ancestors suggesting an overall increase in the rate of gene acquisition via horizontal gene exchange, and this increase in gene acquisition has resulted in an increase in strain-specific SMGC content in NDR. In addition, the presence of NDR-specific core SMGCs (e.g., melanin gene cluster) indicates that some horizontally acquired SMGC have gone to fixation within NDR. At the same time, deletion events in NDR have pruned away SMGCs inherited from ancestral lineages (i.e., those clusters present in SDR and INT). We hypothesize that these changes in SMGC content are likely to have effects on fitness which should act to reinforce lineage divergence either as a result of antagonism or niche differentiation.

3. Materials and Methods

3.1. Streptomyces Isolation and DNA Extraction

We built a culture collection of >1000 *Streptomyces* isolated from grassland soils (pH 3.9–7.3) sampled at 0–5 cm from sites across the United States [27]. Pure *Streptomyces* cultures were obtained from air-dried soils on glycerol-arginine agar (pH 8.7) containing antifungals as previously described [58]. Genomic DNA was extracted using a standard phenol/chloroform/isoamyl alcohol protocol from liquid cultures grown in yeast extract-malt extract medium (YEME) with 0.5% glycine [5] for 72 h shaking at 30 °C.

3.2. Whole Genome Sequencing, Assembly, and Annotation

Streptomyces genomic sequencing libraries were prepped with the Nextera DNA Library Preparation Kit (Illumina, San Diego, CA, USA), and draft genomes were generated using the Illumina HiSeq2500 platform (Illumina, San Diego, CA, USA) and paired-end 2 × 100 bp reads at the Cornell University Biotechnology Resource Center (BRC). Quality control and assembly was performed with the A5 pipeline [59], and genomes were annotated using the online RAST Server [60]. Multiple whole genome alignments were obtained with Mugsy [61], and trimAL v1.2 removed poorly aligned regions [62]. Orthologous genes were identified using ITEP [63] with MCL clustering parameters as follows: inflation value = 2.0, cutoff = 0.04, maxbit score. Average nucleotide identity (ANI) was determined using mother [64]. Genome sequences are available at NCBI under BioProject ID PRJNA401484 accession numbers SAMN07606143–SAMN07606166.

3.3. Phylogenetic Reconstruction

The phylogenetic relationship between genomes was reconstructed from DNA sequences of multiple whole genome alignments using maximum likelihood (ML) with the generalized time reversible nucleotide substitution model [65] with gamma distributed rate heterogeneity among sites (GTRGAMMA) in RAxML v7.3.0 [66]. Bootstrap support was determined using the RAxML rapid bootstrapping algorithm [67].

3.4. Secondary Metabolite Biosynthetic Gene Cluster (SMGC) Identification

Secondary metabolite biosynthetic gene clusters (SMGC) were predicted and annotated using the online server antiSMASH 3.0 [32]. We also used an annotation-independent approach to identify SMGCs shared between genomes. For each SMGC identified by antiSMASH, we used Prodigal [68] to call open reading frames (ORFs) and Parasail with default parameters to identify orthologous genes and orthologous gene groups [69]. We used the R package igraph [70] to cluster similar SMGCs, define cluster membership, and thus determine which SMGCs are shared between genomes. Cluster membership was determined based on gene content using a binary (i.e., Jaccard) dissimilarity distance of ≤4.0 generated from an orthologous group presence/absence table. Dissimilarity distances of >4.0 did not result in an appreciable gain in the number of total clusters. The SMGC network was visualized and analyzed with Cytoscape 3.3.0 [71].

4. Conclusions

We used comparative genomics to examine SMGC diversity within strains of two closely related *Streptomyces* species that recently diverged from a common ancestor. Our objective was to observe and explore the evolutionary dynamics of SMGCs that accompany evolutionary diversification and to assess SMGC conservation within and between closely related species. It is clear that gene gain and loss events drive major differences in SMGC composition, both within and between species. While both species share conserved core SMGCs, each clade has its own species-specific SMGC core, and the majority of SMGCs were strain-specific. This pattern indicates that these SMGCs, not present in shared ancestors, were acquired recently due to horizontal gene exchange.

In addition, we observe that SMGCs that have been inherited from a shared ancestor can vary considerably in gene content, both due to the acquisition and deletion of individual genes within each gene cluster. We observe SMGC gain and loss dynamics that differ between clades and identify SMGC acquisition and deletion events that correspond to ancestral diversification events. These findings show that SMGC modification is associated with lineage divergence, though whether these changes cause or reinforce divergence directly or are an indirect product of evolutionary divergence remains to be seen. A limitation of the comparative genomics approach is that we cannot assess the ecological activity of a pathway from genome sequence data. It is possible that some (or all) of the strain-specific pathways, if acquired by recent horizontal exchange, may be non-functional. It is also possible that changes in SMGC architecture and gene content could alter pathway functionality and that pathways deemed orthologous on the basis of genetic similarity may have different functions in different strains.

Finally, we can conclude that, while strains within a species will share a core set of SMGCs, the number of accessory SMGC within a given species can be quite large, with each strain having its own repertoire of strain-specific SMGCs. Furthermore, the majority of these strain-specific SMGCs remain uncharacterized and lack similarity to SMGCs documented in public databases.

Supplementary Materials:
Figure S1: Each clade has a distinct SMGC network. The network illustrates inter- and intra-clade sharing of SMGC content. Large circles represent the genomes of Streptomyces strains and are labeled with isolate names and colored according to clade affiliation. Smaller circles represent non-redundant distinct SMGCs identified using our annotation-independent approach (see Materials and Methods). Lines connect each SMGC to the strains in which they are found. Network nodes and edges are scaled in proportion to the number of connections and colored according to gene cluster class (see legend). Network is arranged in the organic layout using Cytoscape 3.3.0 [71]. Core SMGCs can be observed as larger central nodes while strain specific and low frequency SMGCs occur around the edges of the graph; Table S1: The 24 Streptomyces genomes were isolated from 11 sites. Isolate names begin with the site code from which they were isolated from followed by strain number; Table S2: Genome and assembly characteristics for 24 Streptomyces genomes. The clade affiliations include the northern-derived (NDR), southern-derive (SDR), and intermediate (INT). Sample site of each isolate can be found in Table S1. Values report assembled draft genome size, genome-wide G+C content, the number of predicted open reading frames (ORFs), and the number of predicted secondary metabolite biosynthetic gene clusters (SMGCs) per genome; Table S3: SMGCs are predicted by antiSMASH [32] in our 24 Streptomyces genomes. For each SMGC, columns report the affiliated genome, clade, gene cluster class (hybrids are indicated by hyphens), gene cluster length (bp), natural product annotation provided by antiSMASH, cluster membership (Clust Memb), MIBiG database identification, the portion of genes with similarity to genes within the most similar known cluster from the MIBiG database (% Genes w/Similarity). Cluster membership was determined using our annotation-independent approach (see Materials and Methods). NA indicates information is not available.

Acknowledgments: This material is based upon work supported by the National Science Foundation under Grant No. DEB-1456821 awarded to Daniel H. Buckley.

Author Contributions: Mallory J. Choudoir and Daniel H. Buckley conceived and designed the study; Mallory J. Choudoir performed the analyses and analyzed the data; Charles Pepe-Ranney contributed to the analyses; Mallory J. Choudoir and Daniel H. Buckley wrote the paper.

References

1. Kossel, A. Ueber die chemische zusammensetzung der zelle. *Arch. Physiol.* **1891**, *4*, 181–186.

2. Doroghazi, J.R.; Metcalf, W.W. Comparative genomics of actinomycetes with a focus on natural product biosynthetic genes. *BMC Genom.* **2013**, *14*, 611. [CrossRef] [PubMed]

3. Karlovsky, P. *Secondary Metabolites in Soil Ecology*; Springer: New York, NY, USA, 2008; pp. 1–19.

4. Davies, J. Where have all the antibiotics gone? *Can. J. Infect. Dis. Med. Microbiol.* **2006**, *17*, 287–290. [CrossRef] [PubMed]

5.   Kieser, T.; Bibb, M.J.; Buttner, M.J.; Charter, K.F.; Hopwood, D.A. *Practical Streptomyces Genetics*; John Innes Foundation: Norwich, UK, 2000.

6.   Bérdy, J. Bioactive microbial metabolites. *J. Antibiot.* **2005**, *58*, 1–26. [CrossRef] [PubMed]

7.   Watve, M.; Tickoo, R.; Jog, M.; Bhole, B. How many antibiotics are produced by the genus *Streptomyces*? *Arch. Microbiol.* **2001**, *176*, 386–390. [CrossRef] [PubMed]

8.   O'Brien, J.; Wright, G.D. An ecological perspective of microbial secondary metabolism. *Curr. Opin. Biotechnol.* **2011**, *22*, 552–558. [CrossRef] [PubMed]

9.   Vaz Jauri, P.; Bakker, M.G.; Salomon, C.E.; Kinkel, L.L. Subinhibitory antibiotic concentrations mediate nutrient use and competition among soil *Streptomyces*. *PLoS ONE* **2013**, *8*, e81064. [CrossRef] [PubMed]

10. Traxler, M.F.; Kolter, R. Natural products in soil microbe interactions and evolution. *Nat. Prod. Rep.* **2015**, *32*, 956–970. [CrossRef] [PubMed]

11. Hopwood, D.A. Soil to genomics: The *Streptomyces* chromosome. *Annu. Rev. Genet.* **2006**, *40*, 1–23. [CrossRef] [PubMed]

12. Kämpfer, P. The family Streptomycetaceae Part I: Taxonomy. In *The Prokaryotes*; Springer: New York, NY, USA, 2006; pp. 538–604.

13. Van der Meij, A.; Worsley, S.F.; Hutchings, M.I.; van Wezel, G.P. Chemical ecology of antibiotic production by actinomycetes. *FEMS Microbiol. Rev.* **2017**, *41*, 392–416. [CrossRef] [PubMed]

14. Bentley, S.D.; Chater, K.F.; Cerdeño-Tárraga, A.M.; Challis, G.L.; Thomson, N.R.; James, K.D.; Harris, D.E.; Quail, M.A.; Kieser, H.; Harper, D.; et al. Complete genome sequence of the model actinomycete *Streptomyces coelicolor* A3(2). *Nature* **2002**, *417*, 141–147. [CrossRef] [PubMed]

15. Blin, K.; Medema, M.H.; Kazempour, D.; Fischbach, M.A.; Breitling, R.; Takano, E.; Weber, T. AntiSMASH 2.0—A versatile platform for genome mining of secondary metabolite producers. *Nucleic Acids Res.* **2013**, *41*, W204–W212. [CrossRef] [PubMed]

16. Jensen, P.R.; Williams, P.G.; Oh, D.-C.; Zeigler, L.; Fenical, W. Species-specific secondary metabolite production in marine actinomycetes of the genus *Salinispora*. *Appl. Environ. Microbiol.* **2007**, *73*, 1146–1152. [CrossRef] [PubMed]

17. Doroghazi, J.R.; Albright, J.C.; Goering, A.W.; Ju, K.S.; Haines, R.R.; Tchalukov, K.A.; Labeda, D.P.; Kelleher, N.L.; Metcalf, W.W. A roadmap for natural product discovery based on large-scale genomics and metabolomics. *Nat. Chem. Biol.* **2014**, *10*, 963–968. [CrossRef] [PubMed]

18. Ziemert, N.; Lechner, A.; Wietz, M.; Millán-Aguiñaga, N.; Chavarria, K.L.; Jensen, P.R. Diversity and evolution of secondary metabolism in the marine actinomycete genus *Salinispora*. *Proc. Natl. Acad. Sci. USA* **2014**, *111*, E1130–E1139. [CrossRef] [PubMed]

19. Wawrik, B.; Kerkhof, L.; Zylstra, G.J.; Kukor, J.J. Identification of unique type II polyketide synthase genes in soil. *Appl. Environ. Microbiol.* **2005**, *71*, 2232–2238. [CrossRef] [PubMed]

20. Charlop-Powers, Z.; Owen, J.G.; Reddy, B.V.B.; Ternei, M.A.; Brady, S.F. Chemical-biogeographic survey of secondary metabolism in soil. *Proc. Natl. Acad. Sci. USA* **2014**, *111*, 3757–3762. [CrossRef] [PubMed]

21. Davelos, A.L.; Kinkel, L.L.; Samac, D.A. Spatial variation in frequency and intensity of antibiotic interactions among *Streptomycetes* from prairie soil. *Appl. Environ. Microbiol.* **2004**, *70*, 1051–1058. [CrossRef] [PubMed]

22. Davelos Baines, A.L.; Xiao, K.; Kinkel, L.L. Lack of correspondence between genetic and phenotypic groups amongst soil-borne *Streptomycetes*. *FEMS Microbiol. Ecol.* **2007**, *59*, 564–575. [CrossRef] [PubMed]

23. Charlop-Powers, Z.; Owen, J.G.; Reddy, B.V.B.; Ternei, M.A.; Guimarães, D.O.; de Frias, U.A.; Pupo, M.T.; Seepe, P.; Feng, Z.; Brady, S.F. Global biogeographic sampling of bacterial secondary metabolism. *Elife* **2015**, *4*, e05048. [CrossRef] [PubMed]

24. Wawrik, B.; Kutliev, D.; Abdivasievna, U.A.; Kukor, J.J.; Zylstra, G.J.; Kerkhof, L. Biogeography of actinomycete communities and type II polyketide synthase genes in soils collected in New Jersey and Central Asia. *Appl. Environ. Microbiol.* **2007**, *73*, 2982–2989. [CrossRef] [PubMed]

25. Reddy, B.V.B.; Kallifidas, D.; Kim, J.H.; Charlop-Powers, Z.; Feng, Z.; Brady, S.F. Natural product biosynthetic gene diversity in geographically distinct soil microbiomes. *Appl. Environ. Microbiol.* **2012**, *78*, 3744–3752. [CrossRef] [PubMed]

26. Choudoir, M.J.; Campbell, A.N.; Buckley, D.H. Grappling with Proteus: Population level approaches to understanding microbial diversity. *Front. Microbiol.* **2012**, *3*. [CrossRef] [PubMed]

27. Andam, C.P.; Doroghazi, J.R.; Campbell, A.N.; Kelly, P.J.; Choudoir, M.J.; Buckley, D.H. A Latitudinal diversity gradient in terrestrial bacteria of the genus *Streptomyces*. *MBio* **2016**, *7*. [CrossRef] [PubMed]

28. Choudoir, M.J.; Doroghazi, J.R.; Buckley, D.H. Latitude delineates patterns of biogeography in terrestrial *Streptomyces*. *Environ. Microbiol.* **2016**, *18*, 4931–4945. [CrossRef] [PubMed]

29. Choudoir, M.J.; Buckley, D.H. Phylogenetic conservatism of thermal traits explains dispersal limitation and genomic differentiation of *Streptomyces* sister-taxa. *ISME J.* **2018**, under review.

30. Rong, X.; Huang, Y. Taxonomic evaluation of the *Streptomyces griseus* clade using multilocus sequence analysis and DNA-DNA hybridization, with proposal to combine 29 species and three subspecies as 11 genomic species. *Int. J. Syst. Evol. Microbiol.* **2010**, *60*, 696–703. [CrossRef] [PubMed]

31. Konstantinidis, K.T.; Ramette, A.; Tiedje, J.M. The bacterial species definition in the genomic era. *Philos. Trans. R. Soc. Lond. B Biol. Sci.* **2006**, *361*, 1929–1940. [CrossRef] [PubMed]

32. Weber, T.; Blin, K.; Duddela, S.; Krug, D.; Kim, H.U.; Bruccoleri, R.; Lee, S.Y.; Fischbach, M.A.; Müller, R.; Wohlleben, W.; et al. AntiSMASH 3.0—A comprehensive resource for the genome mining of biosynthetic gene clusters. *Nucleic Acids Res.* **2015**, *43*, W237–W243. [CrossRef] [PubMed]

33. Ōmura, S.; Ikeda, H.; Ishikawa, J.; Hanamoto, A.; Takahashi, C.; Shinose, M.; Takahashi, Y.; Horikawa, H.; Nakazawa, H.; Osonoe, T.; et al. Genome sequence of an industrial microorganism *Streptomyces avermitilis*: Deducing the ability of producing secondary metabolites. *Proc. Natl. Acad. Sci. USA* **2001**, *98*, 12215–12220. [CrossRef] [PubMed]

34. Ohnishi, Y.; Ishikawa, J.; Hara, H.; Suzuki, H.; Ikenoya, M.; Ikeda, H.; Yamashita, A.; Hattori, M.; Horinouchi, S. Genome sequence of the streptomycin-producing microorganism *Streptomyces griseus* IFO 13350. *J. Bacteriol.* **2008**, *190*, 4050–4060. [CrossRef] [PubMed]

35. Aigle, B.; Lautru, S.; Spiteller, D.; Dickschat, J.S.; Challis, G.L.; Leblond, P.; Pernodet, J.L. Genome mining of *Streptomyces ambofaciens*. *J. Ind. Microbiol. Biotechnol.* **2014**, *41*, 251–263. [CrossRef] [PubMed]

36. Seipke, R.F. Strain-level diversity of secondary metabolism in *Streptomyces albus*. *PLoS ONE* **2015**, *10*, e0116457. [CrossRef] [PubMed]

37. Du, L.; Sánchez, C.; Shen, B. Hybrid peptide–polyketide natural products: Biosynthesis and prospects toward engineering novel molecules. *Metab. Eng.* **2001**, *3*, 78–95. [CrossRef] [PubMed]

38. Medema, M.H.; Blin, K.; Cimermancic, P.; de Jager, V.; Zakrzewski, P.; Fischbach, M.A.; Weber, T.; Takano, E.; Breitling, R. AntiSMASH: Rapid identification, annotation and analysis of secondary metabolite biosynthesis gene clusters in bacterial and fungal genome sequences. *Nucleic Acids Res.* **2011**, *39*, W339–W346. [CrossRef] [PubMed]

39. Olano, C.; García, I.; González, A.; Rodriguez, M.; Rozas, D.; Rubio, J.; Sánchez-Hidalgo, M.; Braña, A.F.; Méndez, C.; Salas, J.A. Activation and identification of five clusters for secondary metabolites in *Streptomyces albus* J1074. *Microb. Biotechnol.* **2014**, *7*, 242–256. [CrossRef] [PubMed]

40. Claesen, J.; Bibb, M.J. Biosynthesis and regulation of grisemycin, a new member of the linaridin family of ribosomally synthesized peptides produced by *Streptomyces griseus* IFO 13350. *J. Bacteriol.* **2011**, *193*, 2510–2516. [CrossRef] [PubMed]

41. Zetterström, R. Selman, A. Waksman (1888–1973) Nobel Prize in 1952 for the discovery of streptomycin, the first antibiotic effective against tuberculosis. *Acta Paediatr.* **2007**, *96*, 317–319. [CrossRef] [PubMed]

42. Waksman, S.A.; Reilly, H.C.; Johnstone, D.B. Isolation of streptomycin-producing strains of *Streptomyces griseus*. *J. Bacteriol.* **1946**, *52*, 393–397. [PubMed]

43. Hotta, K.; Ishikawa, J. Strain- and species-specific distribution of the streptomycin gene cluster and kan-related sequences in *Streptomyces griseus*. *J. Antibiot.* **1988**, *41*, 1116–1123. [CrossRef] [PubMed]

44. Tettelin, H.; Riley, D.; Cattuto, C.; Medini, D. Comparative genomics: The bacterial pan-genome. *Curr. Opin. Microbiol.* **2008**, *11*, 472–477. [CrossRef] [PubMed]

45. Lefébure, T.; Bitar, P.D.P.; Suzuki, H.; Stanhope, M.J. Evolutionary dynamics of complete *Campylobacter* pan-genomes and the bacterial species concept. *Genome Biol. Evol.* **2010**, *2*, 646–655. [CrossRef] [PubMed]

46. Imbert, M.; Béchet, M.; Blondeau, R. Comparison of the main siderophores produced by some species of *Streptomyces*. *Curr. Microbiol.* **1995**, *31*, 129–133. [CrossRef]

47. Roberts, A.A.; Schultz, A.W.; Kersten, R.D.; Dorrestein, P.C.; Moore, B.S. Iron acquisition in the marine actinomycete genus *Salinispora* is controlled by the desferrioxamine family of siderophores. *FEMS Microbiol. Lett.* **2012**, *335*, 95–103. [CrossRef] [PubMed]

48. Antony-Babu, S.; Stien, D.; Eparvier, V.; Parrot, D.; Tomasi, S.; Suzuki, M.T. Multiple *Streptomyces* species with distinct secondary metabolomes have identical 16S rRNA gene sequences. *Sci. Rep.* **2017**, *7*, 11089. [CrossRef] [PubMed]

49. Gogarten, J.P.; Townsend, J.P. Horizontal gene transfer, genome innovation and evolution. *Nat. Rev. Microbiol.* **2005**, *3*, 679–687. [CrossRef] [PubMed]

50. Marri, P.R.; Hao, W.; Golding, G.B. Gene gain and gene loss in *Streptococcus*: Is it driven by habitat? *Mol. Biol. Evol.* **2006**, *23*, 2379–2391. [CrossRef] [PubMed]

51. Reno, M.L.; Held, N.L.; Fields, C.J.; Burke, P.V.; Whitaker, R.J. Biogeography of the *Sulfolobus islandicus* pan-genome. *Proc. Natl. Acad. Sci. USA* **2009**, *106*, 8605–8610. [CrossRef] [PubMed]

52. Mira, A.; Ochman, H.; Moran, N.A. Deletional bias and the evolution of bacterial genomes. *Trends Genet.* **2001**, *17*, 589–596. [CrossRef]

53. Ochman, H.; Lawrence, J.G.; Groisman, E.A. Lateral gene transfer and the nature of bacterial innovation. *Nature* **2000**, *405*, 299–304. [CrossRef] [PubMed]

54. Homma, K.; Fukuchi, S.; Nakamura, Y.; Gojobori, T.; Nishikawa, K. Gene cluster analysis method identifies horizontally transferred genes with high reliability and indicates that they provide the main mechanism of operon gain in 8 species of γ-Proteobacteria. *Mol. Biol. Evol.* **2006**, *24*, 805–813. [CrossRef] [PubMed]

55. Penn, K.; Jenkins, C.; Nett, M.; Udwary, D.W.; Gontang, E.A.; McGlinchey, R.P.; Foster, B.; Lapidus, A.; Podell, S.; Allen, E.E.; et al. Genomic islands link secondary metabolism to functional adaptation in marine Actinobacteria. *ISME J.* **2009**, *3*, 1193–1203. [CrossRef] [PubMed]

56. Bolotin, E.; Hershberg, R. Gene loss dominates as a source of genetic variation within clonal pathogenic bacterial species. *Genome Biol. Evol.* **2015**, *7*, 2173–2187. [CrossRef] [PubMed]

57. Choudoir, M.J.; Panke-Buisse, K.; Andam, C.P.; Buckley, D.H. Genome surfing as driver of microbial genomic diversity. *Trends Microbiol.* **2017**, *25*, 624–636. [CrossRef] [PubMed]

58. Doroghazi, J.R.; Buckley, D.H. Widespread homologous recombination within and between *Streptomyces* species. *ISME J.* **2010**, *4*, 1136–1143. [CrossRef] [PubMed]

59. Tritt, A.; Eisen, J.A.; Facciotti, M.T.; Darling, A.E. An integrated pipeline for de novo assembly of microbial genomes. *PLoS ONE* **2012**, *7*, e42304. [CrossRef] [PubMed]

60. Aziz, R.K.; Bartels, D.; Best, A.A.; DeJongh, M.; Disz, T.; Edwards, R.A.; Formsma, K.; Gerdes, S.; Glass, E.M.; Kubal, M.; et al. The RAST server: Rapid annotations using subsystems technology. *BMC Genom.* **2008**, *9*, 75. [CrossRef] [PubMed]

61. Angiuoli, S.V.; Salzberg, S.L. Mugsy: Fast multiple alignment of closely related whole genomes. *Bioinformatics* **2011**, *27*, 334–342. [CrossRef] [PubMed]

62. Capella-Gutierrez, S.; Silla-Martinez, J.M.; Gabaldon, T. TrimAl: A tool for automated alignment trimming in large-scale phylogenetic analyses. *Bioinformatics* **2009**, *25*, 1972–1973. [CrossRef] [PubMed]

63. Benedict, M.N.; Henriksen, J.R.; Metcalf, W.W.; Whitaker, R.J.; Price, N.D. ITEP: An integrated toolkit for exploration of microbial pan-genomes. *BMC Genom.* **2014**, *15*, 8. [CrossRef] [PubMed]

64. Schloss, P.D.; Westcott, S.L.; Ryabin, T.; Hall, J.R.; Hartmann, M.; Hollister, E.B.; Lesniewski, R.A.; Oakley, B.B.; Parks, D.H.; Robinson, C.J.; et al. Introducing mothur: Open-source, platform-independent, community-supported software for describing and comparing microbial communities. *Appl. Environ. Microbiol.* **2009**, *75*, 7537–7541. [CrossRef] [PubMed]

65. Tavaré, S. Some probabilistic and statistical problems in the analysis of DNA sequences. In *Lectures on Mathematics in the Life Sciences*; American Mathematical Society: Providence, RI, USA, 1986; Volume 17, pp. 57–86.

66. Stamatakis, A. RAxML-VI-HPC: Maximum likelihood-based phylogenetic analyses with thousands of taxa and mixed models. *Bioinformatics* **2006**, *22*, 2688–2690. [CrossRef] [PubMed]

67. Stamatakis, A.; Hoover, P.; Rougemont, J.; Renner, S. A rapid bootstrap algorithm for the RAxML Web Servers. *Syst. Biol.* **2008**, *57*, 758–771. [CrossRef] [PubMed]

68. Hyatt, D.; LoCascio, P.F.; Hauser, L.J.; Uberbacher, E.C. Gene and translation initiation site prediction in metagenomic sequences. *Bioinformatics* **2012**, *28*, 2223–2230. [CrossRef] [PubMed]

69. Daily, J. Parasail: SIMD C library for global, semi-global, and local pairwise sequence alignments. *BMC Bioinform.* **2016**, *17*, 81. [CrossRef] [PubMed]

70. Csardi, G.; Nepusz, T. The Igraph Software Package for Complex Network Research. 2006. Available online: http://www.interjournal.org/manuscript_abstract.php?361100992 (accessed on 6 February 2018).
71. Shannon, P.; Markiel, A.; Ozier, O.; Baliga, N.S.; Wang, J.T.; Ramage, D.; Amin, N.; Schwikowski, B.; Ideker, T. Cytoscape: A software environment for integrated models of biomolecular interaction networks. *Genome Res.* **2003**, *13*, 2498–2504. [CrossRef] [PubMed]

7

Fragment-Based Discovery of Inhibitors of the Bacterial DnaG-SSB Interaction

Zorik Chilingaryan [1], Stephen J. Headey [2], Allen T. Y. Lo [1], Zhi-Qiang Xu [1], Gottfried Otting [3], Nicholas E. Dixon [1] (ID), Martin J. Scanlon [2] (ID) and Aaron J. Oakley [1,*] (ID)

[1] Molecular Horizons and School of Chemistry, University of Wollongong, and Illawarra Health and Medical Research Institute, Wollongong, NSW 2522, Australia; zorik@uow.edu.au (Z.C.); tyl667@uowmail.edu.au (A.T.Y.L.); zhiqiang@uow.edu.au (Z.-Q.X); nickd@uow.edu.au (N.E.D.)
[2] Monash Institute of Pharmaceutical Sciences, Monash University, Parkville, VIC 3052, Australia; stephen.headey@monash.edu (S.J.H.); martin.scanlon@monash.edu (M.J.S.)
[3] Research School of Chemistry, Australian National University, Canberra, ACT 2601, Australia; gottfried.otting@anu.edu.au
*   Correspondence: aarono@uow.edu.au

Abstract: In bacteria, the DnaG primase is responsible for synthesis of short RNA primers used to initiate chain extension by replicative DNA polymerase(s) during chromosomal replication. Among the proteins with which *Escherichia coli* DnaG interacts is the single-stranded DNA-binding protein, SSB. The C-terminal hexapeptide motif of SSB (DDDIPF; SSB-Ct) is highly conserved and is known to engage in essential interactions with many proteins in nucleic acid metabolism, including primase. Here, fragment-based screening by saturation-transfer difference nuclear magnetic resonance (STD-NMR) and surface plasmon resonance assays identified inhibitors of the primase/SSB-Ct interaction. Hits were shown to bind to the SSB-Ct-binding site using ^{15}N–^{1}H HSQC spectra. STD-NMR was used to demonstrate binding of one hit to other SSB-Ct binding partners, confirming the possibility of simultaneous inhibition of multiple protein/SSB interactions. The fragment molecules represent promising scaffolds on which to build to discover new antibacterial compounds.

Keywords: antibacterial agents; fragment-based screening; primase; protein–protein interactions; SSB

1. Introduction

Duplication of chromosomal DNA prior to cell division is a fundamental process in living cells. During initiation of DNA replication in *Escherichia coli*, DnaB helicase is loaded with the assistance of the helicase loader DnaC onto double-stranded DNA and unwinds it [1,2]. DnaB, through direct physical interaction with DnaG primase, forms the primosome [3], which uses its primase activity to synthesize short RNA primers essential for the function of DNA polymerase III [4,5].

DnaG is a DNA-dependent RNA polymerase [6]. In bacteria it is comprised of three distinct domains: an N-terminal zinc-binding domain (ZBD) responsible for DNA template recognition [7], a central catalytic domain (RNA polymerase domain, RPD) [8,9], and a C-terminal helicase-binding domain (HBD or DnaGC), which is responsible for interaction with DnaB helicase and single-stranded DNA-binding protein (SSB) [10–12]. The crystal and solution structures of DnaGC of *E. coli* were determined by X-ray crystallography as a non-physiological domain-swapped dimer [13] and as a monomer in solution by NMR spectroscopy [14].

SSB protects single-stranded DNA during DNA replication. It is an interaction hub known to bind to more than 14 other proteins involved in various stages of DNA replication, repair, and recombination through a highly conserved C-terminal hexapeptide motif (SSB-Ct, sequence: DDDIPF) [15,16]. SSB's binding partners include DnaG [10,12], the Pol lll χ subunit [12,17–22], the PriA replication restart helicase [23], and exonuclease I [24,25].

The SSB-Ct binding site in DnaGC has been identified by NMR. The binding pocket is formed by basic residues K447, R452, and K518, as well as T450, M451, I455, and L519 [26]. Moreover, the DnaGC point mutants K447A, T450A, R452A, and K518A dramatically attenuate SSB-Ct binding. Mutagenesis and NMR experiments, in particular ^{15}N–^{1}H heteronuclear single-quantum correlation (^{15}N–^{1}H HSQC) experiments suggested that the conserved R452 residue forms a salt bridge with the carboxylic acid of the C-terminal Phe residue of the SSB-Ct, whereas the other positively charged residues around the binding pocket interact with the negatively charged residues of SSB-Ct. The SSB-Ct binding pockets in other SSB-binding proteins have characteristics in common with the binding pocket in DnaGC; e.g., those in ExoI [24], RecO [27], Pol lll χ [22], and PriA [23].

The SSB-Ct binding pockets in some or all of these proteins have been suggested to be very good targets for development of new antibacterial agents because many of the interactions are essential for bacterial survival and resistance to compounds that interfere with multiple interactions could not easily develop by target mutagenesis [16]. This argument depends critically on a single compound mimicking the SSB-Ct peptide sufficiently well that it is able to bind tightly to three or more essential binding pockets that are lined with different residues and thus have structures that are more or less distinct. The observed gross structural similarities among pockets in SSB-Ct binding partners, including the ionic interaction with the C-terminal Phe and the basic rim that interacts with the acidic residues suggest such compounds might exist, but the only useful way to establish this for sure is to quantify the binding to multiple potential targets of compounds selected against one of them.

To begin the process of determining whether SSB-Ct binding pockets are actually suitable targets, we report the use of fragment-based screening (FBS) to find compounds binding to *E. coli* DnaGC. FBS uses small (<300 Da) compounds called "fragments" as starting points for drug discovery. Several biophysical methods may be used in fragment screening [28]. Here, we report the use of surface plasmon resonance (SPR) and NMR measurements to screen for binders that target the SSB-binding pocket in DnaGC.

2. Results and Discussion

2.1. Screening of Fragment Libraries

An SPR competition assay (example in Figure S1a) was used as the first-pass screen. It identified six small-molecule fragments that competed with immobilized SSB-Ct peptide for binding to a N-terminally truncated DnaG protein missing just the ZBD; we call this protein DnaG-RCD, comprised of the RPD and DnaGC domains. These fragments were validated by saturation-transfer difference (STD) NMR [29], where transient binding of the ligand to the protein is detected by attenuation of the ligand NMR spectrum (example in Figure S1b). In parallel with the confirmation of SPR hits, cocktails encompassing the complete MIPS library of 1140 structurally diverse fragments [30] were independently screened by STD-NMR. Fragments identified in cocktails were re-tested as pure ligands in the STD-NMR assay. The hits identified were ranked according to STD signal intensity. In total, 56 fragments were identified as top hits (rank 3, clear hit, strong intensity difference) and 62 as rank 2 (clear hit, moderate intensity) [30]. From the final STD rank 3 and 2 compounds together (80 compounds), about 50 fragments were identified as "frequent hits" or "PAINS" [30] and were excluded from further screening.

2.2. Validation of Fragment Binding by 2D NMR

Two-dimensional (2D) ^{15}N–^{1}H HSQC spectra of the uniformly ^{15}N-labeled DnaGC domain were employed to validate STD hits. Buffer conditions were optimized, and no major differences were observed in recorded spectra of the protein alone compared to the original studies [13,14]. We were able to assign some of the missing resonances for residues forming the SSB-Ct binding pocket in the spectrum of the apo-protein reported by Naue et al. [26]; i.e., those of K447, R448, T449, N511, and N565. ^{15}N–^{1}H HSQC spectra were recorded on 0.1 mM solutions of ^{15}N-DnaGC mixed with compounds at 3.3 mM. The compounds were ranked according to the magnitude of the generated weighted chemical shift perturbation (CSP; Section 3.5), and the best four were selected (Figure 1, Figures S2a–c and S3a–d).

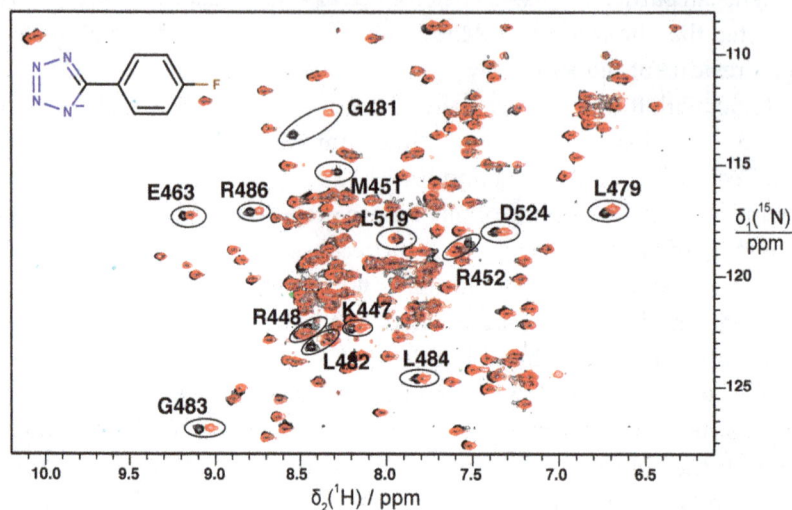

Figure 1. Superimposition of ^{15}N–^{1}H HSQC spectra of DnaGC. The protein spectrum in the absence of fragment in black is compared with its spectrum after addition of fragment **4** (structure shown) in red. Representative assignments of resonances that showed the highest weighted chemical shift perturbation (CSP) (Figure S3d) are shown.

By monitoring the protein chemical shift and peak intensity changes upon addition of compound and mapping the CSP onto the protein surface, the location of the ligand-binding pocket could in each case be identified as the SSB-Ct binding pocket of DnaGC (Figure 2 and Figure S4).

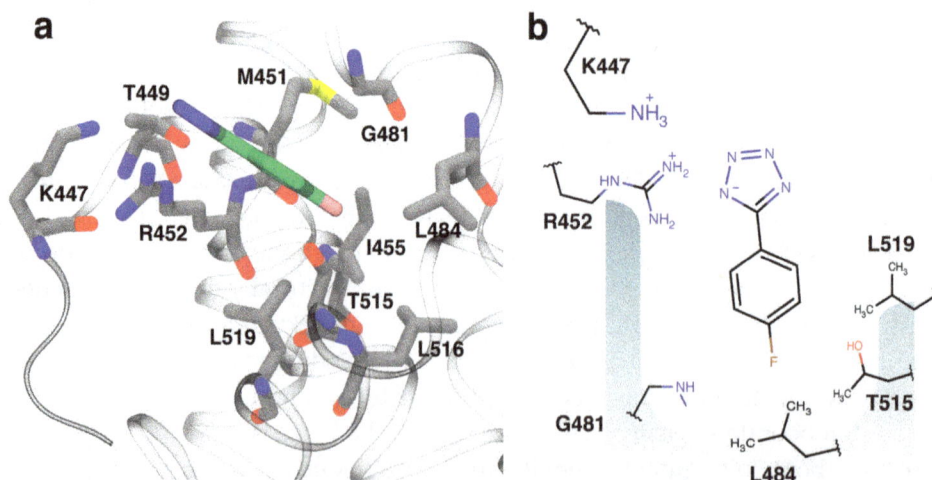

Figure 2. Modeled orientation of fragment **4**. (**a**) The docked orientation of fragment **4** (green carbon atoms) in the single-stranded DNA-binding (SSB)-Ct binding pocket of DnaGC (gray carbon atoms). (**b**) A schematic representation of interactions between fragment **4** and its binding pocket. In all structural figures, the protein was visualized using visual molecular dynamics (VMD) [31].

Comparison of the four hits revealed some similar features such as the presence of indole groups in fragments **1** and **2** or an aliphatic thioether-linked extension in **2** and **3**. In addition, three (**1**–**3**) have a carboxylate attached (Figure 3a) and fragment **4** has a 1*H*-tetrazole group, which is a carboxylate bioisostere [32]. Tetrazoles have pK_a values comparable to carboxylic acids (~5) and are good hydrogen bond acceptors. Modeling studies suggest that deprotonated tetrazoles form stronger hydrogen bonds than carboxylate groups [33].

Affinity measurements of weakly binding ligands are challenging for most biophysical techniques [34,35]. Nevertheless, binding affinities of fragments **1–4** can be roughly estimated to be in the 1–3 mM range by NMR titration experiments that monitored the gradual change in chemical shift of a few well-resolved resonances in HSQC spectra (Figure 3b).

2.3. Orientation of Identified Hits Using Molecular Docking

The docked structure of fragment **4** bound into DnaGC (Figure 2a) is in agreement with the chemical shift perturbation (CSP) data. The tetrazole anion of **4** makes hydrogen bonds and/or a salt bridge with the side chains of K447, T449, and R452. The phenyl ring appears likely to mimic the last phenylalanine residue in the SSB-Ct peptide and makes hydrophobic interactions with P480, G481, T515 and L519 in the binding site. Fluorine is a strong hydrogen-bond acceptor [36], and the model suggests that there is a hydrogen bond to the *para*-fluoro group from the amide proton of G481. Methyl groups from the side chains of L448, L455, T515, L516, and L519 also interact with the *para*-fluoro group.

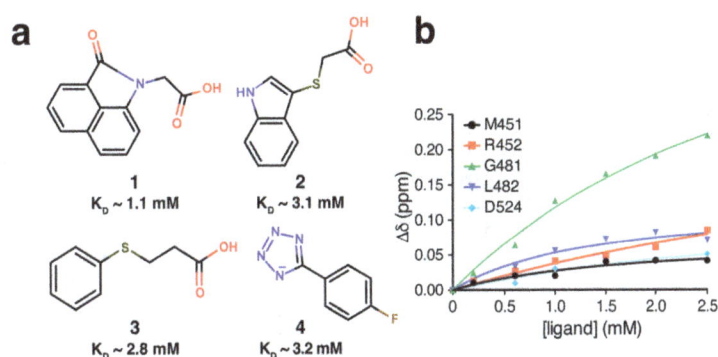

Figure 3. (a) Structure of hits with binding affinities for further optimization. (b) ^{15}N–^{1}H HSQC titration of fragment **4**. Binding affinities (K_D values) were derived from the change in chemical shift, $\Delta\delta$, with incremental additions of ligand.

In the case of fragment **1**, CSP-guided docking predicts that the carbonyl group interacts with the side-chain of R452. The fragment orientation enables favorable contact of the free carboxylate of the fragment and the positively charged side chain of K518 (Figure S4). Its improved binding affinity (~1.1 mM) is most likely explained by its hydrophobic skeleton occupying the shallow binding pocket. Comparison of fragment 1 with an analog where the carboxylate is substituted with a methyl group gave fewer peak shifts in the HSQC spectrum, confirming that the carboxylic acid group improves the binding (Figure S5).

Fragments **2** and **3** have similar aliphatic chains with thioether links to aromatic groups. As with other fragments, the carboxylate moieties are predicted to form electrostatic and hydrogen bond interaction, whereas the main chemical backbone mimics the phenylalanine residue in SSB-Ct. Thioethers may have a strong influence on the conformation of aliphatic chains [37]. In the proposed binding mode of fragment **3**, the sulfur atom interacts with R452 while the carboxylate forms hydrogen bonds with I455 and G481 (Figure S6).

One of the fragments tested, *N*-acetylated L-Phe, is expected to mimic the C-terminal residue (F177) in the SSB-Ct peptide. STD and ^{15}N–^{1}H HSQC experiments confirmed the binding event (data not shown). However, binding affinities measured in titration experiments monitored by HSQC spectra showed that it has about two-fold lower affinity compared to other hits (**3, 4**). The modeled orientations of the fragment show indeed that the phenyl ring forms hydrophobic contacts in the binding site, and the carboxylate interacts with R452 (Figure S7). Substituting the carboxylate with a 1H-tetrazole ring, as found in fragment **4**, increased the affinity 2-fold.

2.4. Fragment-to-Hit Optimization

With the knowledge that the tetrazole moiety might confer improved membrane-crossing properties compared with carboxylates owing to its higher lipophilicity, fragment **4** (Figure 3a) was chosen as a starting point for fragment-to-hit optimization. As docked into DnaGC, **4** has suitable vectors for fragment growth. The in silico analog screen identified 10 tetrazole analogs with favorable binding poses relative to the SSB-Ct peptide (not shown). Nevertheless, STD and 2D NMR experiments showed that most of these analogs did not bind to DnaGC. As an exception, 5-[2-fluoro-6-(4-fluorphenoxy)phenyl]tetrazol-1-ide (**5**) showed a STD signal and significant CSP in 2D NMR experiments (Figure S3e). Mapping of the CSP on the protein surface allowed a binding pose of compound **5** to be calculated (Figure 4).

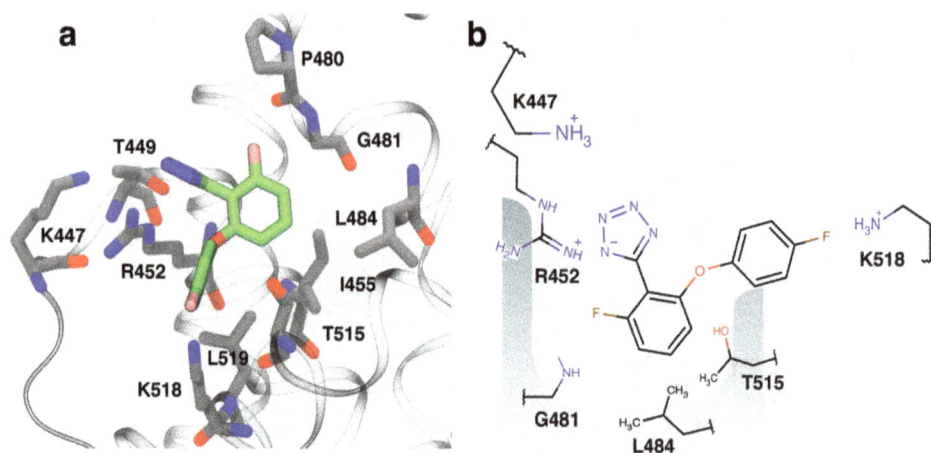

Figure 4. Visualization of binding of compound **5**. (**a**) The lowest energy binding poses of **5** (green carbon atoms) bound to DnaGC (gray carbon atoms). (**b**) Schematic representation of residues involved in interaction with compound **5**.

The observed NMR peak shifts were consistent with the docked orientation. The negatively charged tetrazole is predicted to form favorable electrostatic and hydrogen bond interactions with the side chains of K447 and R452. The methyl groups of L446, M451, L455, L484 T515 and L519 form a hydrophobic pocket accommodating two aromatic rings of the compound. One of the fluorine atoms is about 3 Å from the amide group of G481 while the second at the *para*-position of the phenoxy group points out of the pocket toward K518. In the docked conformation, these fluorine atoms are involved in hydrogen bond formation with these two residues (Figure 4). To test the docked orientation of **5**, 1D ^{19}F-NMR was carried out using a 20-fold excess of compound over protein. Fluorine signals were broadened and shifted slightly downfield, confirming binding of **5** to DnaGC (Figure 5). Nevertheless, the 3D NOESY-^{15}N-HSQC spectrum failed to detect any protein–ligand NOEs.

Compound **5** was shown to bind to DnaGC with about a three-fold improved affinity compared to the starting fragment **4**, as measured by titration experiments monitored by ^{15}N–^{1}H HSQC spectra (K_D = 1.3 mM). Searching the *ZINC* database [38] for ligands structurally similar to **5** indicated that the only available analog was **6**. It is missing the halogen atoms and has a *meta*-phenoxy group (Figure 6). The binding of **6** to DnaGC was also assessed by STD and ^{15}N–^{1}H HSQC experiments (Figure 6).

Compounds **5** and **6** showed similar patterns of CSPs (Figure S3e,f). Compounds that possess similar protein-binding modes are known to induce similar CSPs [39]. Changes in the position of the phenoxy group in **6** relative to **5** increased the magnitude of the CSP as a result of a slightly improved binding affinity, K_D = 1.2 mM.

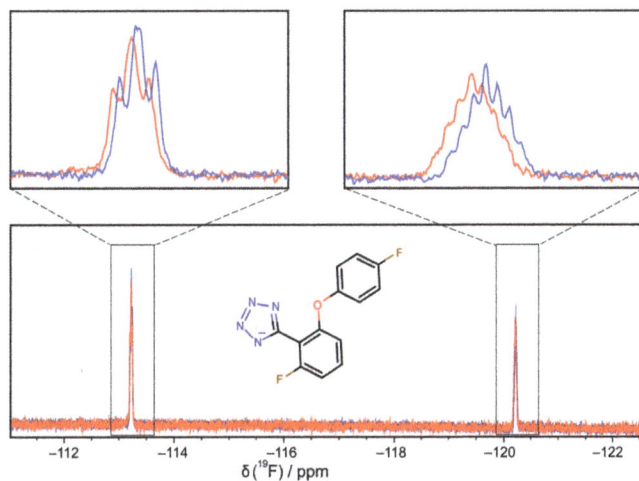

Figure 5. 1D ^{19}F-NMR spectra of compound **5** at 1 mM in the presence (red trace) and absence (blue trace) of 50 μM DnaGC.

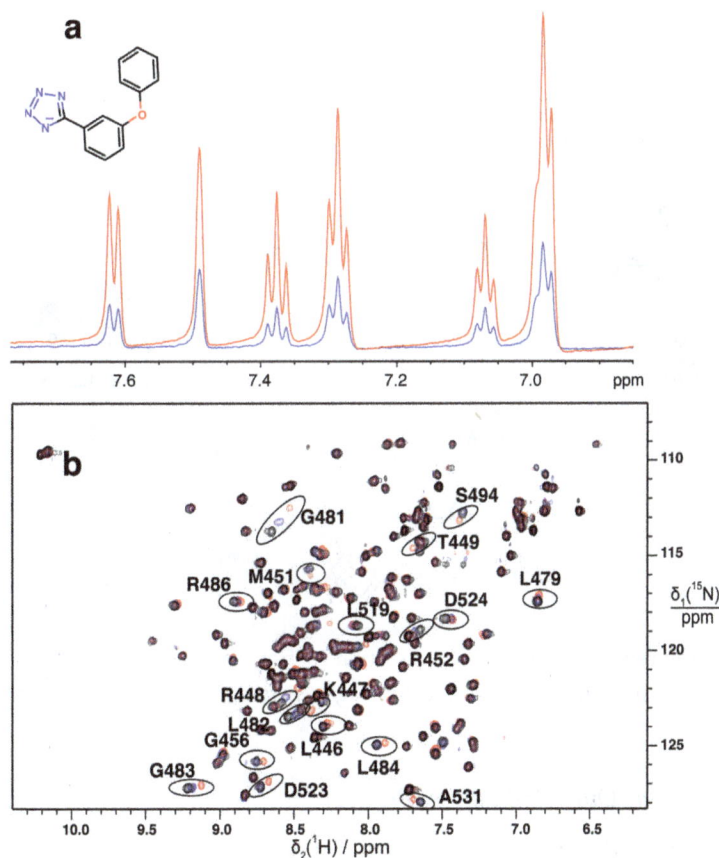

Figure 6. (**a**) Saturation transfer difference (STD) spectrum of compound **6** using DnaG-RCD. In red is a 1D ^{1}H-NMR reference spectrum, overlaid with a STD spectrum (blue). (**b**) Overlay of ^{15}N–^{1}H HSQC spectra of ^{15}N-DnaGC (black) with **5** (blue) and **6** (red), each at 1 mM. The apo-protein spectrum is shown in black. Representative assignments of resonances that showed the highest weighted CSP (Figure S3e,f) are shown.

Compound **6** was in turn docked to DnaGC and is predicted to form electrostatic interactions with the side chains of K447, T449 ad R452 (Figure 7). The central aromatic ring sits in a hydrophobic groove formed by M451, I455 and L484, while the phenoxy oxygen atom forms a hydrogen bond with the side chain –OH of T515. In addition, the phenoxy ring forms a cation–π interaction with the guanidinium group of R452 and hydrophobic contacts with the L446 and W522 side chains.

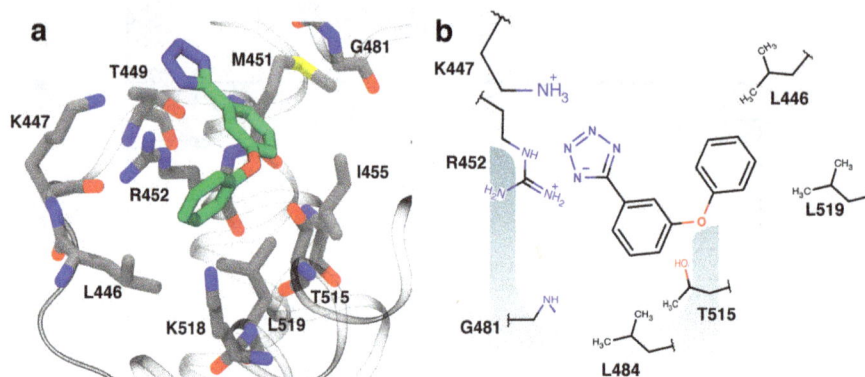

Figure 7. (a) Docked binding pose of **6** (green carbon atoms) bound to DnaGC (gray carbon atoms). (b) Schematic representation of interactions.

To sample the impact of substituents at the *para*-position of the phenyl group of **4**, additional compounds were purchased (compounds **7** and **8**; Figure 8). Molecular docking suggested that *para*-substitutions might dramatically change the orientation of the tetrazole moiety in the binding pocket, and STD and ^{15}N–^{1}H HSQC experiments showed that replacing the *para*-fluorine with a bulky substituent reduced the CSPs substantially.

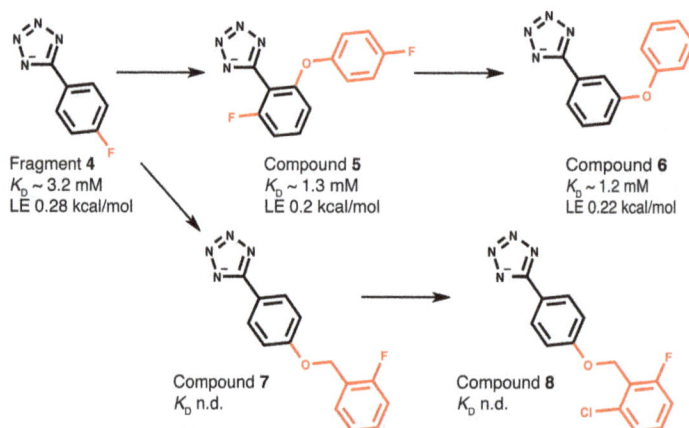

Figure 8. Schematic representation of optimization of fragment **4**. The red labeled groups were added during fragment-to-hit optimization. LE: Ligand efficiency (ΔG/[number of heavy atoms]), n.d.: not determined.

2.5. Binding of Compounds to Other SSB Partner Proteins

The fragments identified here and the first generation of optimized leads for DnaGC were tested against other SSB-Ct binding partners including *E. coli* PriA, *E. coli* RNAse HI, and the χ subunit of *E. coli* and *Acinetobacter baumannii* DNA polymerase III. STD-NMR was used to assess binding. All of the identified fragments showed STD signals, confirming binding (Figure S8). Moreover, the docked orientation of fragment **4** in the binding site of *E. coli* χ showed the possibility of hydrogen bonding with the fluorine atom. 1D ^{19}F NMR (Figure 9) demonstrated binding.

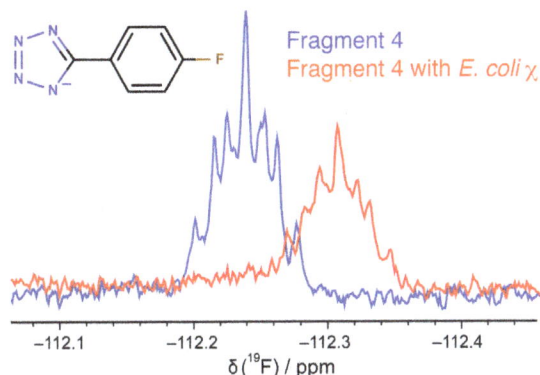

Figure 9. 1D ^{19}F-NMR spectra. The blue spectrum is of fragment **4** alone and its spectrum in the presence of *E. coli* χ is shown in red.

3. Materials and Methods

3.1. Protein Expression and Purification

A phage λ-promoter plasmid (pZX1404) that directs overexpression of a protein comprising the central and C-terminal domains of *E. coli* DnaG primase (residues 111–581, here called DnaG-RCD) was constructed by cloning a PCR fragment between the *Bam*HI and *Eco*RI sites of vector pND706 [40]. PCR was performed using plasmid pPL195 [41] as template and the following primers (restriction sites in italics): dnaG_RCD_F, 5′-GCGGGATCCTAAGAAGGAGATATA*CATATG* ACGCTTTATCAGTTGATG; dnaG_RCD_R, 5′-GCG*GAATTC*TTACTTTTTCGCCAGCTC C. The full sequence of the gene encoding RCD was then verified by nucleotide sequence determination. Another plasmid pZX1399 encoding amino acids 115–581 of *E. coli* DnaG was also constructed in a similar manner. However, the protein was expressed in insoluble form, and therefore was not used. Unlabeled DnaG-RCD and unlabeled and ^{15}N-labeled DnaGC were expressed and purified as described previously for DnaGC [42].

3.2. Fragment Libraries

The "first pass screen" fragment library (Zenobia Therapeutics, San Diego, CA, USA) was used for the SPR competition assay. Each fragment (50 mM in DMSO) was diluted to 1 mM final concentration. Fragment library members were tested for chip surface binding to eliminate false positives.

The Monash Institute of Pharmaceutical Science (MIPS) library comprised of around 1140 fragments purchased from Maybridge was used for STD-NMR experiments. The individual fragments were diluted in ^{2}H$_6$-DMSO to give ~660 mM final stock concentrations [30]. The fragments were mixed in cocktails of up to 6 compounds with well-resolved resonances in their 1D ^{1}H-NMR spectra.

3.3. SPR Competition Assay

SPR measurements utilized a Biacore T200 instrument (GE Healthcare, Little Chalfont, UK) at 20 °C to measure the competition of compounds for the DnaGC/SSB-Ct peptide interaction. The buffer contained 10 mM HEPES (pH 7.4), 3 mM EDTA, 100 mM NaCl, 2% DMSO, 1 mM dithiothreitol and 0.05% (*v/v*) surfactant P20 (GE Healthcare). An N-terminally biotinylated SSB-Ct peptide [Biotin-(Ahx)-GSAPS-NEPPMDFDDDIPF; where Ahx is an amino-hexanoate spacer, followed by the 16 C-terminal residues of SSB highlighted in bold] was immobilized onto a streptavidin (SA) chip surface. RCD at 30 μM and fragments at 1 mM concentrations were used in all SPR experiments. Each sample was mixed for approximately 15 min prior to measurements. Mixtures were injected separately onto two flow cells, one of which served as a reference.

Prior to measurements, each individual fragment was tested for solubility and non-specific binding to an unmodified surface at 1 mM concentration to eliminate false positive responses.

Compounds that bound non-specifically to the chip surface were excluded from screening. A flow rate of 5 µL/min was used during the 60 s injection and 60 s dissociation phases for all experiments.

3.4. Saturation-Transfer Difference (STD) NMR Spectroscopy

STD-NMR experiments were carried out using 5 µM unlabeled DnaG-RCD and mixtures of 6 fragments in each sample, at ~250 µM for each fragment. The sample volume was 500 µL with 98–99% ^2H_2O buffer containing 50 mM phosphate (pH 7.8), 50 mM NaCl and 1 mM dithiothreitol. Spectra were recorded at 283 K using a Bruker Avance 600 MHz spectrometer (Bruker, Karlsruhe, Germany) equipped with a cryoprobe. Saturation of protein was achieved with a 4 s Gaussian pulse sequence train centered at −1 ppm. For reference spectra, a similar saturation pulse was applied 20 kHz off-resonance. A 20 ms spin-lock period was applied before acquisition to allow the residual protein signals to decay. The STD experiments were recorded over 64 scans. All NMR data were processed using TOPSPIN 3.1. Relative intensities were based on the most intense STD signal (I_{max}) identified across all STD spectra. A positive STD signal was categorized as "strong", "moderate" or "weak" where the intensity was >50%, >25% or <25% of I_{max}, respectively [30].

3.5. 2D ^{15}N–^1H HSQC Spectra

Protein binding by compounds identified by SPR and STD screens was confirmed by recording ^{15}N–^1H HSQC spectra on uniformly ^{15}N-labeled DnaGC (100 µM) in the presence of 3.3 mM compounds (from $^2H_6$-DMSO stocks) with HSQC buffer (50 mM MES pH 6.0, 60 mM NaCl, 1 mM dithiothreitol) containing 3% ^2H_2O. The final volume of each sample was 150 µL. The recording time was 30 min for each ^{15}N–^1H HSQC experiment. A standard pulse sequence was used for data acquisition. Spectra were recorded at 298 K with a Bruker Avance 600 MHz NMR spectrometer equipped with cryoprobe and auto-sample changer. Compounds were regarded as hits if chemical shift perturbation was observed in the ^{15}N–^1H HSQC spectra. The spectra were processed with TOPSPIN 3.1 and analyzed using CCPN [43]. Weighted CSP values [44] were calculated as

$$CSP = (\Delta\delta_H{}^2 + 0.2\,\Delta\delta_N{}^2)^{0.5}$$

Binding affinities were estimated by incremental titration of fragments into protein, with recording of a ^{15}N–^1H HSQC experiment at each concentration point. Compound solubilities were tested to determine the highest concentrations of ligands used in assays. Equilibrium dissociation constants from NMR titration data were derived using the "single site-specific binding with ligand depletion" model in GraphPad Prism v.6.0 (La Jolla, CA, USA).

3.6. ^{19}F-NMR Spectroscopy

1D ^{19}F-NMR spectra were recorded on a Bruker Avance III 400 MHz NMR spectrometer (Bruker, Karlsruhe, Germany) equipped with the two-channel BBO probe with z-gradient at 300 K. All ^{19}F-NMR spectra were recorded with 256 scans for fragment and complex samples sequentially. Fragments dissolved in $^2H_6$-DMSO were diluted in HSQC buffer to give final fragment and protein concentrations of 1 mM and 50 µM, respectively.

3.7. Molecular Docking

AutoDock Tools 1.5.6 [45] was used to prepare protein [46] and ligand structures for docking. The protonation state of the titratable groups in the protein were assigned at pH 7.0 using PROPKA 3.1 [47]. Polar hydrogen atoms and atom-based Gasteiger partial charges were added. Nonpolar hydrogen atoms were merged with the parent atom. The DnaGC structure was taken from the previously solved crystal structure (PDB ID: 1T3W) [13]. The protein was treated as a rigid body. The CSP docking calculations were performed using AutoDock Vina 1.1.2 [45]. The calculations utilized an exhaustiveness of 1024 with grid points separated by 1.0 Å and grid size large enough to include the SSB-Ct peptide binding site ($16 \times 16 \times 14$ Å). Ligand data were obtained from the *ZINC* database of commercially available compounds [38].

4. Conclusions

Fragment-based screening has successfully identified compounds targeting the DnaG primase and its SSB-Ct interaction. Compounds containing indole and 1*H*-tetrazole scaffolds were identified as first-generation hits. Based on CSP-guided molecular modeling studies, they are involved in formation of various electrostatic and hydrogen bond networks in the binding pockets, which makes them promising starting points for further optimization. Initial in silico fragment-to-lead optimization was carried out using the *ZINC* Database. *Para*-phenyl substituted tetrazoles were identified. The observation that compounds selected for binding to the C-terminal domain of DnaG primase also bind to other SSB-interacting proteins indicates that compounds may in future be derived that bind to similar binding pockets in multiple protein targets, which is a prerequisite for development of antibacterial compounds with a very low propensity for development of resistance.

Supplementary Materials:
Figure S1. Surface plasmon resonance (SPR) competition sensorgram for one of the SPR hits, and saturation transfer difference (STD)-NMR spectrum of SPR hit **D6**; Figure S2. ^{15}N–^{1}H HSQC spectra of DnaGC protein with and without fragment hits **1–3**; Figure S3. Residue-specific weighted chemical shift perturbations induced in ^{15}N-DnaGC by binding to compounds **1–6**; Figure S4. Modeled orientation of fragment **1**; Figure S5. Comparison of chemical shift perturbation (CSP) induced by fragment **1** and compound **L1C6**; Figure S6. Modeled orientation of fragment **3**; Figure S7. Modeled orientation of *N*-acetyl-L-Phe (green carbon atoms) in the SSB-Ct binding pocket of DnaGC (gray carbon atoms). Figure S8. STD NMR spectrum of fragment **4** with four SSB-Ct binding partners other than DnaG primase.

Acknowledgments: This work was supported in part by an infrastructure grant from the Australian Research Council (LE160100047 to M.J.S., N.E.D., and A.J.O.), an ARC Future Fellowship (FT0990287 to A.J.O.), a project grant from the Australian National Health & Medical Research Council (APP1007947 to N.E.D., G.O., and A.J.O.), and a postgraduate scholarship from the University of Wollongong (to Z.C.).

Author Contributions: Z.C., G.O., N.E.D., M.J.S. and A.J.O. conceived and designed the experiments; Z.C. and S.J.H performed the experiments; Z.C., S.J.H., G.O., M.J.S. and A.J.O. analyzed the data; A.T.Y.L. and Z.-Q.X. contributed reagents and new methods; Z.C., N.E.D. and A.J.O. wrote the paper.

References

1. Kobori, J.A.; Kornberg, A. The *Escherichia coli dnaC* gene product. II. Purification, physical properties, and role in replication. *J. Biol. Chem.* **1982**, *257*, 13763–13769. [PubMed]

2. Kobori, J.A.; Kornberg, A. The *Escherichia coli dnaC* gene product. III. Properties of the dnaB–dnaC protein complex. *J. Biol. Chem.* **1982**, *257*, 13770–13775. [PubMed]

3. Tougu, K.; Marians, K.J. The interaction between helicase and primase sets the replication fork clock. *J. Biol. Chem.* **1996**, *271*, 21398–21405. [CrossRef] [PubMed]

4. Kitani, T.; Yoda, K.; Ogawa, T.; Okazaki, T. Evidence that discontinuous DNA replication in *Escherichia coli* is primed by approximately 10 to 12 residues of RNA starting with a purine. *J. Mol. Biol.* **1985**, *184*, 45–52. [CrossRef]

5. Yoda, K.-Y.; Yasuda, H.; Jiang, X.-W.; Okazaki, T. RNA-primed intitiation sites of DNA replication in the origin region of bacteriophage λ genome. *Nucleic Acids Res.* **1998**, *16*, 6531–6546. [CrossRef]

6. Bouché, J.P.; Zechel, K.; Kornberg, A. dnaG gene product, a rifampicin-resistant RNA polymerase, initiates the conversion of a single-stranded coliphage DNA to its duplex replicative form. *J. Biol. Chem.* **1975**, *250*, 5995–6001. [PubMed]

7. Pan, H.; Wigley, D.B. Structure of the zinc-binding domain of *Bacillus stearothermophilus* DNA primase. *Structure* **2000**, *8*, 231–239. [CrossRef]

8. Keck, J.L.; Berger, J.M. Structure of the RNA polymerase domain of *E. coli* primase. *Science* **2000**, *287*, 2482–2486. [CrossRef] [PubMed]

9. Podobnik, M.; McInerney, P.; O'Donnell, M.; Kuriyan, J. A TOPRIM domain in the crystal structure of the catalytic core of *Escherichia coli* primase confirms a structural link to DNA topoisomerases. *J. Mol. Biol.* **2000**, *300*, 353–362. [CrossRef] [PubMed]

10. Sun, W.; Godson, G.N. Interaction of *Escherichia coli* primase with a phage G4ori_c-E. *coli* SSB complex. *J. Bacteriol.* **1996**, *178*, 6701–6705. [CrossRef] [PubMed]

11. Tougu, K.; Marians, K.J. The extreme C terminus of primase is required for interaction with DnaB at the replication fork. *J. Biol. Chem.* **1996**, *271*, 21391–21397. [CrossRef] [PubMed]

12. Yuzhakov, A.; Kelman, Z.; O'Donnell, M. Trading places on DNA–a three-point switch underlies primer handoff from primase to the replicative DNA polymerase. *Cell* **1999**, *96*, 153–163. [CrossRef]

13. Oakley, A.J.; Loscha, K.V.; Schaeffer, P.M.; Liepinsh, E.; Pintacuda, G.; Wilce, M.C.J.; Otting, G.; Dixon, N.E. Crystal and solution structures of the helicase-binding domain of *Escherichia coli* primase. *J. Biol. Chem.* **2005**, *280*, 11495–11504. [CrossRef] [PubMed]

14. Su, X.-C.; Schaeffer, P.M.; Loscha, K.V.; Gan, P.H.P.; Dixon, N.E.; Otting, G. Monomeric solution structure of the helicase-binding domain of *Escherichia coli* DnaG primase. *FEBS J.* **2006**, *273*, 4997–5009. [CrossRef] [PubMed]

15. Shereda, R.D.; Kozlov, A.G.; Lohman, T.M.; Cox, M.M.; Keck, J.L. SSB as an organizer/mobilizer of genome maintenance complexes. *Crit. Rev. Biochem. Mol. Biol.* **2008**, *43*, 289–318. [CrossRef] [PubMed]

16. Robinson, A.; Causer, R.J.; Dixon, N.E. Architecture and conservation of the bacterial DNA replication machinery, an underexploited drug target. *Curr. Drug Targets* **2012**, *13*, 352–372. [CrossRef] [PubMed]

17. Glover, B.P.; McHenry, C.S. The χψ subunits of DNA polymerase III holoenzyme bind to single-stranded DNA-binding protein (SSB) and facilitate replication of an SSB-coated template. *J. Biol. Chem.* **1998**, *273*, 23476–23484. [CrossRef] [PubMed]

18. Kelman, Z.; Yuzhakov, A.; Andjelkovic, J.; O'Donnell, M. Devoted to the lagging strand–the χ subunit of DNA polymerase III holoenzyme contacts SSB to promote processive elongation and sliding clamp assembly. *EMBO J.* **1998**, *17*, 2436–2449. [CrossRef] [PubMed]

19. Witte, G. DNA polymerase III χ subunit ties single-stranded DNA binding protein to the bacterial replication machinery. *Nucleic Acids Res.* **2003**, *31*, 4434–4440. [CrossRef] [PubMed]

20. Fedorov, R.; Witte, G.; Urbanke, C.; Manstein, D.J.; Curth, U. 3D structure of *Thermus aquaticus* single-stranded DNA-binding protein gives insight into the functioning of SSB proteins. *Nucleic Acids Res.* **2006**, *34*, 6708–6717. [CrossRef] [PubMed]

21. Naue, N.; Fedorov, R.; Pich, A.; Manstein, D.J.; Curth, U. Site-directed mutagenesis of the χ subunit of DNA polymerase III and single-stranded DNA-binding protein of *E. coli* reveals key residues for their interaction. *Nucleic Acids Res.* **2011**, *39*, 1398–1407. [CrossRef] [PubMed]

22. Marceau, A.H.; Bahng, S.; Massoni, S.C.; George, N.P.; Sandler, S.J.; Marians, K.J.; Keck, J.L. Structure of the SSB–DNA polymerase III interface and its role in DNA replication. *EMBO J.* **2011**, *30*, 4236–4247. [CrossRef] [PubMed]

23. Bhattacharyya, B.; George, N.P.; Thurmes, T.M.; Zhou, R.; Jani, N.; Wessel, S.R.; Sandler, S.J.; Ha, T.; Keck, J.L. Structural mechanisms of PriA-mediated DNA replication restart. *Proc. Natl. Acad. Sci. USA* **2014**, *111*, 1373–1378. [CrossRef] [PubMed]

24. Lu, D.; Keck, J.L. Structural basis of *Escherichia coli* single-stranded DNA-binding protein stimulation of exonuclease I. *Proc. Natl. Acad. Sci. USA* **2008**, *105*, 9169–9174. [CrossRef] [PubMed]

25. Lu, D.; Windsor, M.A.; Gellman, S.H.; Keck, J.L. Peptide inhibitors identify roles for SSB C-terminal residues in SSB/exonuclease I complex formation. *Biochemistry* **2009**, *48*, 6764–6771. [CrossRef] [PubMed]

26. Naue, N.; Beerbaum, M.; Bogutzki, A.; Schmieder, P.; Curth, U. The helicase-binding domain of *Escherichia coli* DnaG primase interacts with the highly conserved C-terminal region of single-stranded DNA-binding protein. *Nucleic Acids Res.* **2013**, *41*, 4507–4517. [CrossRef] [PubMed]

27. Ryzhikov, M.; Koroleva, O.; Postnov, D.; Tran, A.; Korolev, S. Mechanism of RecO recruitment to DNA by single-stranded DNA binding protein. *Nucleic Acids Res.* **2011**, *39*, 6305–6314. [CrossRef] [PubMed]

28. Chilingaryan, Z.; Yin, Z.; Oakley, A.J. Fragment-based screening by protein crystallography: Successes and pitfalls. *Int. J. Mol. Sci.* **2012**, *13*, 12857–12879. [CrossRef] [PubMed]

29. Mayer, M.; Meyer, B. Characterization of ligand binding by saturation transfer difference NMR spectroscopy. *Angew. Chem. Int. Ed.* **1999**, *38*, 1784–1788. [CrossRef]

30. Doak, B.C.; Morton, C.J.; Simpson, J.S.; Scanlon, M.J. Design and evaluation of the performance of an NMR screening fragment library. *Aust. J. Chem.* **2013**, *66*, 1465–1472. [CrossRef]

31. Humphrey, W.; Dalke, A.; Schulten, K. VMD: Visual molecular dynamics. *J. Mol. Graph.* **1996**, *14*, 33–38. [CrossRef]

32. Malik, M.A.; Wani, M.Y.; Al-Thabaiti, S.A.; Shiekh, R.A. Tetrazoles as carboxylic acid isosteres: Chemistry and biology. *J. Incl. Phenom. Macrocycl. Chem.* **2014**, *78*, 15–37. [CrossRef]

33. Allen, F.H.; Groom, C.R.; Liebeschuetz, J.W.; Bardwell, D.A.; Olsson, T.S.G.; Wood, P.A. The hydrogen bond environments of 1*H*-tetrazole and tetrazolate rings: The structural basis for tetrazole–carboxylic acid bioisosterism. *J. Chem. Inf. Model.* **2012**, *52*, 857–866. [CrossRef] [PubMed]

34. Fielding, L. NMR methods for the determination of protein–ligand dissociation constants. *Curr. Top. Med. Chem.* **2007**, *3*, 39–53. [CrossRef]

35. Lian, L.-Y. NMR studies of weak protein–protein interactions. *Prog. Nucl. Magn. Reson. Spectrosc.* **2013**, *71*, 59–72. [CrossRef] [PubMed]

36. Dalvit, C.; Vulpetti, A. Intermolecular and intramolecular hydrogen bonds involving fluorine atoms: Implications for recognition, selectivity, and chemical properties. *ChemMedChem* **2012**, *7*, 262–272. [CrossRef] [PubMed]

37. Brameld, K.A.; Kuhn, B.; Reuter, D.C.; Stahl, M. Small molecule conformational preferences derived from crystal structure data. A medicinal chemistry focused analysis. *J. Chem. Inf. Model.* **2008**, *48*, 1–24. [CrossRef] [PubMed]

38. Irwin, J.J.; Shoichet, B.K. *ZINC*—A free database of commercially available compounds for virtual screening. *J. Chem. Inf. Model.* **2005**, *45*, 177–182. [CrossRef] [PubMed]

39. Medek, A.; Hajduk, P.J.; Mack, J.; Fesik, S.W. The use of differential chemical shifts for determining the binding site location and orientation of protein-bound ligands. *J. Am. Chem. Soc.* **2000**, *122*, 1241–1242. [CrossRef]

40. Stamford, N.P.J.; Lilley, P.E.; Dixon, N.E. Enriched sources of *Escherichia coli* replication proteins. The dnaG primase is a zinc metalloprotein. *Biochim. Biophys. Acta* **1992**, *1132*, 17–25. [CrossRef]

41. Love, C.A.; Lilley, P.E.; Dixon, N.E. Stable high-copy-number bacteriophage λ promoter vectors for overproduction of proteins in *Escherichia coli*. *Gene* **1996**, *176*, 49–53. [CrossRef]

42. Loscha, K.; Oakley, A.J.; Bancia, B.; Schaeffer, P.M.; Prosselkov, P.; Otting, G.; Wilce, M.C.J.; Dixon, N.E. Expression, purification, crystallization, and NMR studies of the helicase interaction domain of *Escherichia coli* DnaG primase. *Protein Expr. Purif.* **2004**, *33*, 304–310. [CrossRef] [PubMed]

43. Vranken, W.F.; Boucher, W.; Stevens, T.J.; Fogh, R.H.; Pajon, A.; Llinas, M.; Ulrich, E.L.; Markley, J.L.; Ionides, J.; Laue, E.D. The CCPN data model for NMR spectroscopy: Development of a software pipeline. *Proteins* **2005**, *59*, 687–696. [CrossRef] [PubMed]

44. Ziarek, J.J.; Peterson, F.C.; Lytle, B.L.; Volkman, B.F. Binding site identification and structure determination of protein–ligand complexes by NMR: A semiautomated approach. *Methods Enzymol.* **2011**, *493*, 241–275. [PubMed]

45. Trott, O.; Olson, A.J. AutoDock Vina: Improving the speed and accuracy of docking with a new scoring function, efficient optimization, and multithreading. *J. Comput. Chem.* **2010**, *31*, 455–461. [CrossRef] [PubMed]

46. Lo, A.T.Y.; Oakley, A.J.; Dixon, N.E. The DnaG primase interaction with single-stranded DNA-binding protein (SSB). Manuscript in preparation.

47. Li, H.; Robertson, A.D.; Jensen, J.H. Very fast empirical prediction and rationalization of protein pK_a values. *Proteins* **2005**, *61*, 704–721. [CrossRef] [PubMed]

8

Protective Effects of Bacteriophages against *Aeromonas hydrophila* Causing Motile Aeromonas Septicemia (MAS) in Striped Catfish

Tuan Son Le [1,2], Thi Hien Nguyen [3], Hong Phuong Vo [3], Van Cuong Doan [3], Hong Loc Nguyen [3], Minh Trung Tran [3], Trong Tuan Tran [3], Paul C. Southgate [4] and D. İpek Kurtböke [1,*] ⓘ

[1] GeneCology Research Centre, Faculty of Science, Health, Education and Engineering, University of the Sunshine Coast, 90 Sippy Downs Drive, Sippy Downs, QLD 4556, Australia; tuan.son.le@research.usc.edu.au
[2] Research Institute for Marine Fisheries, 224 Le Lai, Ngo Quyen, Hai Phong 180000, Vietnam
[3] Research Institute for Aquaculture No. 2, 116 Nguyen Dinh Chieu, District 1, Ho Chi Minh 700000, Vietnam; nguyenhien05@gmail.com (T.H.N.); vohongphuong@gmail.com (H.P.V.); vancuongdisaqua@gmail.com (V.C.D.); hongloc@gmail.com (H.L.N.); trung16893@yahoo.com.vn (M.T.T.); tuantran_695@yahoo.com.vn (T.T.T.)
[4] Australian Centre for Pacific Islands Research and Faculty of Science, Health, Education and Engineering, University of the Sunshine Coast, Maroochydore, QLD 4556, Australia; psouthgate@usc.edu.au
* Correspondence: ikurtbok@usc.edu.au

Abstract: To determine the effectivity of bacteriophages in controlling the mass mortality of striped catfish (*Pangasianodon hypophthalmus*) due to infections caused by *Aeromonas* spp. in Vietnamese fish farms, bacteriophages against pathogenic *Aeromonas hydrophila* were isolated. *A. hydrophila*-phage 2 and *A. hydrophila*-phage 5 were successfully isolated from water samples from the Saigon River of Ho Chi Minh City, Vietnam. These phages, belonging to the *Myoviridae* family, were found to have broad activity spectra, even against the tested multiple-antibiotic-resistant *Aeromonas* isolates. The latent periods and burst size of phage 2 were 10 min and 213 PFU per infected host cell, respectively. The bacteriophages proved to be effective in inhibiting the growth of the *Aeromonas* spp. under laboratory conditions. Phage treatments applied to the pathogenic strains during infestation of catfish resulted in a significant improvement in the survival rates of the tested fishes, with up to 100% survival with MOI 100, compared to 18.3% survival observed in control experiments. These findings illustrate the potential for using phages as an effective bio-treatment method to control Motile Aeromonas Septicemia (MAS) in fish farms. This study provides further evidence towards the use of bacteriophages to effectively control disease in aquaculture operations.

Keywords: *Aeromonas hydrophila*; Motile Aeromonas Septicemia; MAS; multiple-antibiotic-resistance; bacteriophage; biological control; striped catfish (*Pangasianodon hypophthalmus*)

1. Introduction

Striped catfish (*Pangasianodon hypophthalmus*) is one of the most important farmed fish species, especially in Vietnam, Thailand, Cambodia, Laos and, more recently, the Philippines and Indonesia [1]. Vietnam supplied 90% of catfish production with a value of US$1.1 to 1.7 billion in 2015. Motile Aeromonas Septicemia (MAS), also called haemorrhage disease or red spot disease, causes great losses for farmers (up to 80% mortality) and presents in fish with clinical signs of haemorrhages on the head, mouth, and at the base of fins, a red, swollen vent, and the presence of pink to yellow ascitic fluid [2]. *Aeromonas hydrophila*, *Aeromonas caviae*, and *Aeromonas sobria* species were often isolated from diseased catfish, and new species such as *Aeromonas dhakensis* and *Aeromonas veronii* were also reported by using molecular methods based on the sequencing of the *rpoD* gene [3].

Multiple antibiotic resistance (MAR) of *A. hydrophila* strains has been reported in different countries. Vivekanandhan et al. [4] tested 319 strains of *A. hydrophila* isolated from fish and prawns in South India and indicated that all of them were resistant to methicillin, rifampicin, bacitracin, and novobiocin (99%). Moreover, 21 *Aeromonas* spp. isolated from carp showed resistance to ampicillin and penicillin [5]. Recently, Thi et al. [6] tested antibiotic resistance of 30 strains of *A. hydrophila* isolated from diseased striped catfish in the Mekong Delta from January 2013 to March 2014. The study found that *A. hydrophila* isolates were highly resistant to tetracycline and florfenicol and were completely resistant to trimethoprim, sulfamethoxazole, ampicillin, amoxicillin, and cefalexine.

ALPHA JECT ® Panga 2 vaccine, protecting against *Edwardsiella ictaluri* and *A. hydrophila*, has been approved for market in Vietnam since the early 2017 (https://www.pharmaq.no/updates/pharmaq-fish-va/). However, the cost-effectiveness of vaccine use in catfish production is another obstacle in intensive catfish production. Moreover, the development of a commercial vaccine against *A. hydrophila* has been slow because *A. hydrophia* is biochemically and serologically heterogeneous [7]. Therefore, there is a need for effective, environmentally safe control measures for managing MAS in catfish.

One approach has been the use of bacteriophages (phages) to control pathogenic bacteria in aquaculture operations. Recently, studies related to the use of phages specific to *A. hydrophila* in aquaculture have gained attention. Hsu et al. [8] isolated two *A. hydrophila* phages and three *Edwardsiella tarda* phages to treat disease in eels (*Anguilla japonica*) in vitro. The phages reduced bacterial density by about 1000 times after 2 h when the MOI was 11.5 at 25 °C in the fluid environment. El-Araby et al. [9] demonstrated the effectiveness of bacteriophage ZH1 and ZH2 treatment against *A. hydrophila* in Tilapia, improving the survival rates by up to 82%.

However, so far, treatments using bacteriophages against pathogens causing MAS in catfish have not been studied extensively. The objective of this study was, therefore, to isolate bacteriophages infective in pathogenic *A. hydrophila* with a long-term objective to eradicate this disease-causing pathogen in aquaculture operations.

2. Results

2.1. Prophage Induction

No reduction in the optical density of bacterial suspension treated with Mitomycin C (Table S1, Supplementary Materials) and no clear zones from the spot technique were observed. Therefore, it was concluded that there was no prophage in *A. hydrophila* N17.

2.2. Antibiotic Susceptibility

All isolates were completely (100%) resistant to oxytetracycline, ampicillin, gentamycin and amoxicillin/clavulanic acid, enrofloxacin, and bactrim. Nearly all isolates (83.3%) were resistant to kanamycin and 33.3% were resistant to tetracycline, doxycycline, and ciprofloxacin (Table 1).

Table 1. Antibiogram profile of the *Aeromonas hydrophila* strains tested.

Antibiotics	Number of Resistant Isolates ($n = 6$)
Tetracycline	2
Oxytetracycline	6
Gentamycin	6
Kanamycin	5
Bactrim (SMX/TMP)	6
Doxycycline	2
Enrofloxacin	6
Amoxicillin/clavulanic acid	6
Ampicillin	6
Ciprofloxacin	2

2.3. Isolation and Characterization of Bacteriophages

The A. hydrophila-phage 2 (or Φ2) and A. hydrophila-phage 5 (or Φ5) were successfully isolated against the propagation hosts used (Figure 1 and Table 2).

Φ2 had an isometric head of 129 nm in diameter with a tail sheath 173 nm long and 15 nm wide. Φ5 was composed of: (i) an isometric head of 120 nm in diameter, (ii) a tail sheath of 198 nm in length and 15 nm in width. All of the phages had contractile tails (Figure 1 and Table 2).

Table 2. Characteristics of bacteriophages against *A. hydrophila* strains.

Φ	Concentration PFU/mL	Head (nm)		Neck (nm)		Tail Sheath (nm)		Genus
		L	W	L	W	L	W	
2	10^9		129	10	15	173	15	*Spounalikevirus*
5	10^{10}		120	15	15	198	15	*Spounalikevirus*

W: width; L: length.

Both phages produced clear plaques with diameters of 0.1 mm (Figure 1).

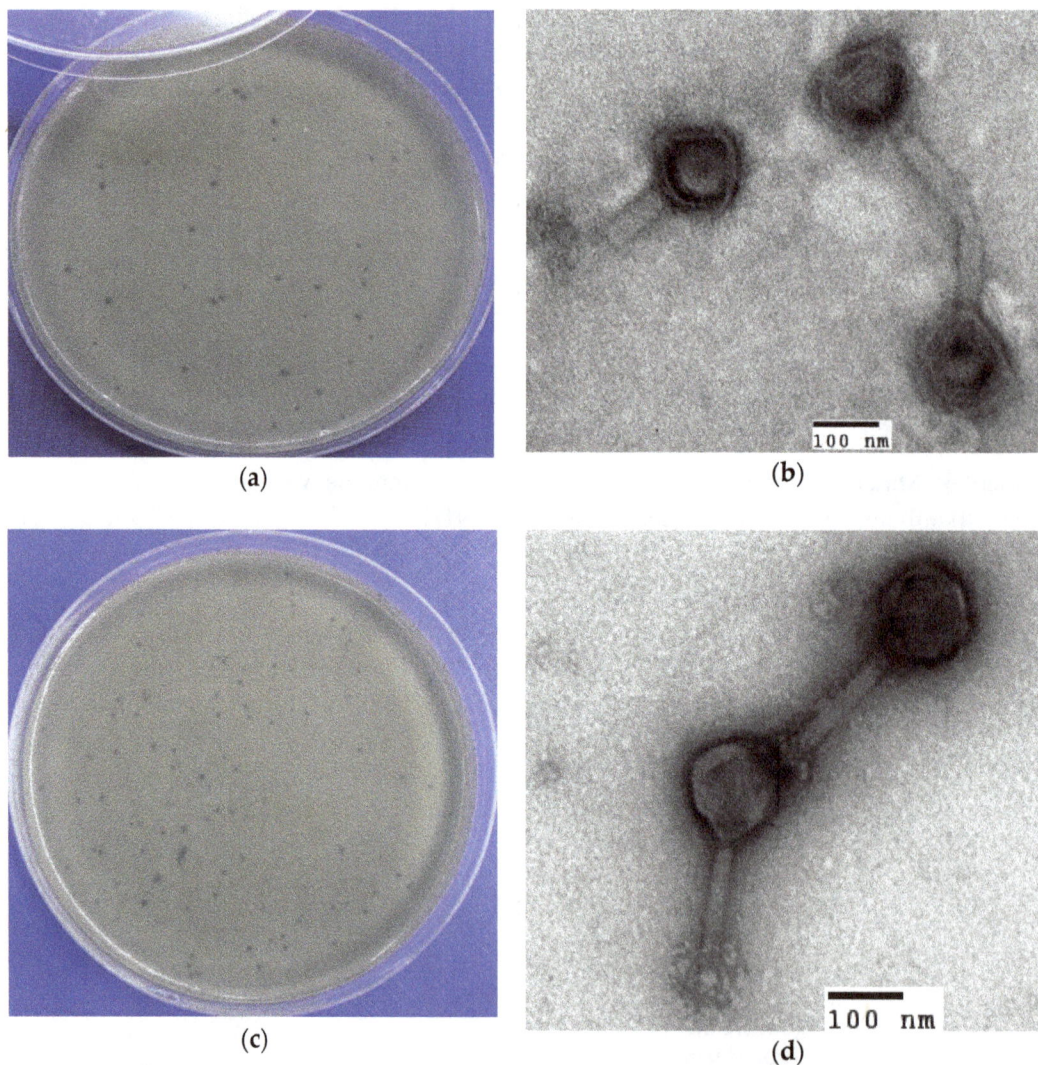

Figure 1. Plaque formation and microphotograph of *A. hydrophila* phages. (**a**,**b**) Φ2 and (**c**,**d**) phage Φ5.

The genome size of the phage isolates was above 20 kb. The genomic material of the isolated phages was not digested by Mung bean nuclease and RNase A. Since Mung bean nuclease specifically cuts single-stranded nucleic acids of both DNA and RNA, it was concluded that the genomic DNA of both phages was double-stranded. RNA nucleic acids are degraded by RNase A, therefore, the nucleic acids of Φ2 and Φ5 were determined as double-stranded DNA (dsDNA) (Figure 2). The phages Φ2 and Φ5 belong to the Myoviridae family.

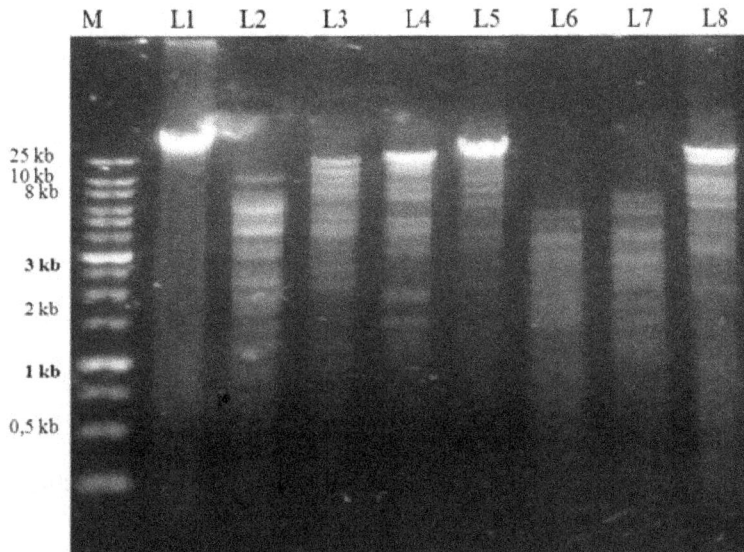

Figure 2. Restriction enzyme-digested fragments of the genomic DNA of *A. hydrophila*-phage 2. Footnote: Lane M: 1kb Plus Opti-DNA Marker (ABM, Canada); Lane L1: genomic DNA of Φ2; Lanes L2–L8: genomic DNA of Φ2 digested with EcoRV; EcoRI; Ncol; SalI; MspI; XmnI; KpnI, restriction enzymes respectively.

2.4. Host Range

Phage 2 and phage 5 were found to inhibit the growth of all *A. hydrophila* strains tested. None of the other 27 species was found to be susceptible to these phages (Table S2, Supplementary Materials).

2.5. Adsorption Rate of Phages and One-Step Growth Curve

The number of free phages in suspension decreased over time, as illustrated in the adsorption curve (Figure 3a). At 40 min, the percentage of Φ2-infected bacteria was over 90%.

The one-step growth experiment (Figure 3b) results revealed that the latent period and burst size of Φ2 were 10 and 213 PFU per infected host cell, respectively.

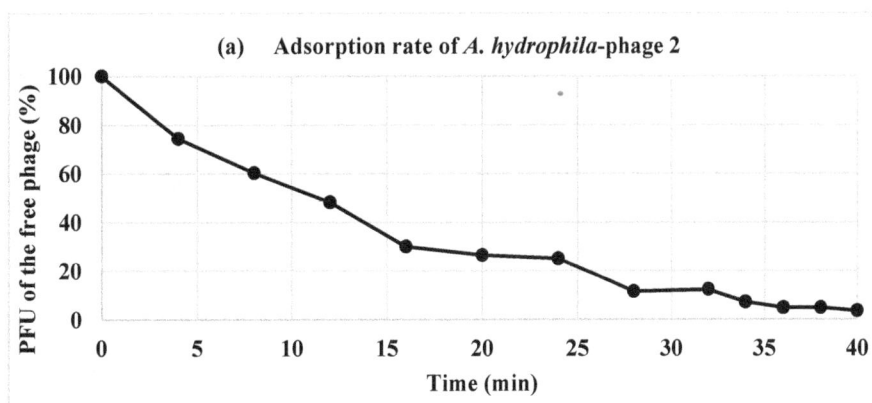

Figure 3. *Cont.*

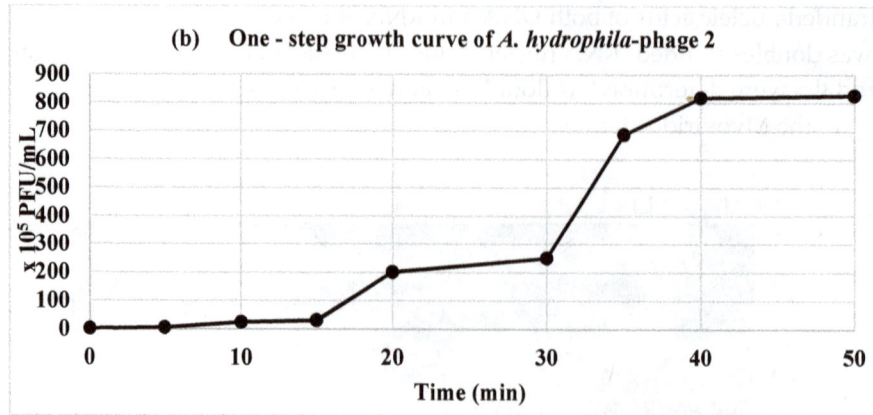

Figure 3. (**a**) Adsorption rate and (**b**) one-step growth curves of Φ2.

2.6. Inactivation of Aeromonas Species in Vitro

The bacterial concentration (OD_{550nm} values) of the uninfected control (only *A. hydrophila* N17) increased continuously during 18 h of incubation. In contrast, during the infection with Φ2 at MOI 1, MOI 0.1, and MOI 0.01 bacterial growth began to be inhibited at 1, 2, and 2.5 h, respectively, and the inhibition was maintained up to 8 h (Figure 4a). Then, the bacterial concentration increased as a consequence of the development of phage-resistant *A. hydrophila* cells.

The lowest OD_{550nm} value was 0.177 ± 0.023 after 4 h of incubation of Φ5 at MOI 0.1. There was a significant decline in the bacterial concentration (MOI 0.01, 0.1, and 1) in the first 3 h, followed by low level stabilization in the next 1, 2, and 4 h for MOI 1, 0.1, and 0.01, respectively (Figure 4b). Then, the bacterial concentration underwent a turnaround because of the development of phage-resistant *A. hydrophila* cells.

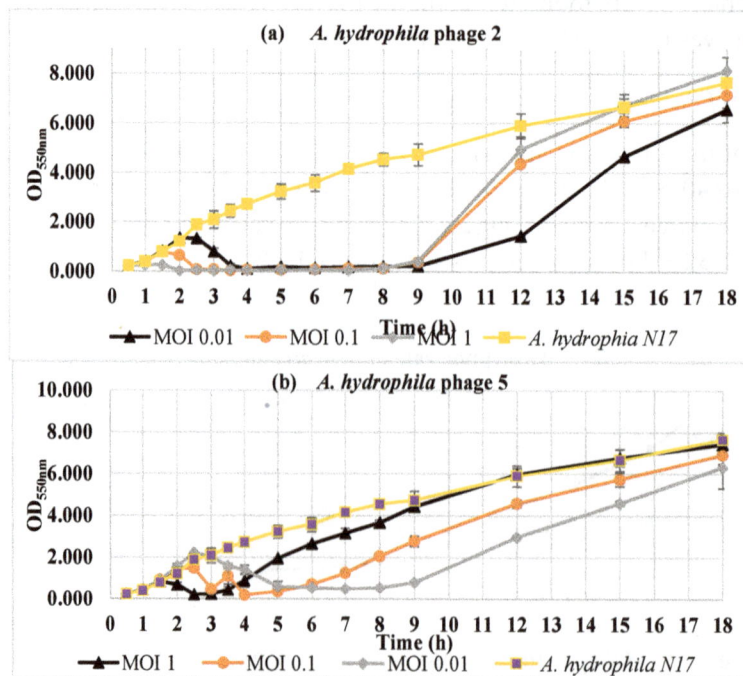

Figure 4. Inactivation of *A. hydrophila* N17 by the phages (**a**) Φ2 and (**b**) Φ5 at different MOI (0.01, 0.1 and 1).

2.7. Phage Treatment of Infected Fish

The negative control 1 (fishes with no injection) and negative control 2 (fishes injected with the growth medium filtered to remove bacterial cells) showed no mortality of catfish (Figure 5), indicating that the uninfected, control medium did not have any detrimental effect on fish health.

Catfish in the positive control groups (infected with *A. hydrophila* N17) that were not treated with bacteriophages started to die at a constant rate starting from post-infection day two, with a cumulative mortality rate of $81.67 \pm 2.36\%$ (Figure 5).

In contrast, the fish treated with the phages showed lower mortality rates at each different MOI ($p < 0.01$). While no mortality was observed in the groups treated with MOI 100, the cumulative mortalities in the other groups were 45% (MOI 1) and $68.33 \pm 2.36\%$ (MOI 0.01) at the end of the eight-day experiment (Figure 5).

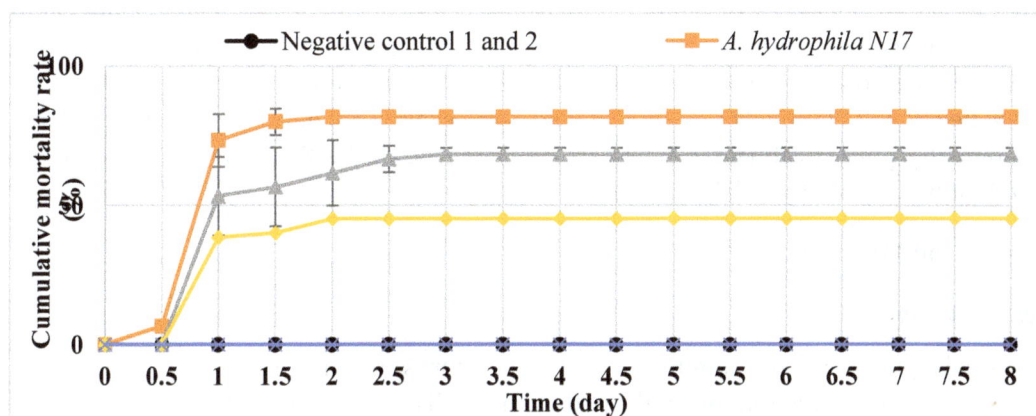

Figure 5. Cumulative mortality rates (%) of striped catfishes obtained in challenging experiments using *A. hydrophia* N17 and the phage cocktail at the different MOIs (0.01, 0.1, and 1). The ratio of Φ2 to Φ5 in a phage cocktail was 1:1.

3. Discussion

The findings of this study demonstrate that the examined *Aeromonas* spp. were resistant to multiple antibiotics and were thus able to cause high mortality rates in catfish in Vietnam, in spite of the use of various antibiotic treatments. In the bacteriophage treatments, however, Φ2 and Φ5 were able to lyse all tested *A. hydrophila* strains, displaying strong inhibition also of the virulent *A. hydrophila* strains carrying many virulence genes. Therefore, Φ2 and Φ5 are promising candidates for the application of a phage therapy to control *Aeromonas* infection in catfish.

Phage Φ2 and Φ5 were found to belong to the *Myoviridae* family, and our findings are in line with those of Ackermann [10] who indicated that 33 of a total of 43 *Aeromonas* phages he investigated were tailed and belonged to the *Myoviridae* family. Recently, other *Aeromonas* phage studies against different *Aeromonas* species by Haq et al. [11], Jun et al. [12], and Kim et al. [13] also reported that all phages they identified belonged to the *Myoviridae* family. Therefore, *Myoviridae* family members are most likely to be abundant in natural environments.

There was a correlation between the diameter of the plaques observed and the latent period and burst size for the *A. hydrophila* phage. The Φ2 had a short latent period (10 min), and these findings are in line with another study conducted by Anand et al. [14] who found that *Aeromonas* phage BPA 6 had a latent period of 10 min and a burst size of 244 PFU/cell.

The different MOI of Φ2 and Φ5 caused different bacterial growth patterns. The higher the MOI value, the sooner phage-resistant bacterial cells appeared. A similar result was noted by Kim et al. [13] for the phage PAS 1 against an *Aeromonas salmonicida* strain, indicating that bacterial resistance appeared after 3, 6, and 24 h at MOIs 10, 1, and 0.1, respectively.

Several *Aeromonas* phages, such as Aeh1, Aeh2, AH1 have also been reported [12,15,16]. However, there have been few reports demonstrating the successful use of phages for the treatment of *Aeromonas* infections in catfish. The treatment of catfish by an intraperitoneal (IP) injection illustrated significant protective effects, which increased the relative percentages of the survival rates observed for fish compared to the controls when the MOI increased. Our study revealed that in the MOI-100 experiment the relative percentage survival was 100%. The study of Jun et al. [12] showed that the relative percentage survival of fish treated with *A. hydrophila* phages pAh6-C and pAh1-C was $16.67 \pm 3.82\%$ and $43.33 \pm 2.89\%$, respectively, when the fish were injected with the bacterium (2.6×10^7 CFU/fish). However, the labour-intensive and time-consuming mode of delivery of bacteriophages can constitute a disadvantage for the treatment of fish by IP injection in catfish farms. Therefore, further studies should be conducted into whether phage treatments are effective when an on-farm oral method of administration is evaluated. With the use of bioreactors, large volumes of bacteriophages can be produced for bacteriophage incorporation into fish feed. Moreover, the survival of phages and their persistent survival on or in fish, as well as in phage-coated feed preparations should be studied under different environmental factors (e.g., temperature, salt concentration) to determine whether phages are able to persist and effectively reduce *Aeromonas* spp. levels in fish farms. In conclusion, this study demonstrates that phage treatment of *Aeromonas* spp. might be an effective tool to improve the survival of farmed catfish affected by MAS.

4. Materials and Methods

4.1. Aeromonas Species

Bacterial isolates stored at the Research Institute for Aquaculture No. 2 (Ho Chi Minh City, Vietnam) and the ATCC type strains of the pathogens are listed in Table S2. Isolates were previously obtained from diseased catfish in farms in the south of Vietnam (Table S2).

4.2. Prophage Induction

In order to choose an *Aeromonas* species as a propagation host for phage isolation, *A. hydrophila* N17 was subjected to a prophage induction test. The *Aeromonas* species was cultured in 10 mL fresh Luria-Bertani (or LB) broth (Sigma-Aldrich, St. Louis, MO, USA) and incubated at 30 °C on an orbital shaker operating at 150 rpm until reaching an OD_{550nm} of 0.2. Mitomycin C (Sigma-Aldrich) was added to a final concentration of 1 μg/mL and 5 μg/mL, and again the bacterial suspension was incubated at 30 °C on an orbital shaker operating at 150 rpm. The cell density of the bacteria (OD_{550nm}) was monitored every 1 h for a 6 h period. At the end of the incubation, the bacterial suspension was centrifuged at 10,000 g for 15 min and filtered through a nitrocellulose filter (0.45 μm, Merck Millipore, Burlington, MA, USA) before spotting the filtrate onto an agar plate seeded with the host bacterium to confirm the presence of viable phage particles. A significant decrease in the cell density (OD_{550nm}) suggested that prophages were released [17,18].

4.3. Antibiotic Susceptibility

Antibiotic susceptibility tests of six *A. hydrophila* strains [3] were conducted against 10 different antimicrobial susceptibility discs (OXOID, Hampshire, UK) by the method recommended by the Clinical and Laboratory Standards Institute [19]. The antimicrobial agents tested included tetracycline (30 μg), doxycycline (30 μg), oxytetracycline (30 μg), bactrim (SMX/TMP) (23.75/1.25 μg), gentamycin (40 μg), kanamycin (30 μg), ciprofloxacin (10 μg), enrofloxacin (10 μg), ampicillin (33 μg), and amoxicillin-clavulanic acid (20/10 μg).

The antimicrobial susceptibility of *Aeromonas* species is usually recorded using Enterobacteriaceae breakpoints [20]. Susceptible (S), intermediate resistance (I), and resistant (R) were evaluated according the criteria given in the Performance Standards for Antimicrobial Susceptibility Testing M100-S21

(2017, Table 2A-1, pages 33–39) [19]. Multi-antibiotic resistance (MAR) was recorded when the bacteria resisted to three or more antibiotics [21].

4.4. Isolation and Characterization of Bacteriophages

Phages were isolated from water samples from the Saigon River in the south of Vietnam against *A. hydrophila* N17 and they were purified following the methods described by Jun et al. [12].

Phage titres were determined using both surface spread [22,23] and double-layer [24] agar plaque assay techniques where agar plates were previously seeded with the *Aeromonas* sp. ($\times 10^6$ CFU/mL).

For transmission electron microscopy (TEM): A 200 mesh copper grid was immersed in 40 μL of phage solution for five min before fixing the phage with glutaraldehyde solution (1%) for five min. Then, the phage samples were negatively stained with 5% (*w/v*) uranyl acetate and observed by TEM (JEOL JEM-1010) operating at a voltage of 80 kV at the Vietnam National Institute of Hygiene and Epidemiology. The phage morphology was determined using the criteria of the International Committee on Taxonomy of Viruses (ICTV) (http://www.ictvonline.org/) and Ackermann et al. [25].

Phage genomic DNA extraction and restriction analyses: Phage genomic DNA was extracted using the Phage DNA Isolation Kit (Norgen Biotek Corp, Thorold, Canada). The nature of the nucleic acids was determined by digestion with Mung bean nuclease and RNase A (ThermoFisher Scientific, Waltham, MA, USA) as per the manufacturer's protocols. The genomic DNA phages were digested using the restriction enzymes: EcoRV, EcoRI, Ncol, SalI, MspI, XmnI, and KpnI, as per the manufacturer's instruction (ThermoFisher Scientific). The DNA fragments were then electrophoresed at 120 V for 40 min.

4.5. Host Range

The method was adapted from Le et al. [23] and Goodridge et al. [26] with some modifications described below. The *Aeromonas* spp. (Table S2) were incubated overnight. Then, a 100 μL aliquot of each *Aeromonas* spp. culture (optical density of 0.5 at 550 nm) was spread on brain heart infusion agar (BHIA) (OXOID, UK) and dried for 20 min in a biological safety cabinet Class II. The host range of the phage was determined by pipetting 10 μL of phage preparation (~10^8 PFU/mL) on lawn cultures of the strains. The plates were observed for the appearance of clear zones after incubation at 30 °C after 18 h.

4.6. Adsorption Rate of Phages

Phage adsorption was studied using the method described previously [27]. A phage solution was added to 100 mL of log-phase growing *Aeromonas hydrophila* N17 culture ($\times 10^7$ CFU/mL) in LB broth to get a final MOI of 0.1. The mixture was incubated at 30 °C. An aliquot of 1 mL was collected from the sample every two min over a period of 60 min. The sample was then centrifuged at 4000 g for 15 min, and then the supernatant was diluted with SM buffer + 1% chloroform (http://cshprotocols.cshlp.org/content/2006/1/pdb.rec8111.full?text_only=true). Then, the titers of unabsorbed free phages in the supernatant were determined by the double-layer agar technique, and the results were recorded as percentages of the initial phage counts. The percentages of free phages and the adsorption rates were calculated following the formula of Haq et al. [11].

4.7. One-Step Growth Curve

The phage and bacteria were prepared in the same way as in the adsorption method described above. At 40 min, when the adsorption rate was maximal, the mixture was further incubated at 30 °C with 150 rpm. Samples were collected every 5 min for 120 min and phage titers were determined by the double-layer agar technique. Then, the latent period and burst size were calculated [28].

4.8. Inactivation of Aeromonas hydrophila N17 in Vitro

The method used in this study was adapted from Jun et al. [12] and Le et al. [23] with some modifications described below. *A. hydrophila* N17 was streaked onto sheep blood agar (OXOID, UK), incubated at 30 °C overnight, and harvested on LB to have a final concentration of 10^7 CFU/mL. A 10 mL suspension of the *Aeromonas* sp. in LB (around 10^7 CFU/mL) was then mixed with same volume of a phage preparation (concentration of 10^5 to 10^7 PFU/mL) to reach multiplicity of infection (MOI) of 0.01, 0.1, 1 (http://www.bio-protocol.org/e1295). A 20 mL sample of *Aeromonas* sp. in LB ($\sim \times 10^7$ CFU/mL) was used as a control. The mixture was incubated at 30 °C and 150 rpm. Samples were taken every 30 min for 8 h to determine the exact time of the appearance of phage-resistant bacteria, and every 60 min for the next 6 h to determine the increase in the concentration of phage-resistant bacteria. Then, samples were withdrawn every 3 h to the end of the experiment. The concentration of the *Aeromonas* sp. was measured by optical density determination at 550 nm using a spectrophotometer (Thermo Scientific Genesys 20, Waltham, MA, USA).

4.9. Phage Treatment of Infected Fish

A total of 360 healthy catfish (*Pangasianodon hypophthalmus*) (30 g/fish) were divided into 12 groups in 50 L plastic tanks at 30 $\pm$ 1 °C. All treatment fishes were infected intraperitoneally with *A. hydrophila* N17 (final concentration: 3.2×10^6 CFU/fish) and were then immediately injected with a phage cocktail (MOI 0.01, 1 and 100). A positive control was composed of fishes injected with *A. hydrophila* N17 only. Negative controls 1 and 2 were fishes with no injection and fishes injected with fluid separated from the broth containing bacteria and medium, respectively. The mixed phage preparation consisted of Φ2 and Φ5.

The mortality rates of the fishes were recorded every 12 h for eight days, and the kidneys of both the dead and surviving fishes were subjected to a bacterial isolation study [3]. Bacteria isolation was carried out from all dead fishes, indicating that the deaths were caused by *A. hydrophila* [3]. All treatments were performed in duplicates.

The animal experiment was conducted according to the animal ethical guidelines of the Vietnamese government (project supported by Vietnam Ministry of Agriculture and Rural Development, 2016–2018, number: 04/TCTS-KHCN-HTQT-DT 2016).

4.10. Statistical analysis

IBM SPSS Statistics 20 software was used to analyze the data. Single factor ANOVA was applied to test for differences in the fish numbers in the *Aeromonas*-infected fishes receiving or not the phage therapy ($p < 0.05$). Standard deviations were calculated in all experiments.

5. Conclusions

The phages Φ2 and Φ5, belonging to the *Myoviridae* family, were successfully isolated and displayed inhibition of the growth of the *A. hydrophila* strains tested. The results obtained from the use of a phage cocktail indicate that phages can be used successfully for the treatment of *Aeromonas* infections in catfish via intraperitoneal injection. Phages may therefore be considered as potential biocontrol agents to combat *Aeromonas* infections in fish farms.

Acknowledgments: Authors would like to acknowledge the financial support from the Vietnam Ministry of Agriculture and Rural Development (2016–2018, number: 04/TCTS-KHCN-HTQT-DT). Son Le Tuan gratefully acknowledges MOET-VIED/USC PhD scholarship.

Author Contributions: Tuan Son Le analysed the data and drafted the manuscript. Thi Hien Nguyen, Hong Phuong Vo, Trong Tuan Tran, Hong Loc Nguyen, Van Cuong Doan, Minh Trung Tran and Tuan Son Le conducted the experiments under the guidance of Ipek Kurtböke, Thi Hien Nguyen, and Hong Phuong Vo, D. Ipek Kurtböke and Paul C. Southgate oversaw the preparation of the manuscript.

References

1. Nguyen, N. Improving Sustainability of Striped Catfish (*Pangasianodon hypophthalmus*) Farming in the Mekong Delta, Vietnam through Recirculation Technology. Ph.D. Thesis, Wageningen University, Wageningen, The Netherlands, 2016.

2. Dung, T.; Ngoc, N.; Thinh, N.; Thy, D.; Tuan, N.; Shinn, A.; Crumlish, M. Common diseases of pangasius catfish farmed in Viet Nam. *GAA* **2008**, *11*, 77–78.

3. Hien, N.T.; Lan, M.T.; Anh, P.V.N.; Phuong, V.H.; Loc, N.H.; Trong, C.Q.; Trung, C.T.; Phuoc, L.H. Report "Genetics of *Aeromonas hydrophila* on Catfish". *Research Institute for Aquaculture No. 2*. 2014. Available online: http://www.sinhhoctomvang.vn/ban-tin/chi-tiet/Phat-hien-gen-gay-doc-cua-vi-khuan-Aeromonas-hydrophila-gay-benh-xuat-huyet-tren-ca-tra-106/ (accessed on 7 August 2017). (in Vietnamese).

4. Vivekanandhan, G.; Savithamani, K.; Hatha, A.; Lakshmanaperumalsamy, P. Antibiotic resistance of *aeromonas hydrophila* isolated from marketed fish and prawn of south India. *Int. J. Food Microbiol.* **2002**, *76*, 165–168. [CrossRef]

5. Guz, L.; Kozinska, A. Antibiotic susceptibility of *Aeromonas hydrophila* and *A. sobria* isolated from farmed carp (*cyprinus carpio l.*). *Bull. Vet. Inst. Pulawy* **2004**, *48*, 391–395.

6. Thi, Q.V.C.; Dung, T.T.; Hiep, D.P.H. The current status antimicrobial resistance in *Edwardsiella ictaluri* and *Aeromonas hydrophila* cause disease on the striped catfish farmed in the mekong delta. *Cantho Univ. J. Sci.* **2014**, *2*, 7–14. (In vietnamese)

7. Pridgeon, J.W.; Klesius, P.H. Major bacterial diseases in aquaculture and their vaccine development. *CAB Rev.* **2012**, *7*, 1–16. [CrossRef]

8. Hsu, C.-H.; Lo, C.-Y.; Liu, J.-K.; Lin, C.-S. Control of the eel (*anguilla japonica*) pathogens, *Aeromonas hydrophila* and *Edwardsiella tarda*, by bacteriophages. *J. Fish. Soc. Taiwan* **2000**, *27*, 21–31.

9. El-Araby, D.; El-Didamony, G.; Megahed, M. New approach to use phage therapy against *Aeromonas hydrophila* induced Motile Aeromonas Septicemia in nile tilapia. *J. Mar. Sci. Res. Dev.* **2016**, *6*. [CrossRef]

10. Ackermann, H.-W. 5500 phages examined in the electron microscope. *Arch. Virol.* **2007**, *152*, 227–243. [CrossRef] [PubMed]

11. Haq, I.U.; Chaudhry, W.N.; Andleeb, S.; Qadri, I. Isolation and partial characterization of a virulent bacteriophage ihq1 specific for *Aeromonas punctata* from stream water. *Microb. Ecol.* **2012**, *63*, 954–963. [CrossRef] [PubMed]

12. Jun, J.W.; Kim, J.H.; Shin, S.P.; Han, J.E.; Chai, J.Y.; Park, S.C. Protective effects of the *Aeromonas* phages pah1-c and pah6-c against mass mortality of the cyprinid loach (*misgurnus anguillicaudatus*) caused by *Aeromonas hydrophila*. *Aquaculture* **2013**, *416*, 289–295. [CrossRef]

13. Kim, J.; Son, J.; Choi, Y.; Choresca, C.; Shin, S.; Han, J.; Jun, J.; Kang, D.; Oh, C.; Heo, S. Isolation and characterization of a lytic *Myoviridae* bacteriophage pas-1 with broad infectivity in *Aeromonas salmonicida*. *Curr. Microbiol.* **2012**, *64*, 418–426. [CrossRef] [PubMed]

14. Anand, T.; Vaid, R.K.; Bera, B.C.; Singh, J.; Barua, S.; Virmani, N.; Yadav, N.K.; Nagar, D.; Singh, R.K.; Tripathi, B. Isolation of a lytic bacteriophage against virulent *Aeromonas hydrophila* from an organized equine farm. *J. Basic Microb.* **2016**, *56*, 432–437. [CrossRef] [PubMed]

15. Chow, M.S.; Rouf, M. Isolation and partial characterization of two *Aeromonas hydrophila* bacteriophages. *Appl. Environ. Microbiol.* **1983**, *45*, 1670–1676. [PubMed]

16. Wu, J.-L.; Lin, H.-M.; Jan, L.; Hsu, Y.-L.; Chang, L.-H. Biological control of fish bacterial pathogen, *Aeromonas hydrophila*, by bacteriophage ah 1. *Fish Pathol.* **1981**, *15*, 271–276. [CrossRef]

17. Fortier, L.-C.; Moineau, S. Morphological and genetic diversity of temperate phages in clostridium difficile. *Appl. Environ. Microbiol.* **2007**, *73*, 7358–7366. [CrossRef] [PubMed]

18. Walakira, J.; Carrias, A.; Hossain, M.; Jones, E.; Terhune, J.; Liles, M. Identification and characterization of bacteriophages specific to the catfish pathogen, *Edwardsiella ictaluri*. *J. Appl. Microbiol.* **2008**, *105*, 2133–2142. [CrossRef] [PubMed]

19. CLSI. Performance standards for antimicrobial susceptibility testing 27th ed. CLSI supplement m100. *Clinical and Laboratory Standards Institute.* 2017. Available online: http://www.facm.ucl.ac.be/intranet/CLSI/CLSI-2017-M100-S27.pdf (accessed on 10 November 2017).

20. Lamy, B.; Laurent, F.; Kodjo, A.; Roger, F.; Jumas-Bilak, E.; Marchandin, H.; Group, C.S. Which antibiotics and breakpoints should be used for *Aeromonas* susceptibility testing? Considerations from a comparison of agar dilution and disk diffusion methods using Enterobacteriaceae breakpoints. *Eur. J. Clin. Microbiol. Infect. Dis.* **2012**, *31*, 2369–2377. [CrossRef] [PubMed]

21. Daka, D.; Yihdego, D. Antibiotic-resistance *Staphylococcus aureus* isolated from cow's milk in the hawassa area, south Ethiopia. *Ann. Clin. Microbiol. Antimicrob.* **2012**, *11*. [CrossRef] [PubMed]

22. Cerveny, K.E.; DePaola, A.; Duckworth, D.H.; Gulig, P.A. Phage therapy of local and systemic disease caused by *Vibrio vulnificus* in iron-dextran-treated mice. *Infect. Immun.* **2002**, *70*, 6251–6262. [CrossRef] [PubMed]

23. Le, T.S.; Southgate, P.C.; O'Connor, W.; Poole, S.; Kurtböke, D.I. Bacteriophages as biological control agents of enteric bacteria contaminating edible oysters. *Curr. Microbiol.* **2017**. [CrossRef] [PubMed]

24. Paterson, W.; Douglas, R.; Grinyer, I.; McDermott, L. Isolation and preliminary characterization of some *Aeromonas salmonicida* bacteriophages. *J. Fish. Board Canada* **1969**, *26*, 629–632. [CrossRef]

25. Ackermann, H.-W.; Dauguet, C.; Paterson, W.; Popoff, M.; Rouf, M.; Vieu, J.-F. *Aeromonas* bacteriophages: Reexamination and classification. *Ann. Inst. Pasteur Virol.* **1985**, *136*, 175–199. [CrossRef]

26. Goodridge, L.; Gallaccio, A.; Griffiths, M.W. Morphological, host range, and genetic characterization of two coliphages. *Appl. Environ. Microbiol.* **2003**, *69*, 5364–5371. [CrossRef] [PubMed]

27. Phumkhachorn, P.; Rattanachaikunsopon, P. Isolation and partial characterization of a bacteriophage infecting the shrimp pathogen *Vibrio harveyi. Afr. J. Microbiol. Res.* **2010**, *4*, 1794–1800.

28. Hyman, P.; Abedon, S.T. Practical methods for determining phage growth parameters. *Methods Mol. Boil.* **2009**, *501*, 175–202.

9

Novel Aspects of Polynucleotide Phosphorylase Function in *Streptomyces*

George H. Jones

Department of Biology, Emory University, Atlanta, GA 30322, USA; george.h.jones@emory.edu

Abstract: Polynucleotide phosphorylase (PNPase) is a 3′–5′-exoribnuclease that is found in most bacteria and in some eukaryotic organelles. The enzyme plays a key role in RNA decay in these systems. PNPase structure and function have been studied extensively in *Escherichia coli*, but there are several important aspects of PNPase function in *Streptomyces* that differ from what is observed in *E. coli* and other bacterial genera. This review highlights several of those differences: (1) the organization and expression of the PNPase gene in *Streptomyces*; (2) the possible function of PNPase as an RNA 3′-polyribonucleotide polymerase in *Streptomyces*; (3) the function of PNPase as both an exoribonuclease and as an RNA 3′-polyribonucleotide polymerase in *Streptomyces*; (4) the function of (p)ppGpp as a PNPase effector in *Streptomyces*. The review concludes with a consideration of a number of unanswered questions regarding the function of *Streptomyces* PNPase, which can be examined experimentally.

Keywords: polynucleotide phosphorylase; *Streptomyces*; ribonuclease; regulation; promoter; RNA decay; polyadenylation; (p)ppGpp; antibiotic

1. Introduction

Polynucleotide phosphorylase (PNPase, EC 2.7.7.8) was the first enzyme shown to synthesize polyribonucleotides [1], and for some time, it was thought to be the bacterial RNA polymerase. The enzyme was subsequently characterized in *Escherichia coli* and other bacteria, and was shown to catalyze the following reaction:

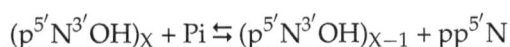

$$(p^{5'}N^{3'}OH)_X + Pi \leftrightarrows (p^{5'}N^{3'}OH)_{X-1} + pp^{5'}N$$

where N is any of the four bases found in RNA [2,3]. As written, the reaction depicts the phosphorolytic degradation of RNA chains, and this activity appears to reflect the major function of PNPase in vivo. The reaction is reversible, however, and PNPase will synthesize polyribonucleotide chains, using nucleoside diphosphates (NDPs), rather than triphosphates, as substrates. The polymerizing activity of PNPase played an important role in the synthesis of polyribonucleotides used to unravel the genetic code [4,5].

PNPase is found in all bacteria examined to date, except *Mycoplasma*, and is also present in eukaryotic organelles [6]. The enzyme has not been identified in Archaea [7]. In *E. coli*, PNPase and RNase II are the major 3′-exonucleases involved in RNA degradation [8]. In addition to its degradative function, PNPase plays a role in the bacterial response to environmental stresses, such as cold shock [9–11], is involved in biofilm formation [12,13] and virulence determination [14,15], and the activity of the enzyme is modulated by a number of small molecule effectors, at least in vitro [16–19].

Streptomyces are Gram-positive, soil-dwelling bacteria, notable for their ability to form spores and for their capacity to produce antibiotics [20,21]. Nearly 70% of all antibiotics used in clinical and veterinary medicine worldwide are synthesized as natural products by members of the genus [22]. Of particular relevance to this review, a number of biochemical and genetic features of *Streptomyces*

PNPase distinguish it from its counterparts in other bacteria. In what follows, the functions of PNPase in *Streptomyces* will be explored. The reader is referred to several excellent reviews as sources of additional information on PNPase from *E. coli* and other bacteria [2,3,23,24].

2. Organization and Expression of the PNPase Gene in *Streptomyces*

In *E. coli*, and other organisms that have been studied, the PNPase gene, *pnp*, is a part of an operon that also includes *rpsO*, the gene for ribosomal protein S15 [9,25,26]. That operon is transcribed from two promoters in *E. coli*, designated P*rpsO* and P*pnp* [25,27]. P*rpsO* is situated upstream of the *rpsO* gene, and P*pnp* is located in the intergenic region between the two genes. Transcription from P*rpsO* ends at a rho-independent terminator and produces the *rpsO* transcript, but transcription through this terminator occurs with significant frequency and produces a readthrough transcript, containing both *rpsO* and *pnp*. Transcription from the intergenic promoter, P*pnp*, produces a transcript containing *pnp* only [25,27]. In addition to the *rpsO* terminator, the *rpsO*–*pnp* intergenic region contains a second stem–loop that functions as a processing site for the double strand specific endoribonuclease, RNase III. RNase III processing plays an important role in *pnp* expression [25,28–30].

Our interest in the mechanisms of RNA decay in *Streptomyces* led to an examination of the transcriptional organization of the *rpsO*–*pnp* operon in *Streptomyces coelicolor*, the paradigm for biological studies in the genus. To our surprise, primer extension analysis of RNAs isolated from a parental strain of *S. coelicolor* and from an RNase III null mutant revealed not two, but four extension products, suggesting the presence of four promoters within the *rpsO*–*pnp* operon [31]. A visual inspection of 162 putative *Streptomyces* promoters from Strohl [32] and Yamazaki et al. [33], and a group of synthetic promoters generated by Seghezzi et al. [34], indicated that all four of the 5′-ends identified by primer extension in our studies were preceded by sequences similar to the −10 and −35 regions of characterized streptomycete promoters. Promoter probe cloning of DNA fragments containing these putative promoter sequences verified that the *rpsO*–*pnp* operon of *S. coelicolor* is transcribed from four promoters, two situated upstream of *rpsO* (P*rpsO*A and P*rpsO*B) and two situated in the intergenic region, upstream of *pnp* (P*pnp*A and P*pnp*B, Figure 1).

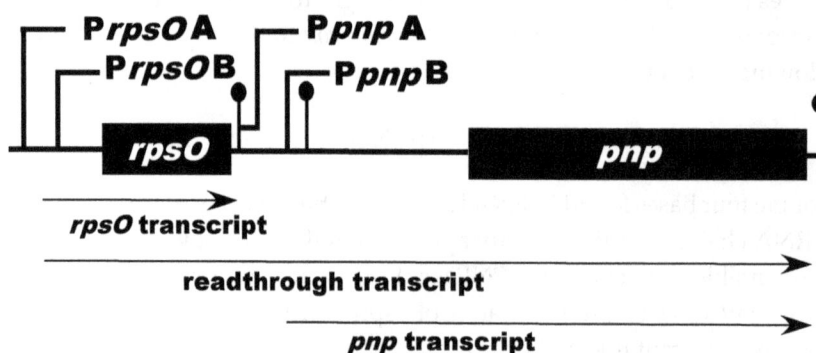

Figure 1. Schematic representation of the *Streptomyces coelicolor rpsO*–*pnp* operon. P*rpsO*A, B and P*pnp*A, B represent the upstream and intergenic promoters found in *S. coelicolor*, respectively. The ball-and-stick structures immediately following *rpsO* and *pnp* represent rho-independent transcription terminators. The ball-and-stick structure just upstream of *pnp* represents the intergenic hairpin which is cleaved by RNase III. The diagram is not drawn to scale.

Of particular interest in this analysis was the observation that the four promoters were temporally regulated. That is, the activity of the four promoters varied with time after inoculation of liquid cultures and the variations were promoter-specific, as shown in Figure 2. In terms of maximal activity, P*pnp*B was most active followed by P*rpsO*B, P*pnp*A, and P*rpsO*A.

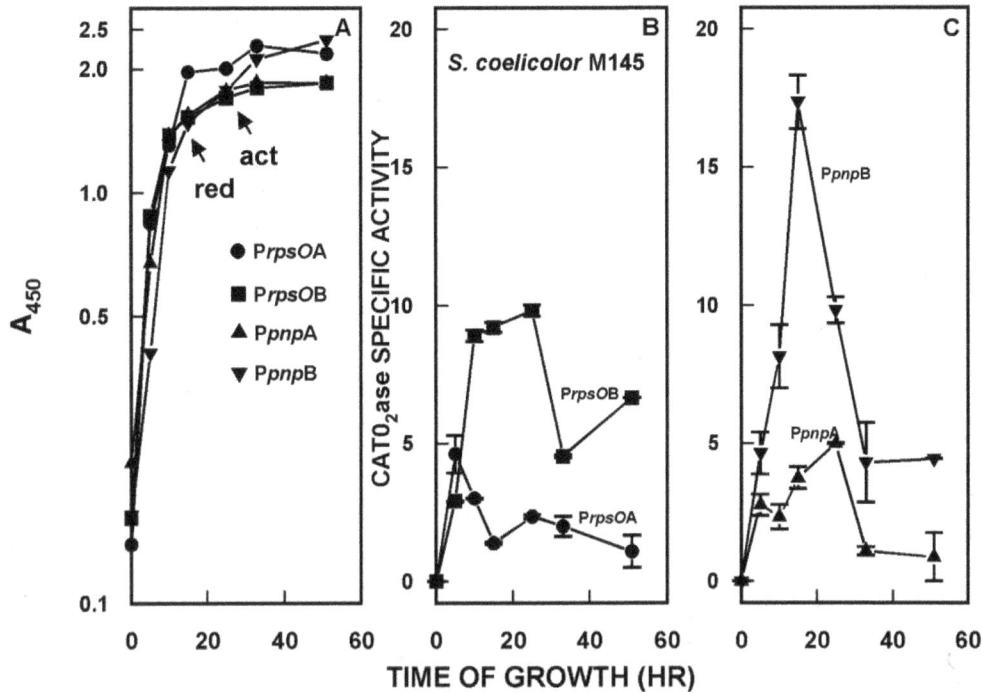

Figure 2. (**A**) Growth of the *S. coelicolor* strains containing promoter probe constructs. Growth was measured as the increase in optical density at 450 nm. The arrows in the figure indicate the onset of the production of two of the secondary metabolites synthesized by *S. coelicolor*, undecylprodigiosin (red) and actinorhodin (act). (**B**) Catechol dioxygenase (CATO$_2$ase) activity of mycelial extracts of *S. coelicolor* derivatives containing the putative *rpsO*A and *rpsO*B promoters, cloned in the promoter probe vector pIPP2 [35]. Mycelium was harvested at the indicated times, disrupted by sonication, and following centrifugation, supernatants were assayed for catechol dioxygenase, as described previously [31,35]. The catechol dioxygenase gene is the reporter in the promoter probe vector [35]. (**C**) CATO$_2$ase activities of extracts of strains containing the putative *pnp*A and *pnp*B promoters. The results shown are the averages of duplicate assays from two independent experiments ± SEM. This figure is reprinted from *Gene*, 536, Patricia Bralley, Marcha L. Gatewood, George H. Jones, Transcription of the *rpsO–pnp* operon of *Streptomyces coelicolor* involves four temporally regulated, stress responsive promoters.

A major mechanism for the modulation of promoter activity in bacterial systems involves the use of alternative sigma factors by RNA polymerase. The *S. coelicolor* genome encodes over sixty alternative sigma factors, many of which play roles in differentiation and responses to stress (reviewed in [36]). It was of considerable interest to determine whether the four *rpsO–pnp* promoters might require alternative sigma factors for transcription in *S. coelicolor*.

To this end, we obtained null mutants for a number of sigma factors, including σ^B, σ^H, and σ^L [36], and their corresponding parental strains. We transferred the *rpsO–pnp* promoter probe constructs to each strain and measured promoter activity. The results obtained for the σ^H and σ^L mutants were quite similar to those for the parental strain of *S. coelicolor*, that is, the same pattern of temporal regulation was observed in both of these sigma factor mutants as in the parental strain (cf. Figure 2). In marked contrast, the P*rpsO*A, P*rpsO*B, and P*pnp*B promoters were completely inactive in the σ^B mutant. P*pnp*A, however, was as active in the σ^B mutant as in the parental strain, and showed a similar pattern of temporal expression [31]. This result indicates that P*rpsO*A and B and P*pnp*B are dependent on σ^B for activity, and suggests that these promoters are transcribed by an RNA polymerase holoenzyme containing σ^B.

PNPase is a cold shock protein in many bacteria, and it has been shown that cold shock leads to an increase in PNPase levels in *E. coli* and other organisms [9–11]. It was of interest to determine whether PNPase levels increased in cold shock in *S. coelicolor*, and whether any such increase reflected changes in the activity of the *rpsO–pnp* promoters. As shown in Figure 3C, PNPase activity increased significantly (two-fold) in *S. coelicolor* over three hours of cold shock at 10 °C. This increase in activity was accompanied by an increase in the activities of all four of the *rpsO–pnp* promoters (Figure 3A,B) as compared with their activities at the normal growth temperature, 30 °C.

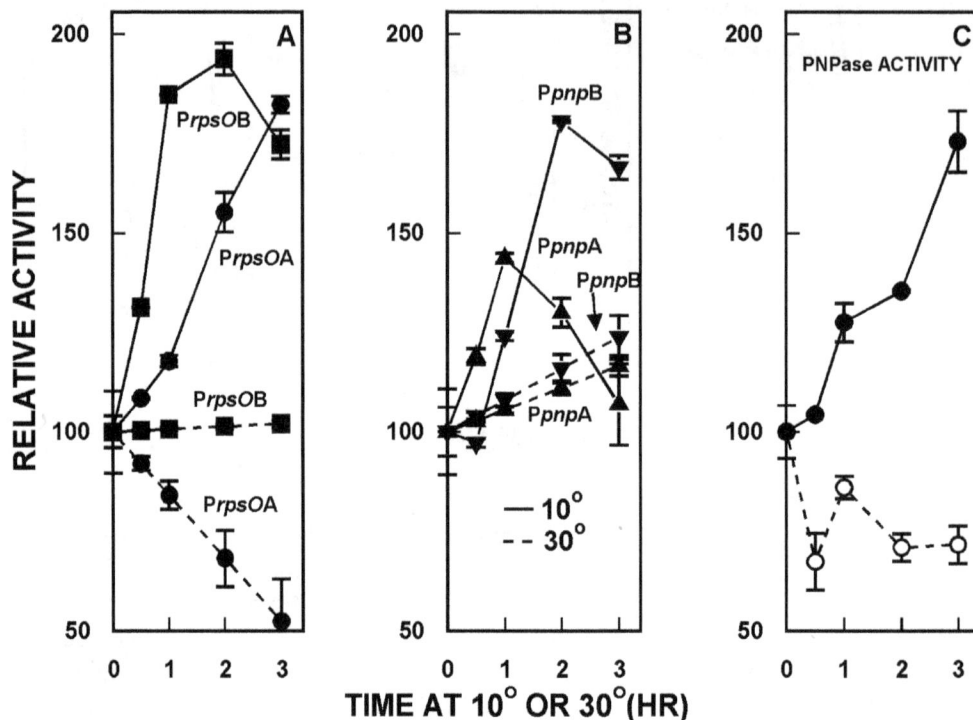

Figure 3. Cold shock responses of *S. coelicolor*. Derivatives containing the *rpsO–pnp* promoter probe constructs were grown and 30 °C, and half of each culture was then shifted to 10 °C. Mycelium was harvested at the indicated times, disrupted by sonication, and following centrifugation, supernatants were assayed for promoter activity, as described [31,35]. Panel **C** shows the results of PNPase polymerization assays. In Panels **A** and **B**, PNPase promoter activities are expressed relative to the activity measured at 30 °C at zero time, immediately before the shift to 10 °C. The results shown are the averages of duplicate assays from two independent experiments ± SEM. In the first experiment, PNPase levels were measured in *S. coelicolor* containing P*rpsO*A and in the second, PNPase levels were measured in the derivative containing P*pnp*B. This figure is reprinted from Gene, 536, Patricia Bralley, Marcha L. Gatewood, George H. Jones, Transcription of the *rpsO-pnp* operon of *Streptomyces coelicolor* involves four temporally regulated, stress responsive promoters.

Thus, PNPase is a cold shock protein in *Streptomyces*, and the cold shock response involves changes in the activities of the promoters responsible for transcription of the *rpsO–pnp* operon [31].

3. PNPase Function as an RNA 3′-Polyribonucleotide Polymerase in *Streptomyces*

As is the case in eukaryotes, bacterial RNAs have oligo- and polyribonucleotide tails at their 3′-ends, and these tails are added post-transcriptionally (reviewed in [37]). In *E. coli*, the primary enzyme responsible for the synthesis of these tails is poly(A) polymerase I (PAP I), and the tails are composed primarily of A residues [38]. In bacteria, poly(A) tails function to facilitate RNA degradation as the major 3′-exoribonucleases, viz. RNase II and PNPase in *E. coli*, digest these tails processively in vitro and in vivo [8,39].

It was shown some years ago by Mohanty and Kushner that an *E. coli* mutant lacking PAP I still added tails to the 3′-ends of its RNAs. However, these tails were not composed exclusively of A residues; the tails contained G, C, and U residues as well, i.e., they were heteropolymeric [40]. Mohanty and Kushner demonstrated that the enzyme responsible for the synthesis of these heteropolymeric tails was none other than PNPase [40]. Thus, even in the absence of PAP I, PNPase can add 3′-tails to facilitate the degradation of cellular RNAs.

Streptomyces do not contain PAP I. Yet the 3′-ends of streptomycete RNAs do possess tails. Moreover, the tails are heteropolymeric in composition, like those synthesized by PNPase in *E. coli* in the absence of PAP I [41,42]. These observations, and the report that PNPase functions as the RNA 3′-polyribonucleotide polymerase in plant chloroplasts and in cyanobacteria [43,44], led to the hypothesis that PNPase played the same role in *Streptomyces* [45]. The straightforward way to test this hypothesis would be to create a *pnp* null mutant, e.g., in *S. coelicolor*, and to determine whether the mutant was still capable of adding 3′-tails to its RNAs. However, attempts to disrupt *pnp* in *S. coelicolor* and in the sister species, *Streptomyces antibioticus*, were only successful when a second copy of *pnp* was added to the genome. In other words, gene disruption attempts revealed that, unlike the situation in *E. coli* and in the Bacilli, *pnp* is an essential gene in *Streptomyces* [42].

A model for the function of PNPase as an RNA 3′-polyribonucleotide polymerase is presented in detail below.

4. Function of PNPase as Both an Exoribonuclease and as an RNA 3′-Polyribonucleotide Polymerase

PNPase activity is highly processive and the enzyme is impeded by stem–loop structures [46]. Streptomycete genomes are GC rich, so that enzymes involved in RNA decay may have evolved to degrade the RNAs derived from these genomes efficiently. A possible strategy for facilitating this degradation was suggested by the observation that PNPase appears to utilize its polymerizing activity to add 3′-tails to streptomycete RNAs [42,45]. It seemed possible that the enzyme might add such tails during phosphorolysis to create single stranded 3′-ends that would then function as the substrates for that phosphorolysis. If this were the case, it might be expected that nucleoside diphosphates, the substrates for polymerization, would stimulate phosphorolysis. To test this hypothesis, two model PNPase substrates were constructed from the sequence of the *rpsO–pnp* operon of *S. coelicolor*. Both substrates contained the *rpsO–pnp* terminator and the intergenic hairpin. Thus, both model substrates contained secondary structure that would be expected to impede phosphorolysis by PNPase. One substrate, designated 5601, also possessed a single stranded 3′-tail, 33 bases in length, while the other substrate, 5650, terminated at the base of the intergenic hairpin, and did not have a single stranded tail [47].

The phosphorolysis of these two substrates was studied in the absence and presence of a mixture of all four nucleoside diphosphates (NDPs) with the interesting result, predicted by our hypothesis, that the NDPs, normally the substrates for the polymerizing activity of PNPase, did stimulate RNA degradation by phosphorolysis. Figure 4 shows the results of phosphorolysis of the 5650 transcript (labeled RP3 in the figure).

Analysis of the results shown in Figure 4 revealed that NDPs at 20–30 μM in phosphorolysis mixtures stimulated that reaction by 2–3 fold as compared with controls, but only when the structured RNA, 5650 (RP3) was used as the substrate [47]. NDPs had no effect on the phosphorolysis of the 5601 substrate, possessing the single stranded tail. Kinetic analyses showed that NDPs affected the K_m for phosphorolysis. Thus, the K_m value for phosphorolysis of the 5650 substrate in the absence of NDPs was 3.1 μM. This value decreased to 0.65 μM in the presence of all four NDPs at 20 μM. This latter K_m was almost identical to that obtained in the absence of NDPs for the 5601 substrate, which has a single stranded 3′-tail (0.62 μM). NDPs did not further decrease the K_m for the 5601 substrate. It is noteworthy as well, that NDPs had no effect on the phosphorolysis of either substrate by *E. coli*

PNPase, and that the *E. coli* enzyme was intrinsically less active with the structured substrate than was its counterpart from *S. coelicolor* [47].

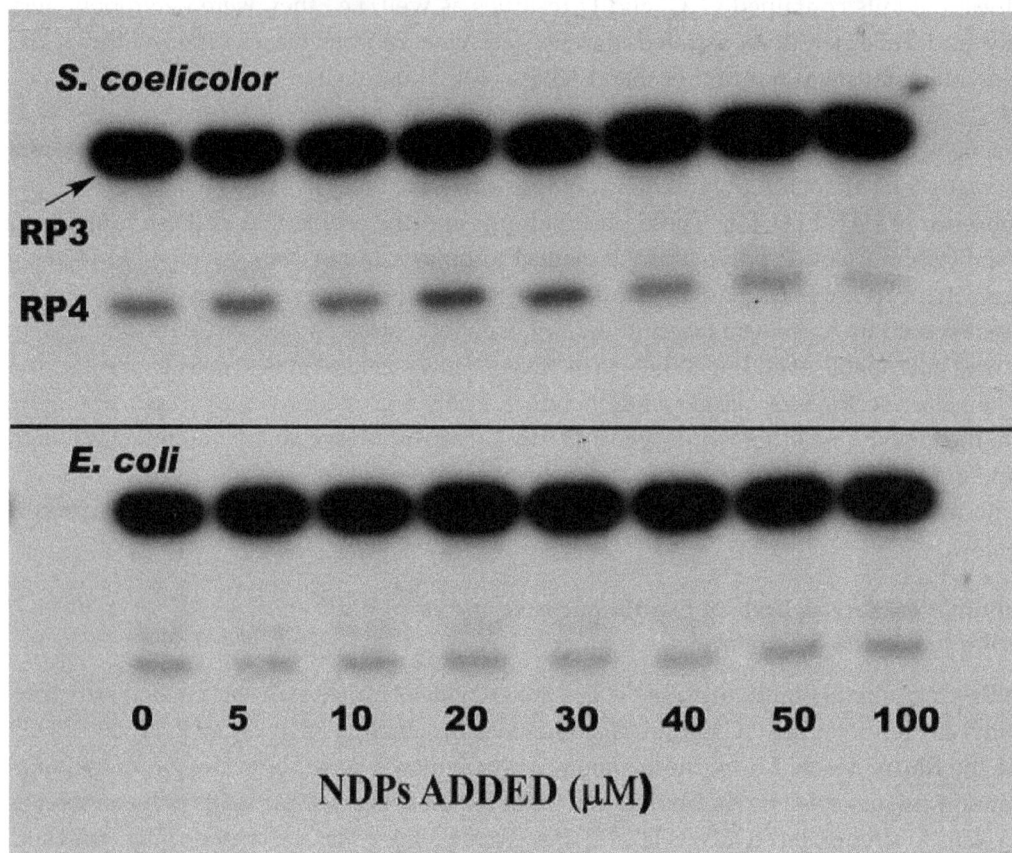

Figure 4.   Effects of nucleoside diphosphates on the phosphorolysis of the 5650 transcript. Phosphorolysis reactions were performed as described in [47], and reaction products were separated by gel electrophoresis. The top panel shows the results obtained with *S. coelicolor* PNPase and the bottom panel results using *E. coli* PNPase. Reactions were conducted in the presence of increasing concentrations of a mixture of ADP, CDP, UDP, and GDP (nucleoside diphosphates (NDPs)) as indicated. RP3 is the 5650 transcript, and RP4 represents the product obtained by complete digestion of the intergenic hairpin in RP3 by PNPase. Note that as PNPase is highly processive [48], no intermediates with mobilities between those of RP3 and RP4 were observed.

Our model for the explanation of the foregoing observations is shown in Figure 5 [49].

We posit that the stem–loops of structured substrates, like 5650, block PNPase action. The addition of short 3'-tails during phosphorolysis, or the presence of naturally occurring tails on substrates like 5601, allows for the breathing of stems and thus permits PNPase, which might otherwise stall at the stem–loops in structured substrates, to continue phosphorolysis through those structures. As indicated above, this mechanism may represent an evolutionary adaptation occasioned by the high GC content of streptomycete genomes and their transcripts.

It must be noted, however, that the evidence for the function of PNPase as a 3'-polyribonucleotide polymerase in *Streptomyces* is indirect. In vivo evidence for this function remains to be uncovered.

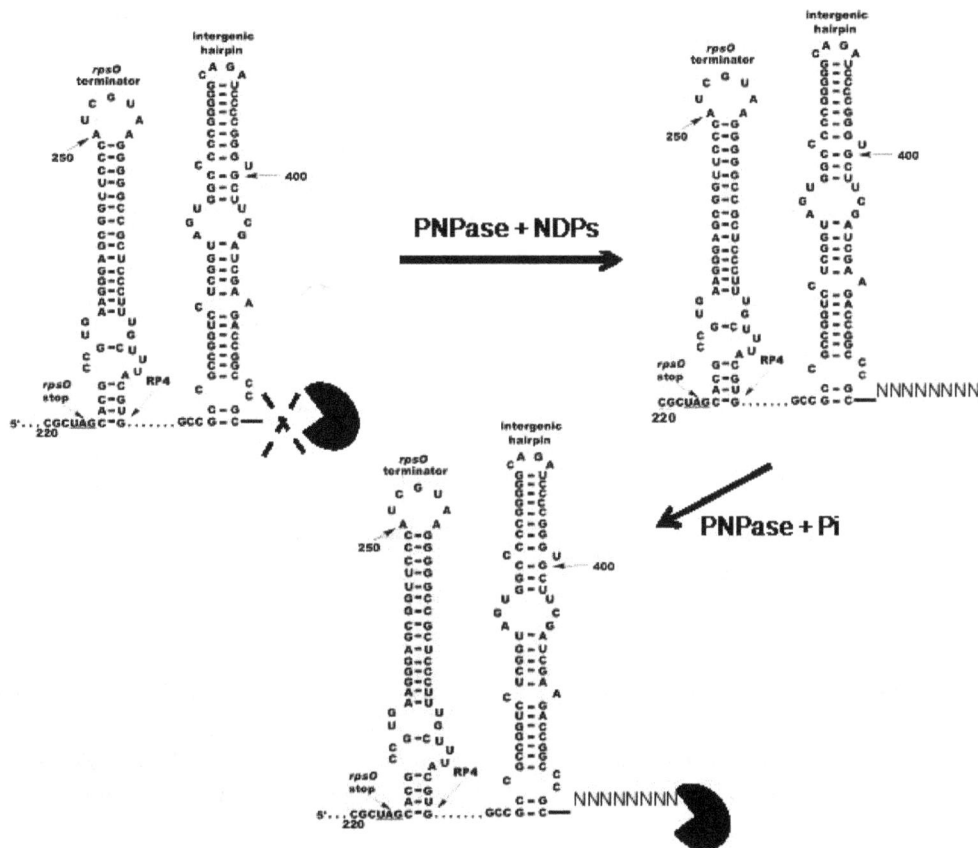

Figure 5. Model for the effects of NDPs on the activity *S. coelicolor* PNPase. The model posits that *S. coelicolor* PNPase (PacMan symbol) is able to phosphorolyze 5650 and other structured substrates to a limited extent in the absence of NDPs, as indicated by the dashed X. In the presence of NDPs, PNPase synthesizes unstructured 3′-tails in vivo, and these tails then provide an anchor for the enzyme, thus facilitating the digestion of structured substrates.

5. (p)ppGpp as a PNPase Effector

Highly phosphorylated guanine nucleotides, (p)ppGpp, guanosine pentaphosphate, and guanosine tetraphosphate, are alarmones that play a number of roles in the regulation of bacterial metabolism (reviewed in [50,51]). (p)ppGpp is synthesized by the product of the *relA* gene in *E. coli* [52], and that gene is found in *S. coelicolor* [53,54], *S. antibioticus* [55], and other streptomycetes [56]. In *Streptomyces*, ppGpp plays an important role in the regulation of antibiotic synthesis [53–56].

PNPase from *S. antibioticus* was shown to synthesize pppGpp in vitro [57,58]. While this activity may be an in vitro artifact, as no other PNPases are known to possess it, the observation suggested a possible relationship between (p)ppGpp and RNA decay in *Streptomyces*. To begin to examine this relationship, the effects of (p)ppGpp on polymerization and phosphorolysis by *S. coelicolor*, *S. antibioticus*, and *E. coli* PNPases were measured in the absence and presence of (p)ppGpp [59]. As shown in Figure 6, both guanosine penta- and tetraphosphates inhibited the activity of *S. coelicolor* PNPase, in both phosphorolysis and polymerization, though ppGpp was a more potent inhibitor than pppGpp.

Essentially identical results were obtained for *S. antibioticus* PNPase (not shown). By contrast, neither ppGpp nor pppGpp were effective inhibitors of the activity of *E. coli* PNPase. Indeed, at concentrations up to 1 mM, pppGpp actually stimulated the polymerizing activity of the *E. coli* enzyme.

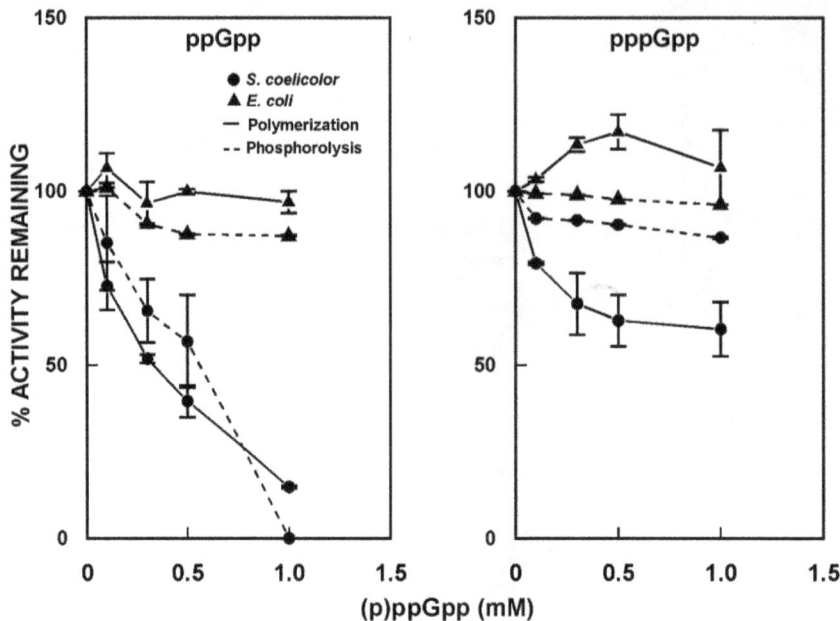

Figure 6. Effects of (p)ppGpp on the activity of PNPase. Polymerization and phosphorolysis reactions were performed in the absence and presence of guanosine tetraphosphate (ppGpp) or guanosine pentaphosphate (pppGpp), using purified PNPase from *S. coelicolor* and *E. coli* [59]. Results are expressed relative to the activities measured in the absence of (p)ppGpp, set arbitrarily to 100%.

In the same study, the effects of (p)ppGpp on the stability of bulk mRNA in *S. coelicolor* were examined [59]. It was initially observed that the half-life of bulk mRNA increased by 1.8-fold in stationary phase cultures as compared with exponential phase. That this increase might be related to the effects of (p)ppGpp was suggested by studies with an *S. coelicolor relA* mutant, and a strain containing an inducible *relA* gene. While the half-life of bulk mRNA was longer in the *relA* mutant than in the parental strain (e.g., 8.9 min vs 3.2 min in exponential phase), the half-life decreased slightly in the *relA* mutant in stationary phase (to 7.2 min). In the strain containing an inducible *relA* gene, producing increased levels of (p)ppGpp, induction occasioned a ca. two-fold increase in the half-life of bulk mRNA, from 6.6 to 11.8 min. Taken together, these observations suggest that (p)ppGpp may stabilize mRNAs in stationary phase *S. coelicolor* cells, as compared with cells growing exponentially.

Why and how might this stabilization occur? It is well established that although levels of RNA and protein synthesis decrease dramatically as *Streptomyces* cultures move from the exponential to the stationary phase of growth, a basal level of synthesis is maintained throughout stationary phase [60,61]. This basal level of macromolecular synthesis is presumably required to produce enzymes and other proteins involved in the synthesis of the secondary metabolites these organisms produce in stationary phase. Stabilization of the transcripts for these proteins would represent one strategy the organisms could employ to ensure the persistence of macromolecular synthesis to support secondary metabolite production. It is known that (p)ppGpp is present in significant amounts, even in stationary phase streptomycete cultures [62,63]. Thus, the inhibition of PNPase by (p)ppGpp might represent a strategy used by *Streptomyces* to stabilize essential mRNAs during stationary phase. It would be interesting to determine whether (p)ppGpp inhibits the activity of other exo- and endonucleases and while such analyses have yet to be performed, it is noteworthy that ppGpp inhibits PNPase from another actinomycete, *Nonomuraea* sp. [64].

6. Conclusions and Unanswered Questions

It is apparent from the brief analysis above that PNPase is a multitalented enzyme that plays a critical role in the metabolic activities of bacterial cells. Despite the wealth of information that has been accumulated about PNPase, a number of important biological questions remain unanswered, particularly as they relate to the functions of *Streptomyces* PNPase.

First, why is the *rpsO–pnp* operon of *S. coelicolor* transcribed from four promoters? The answer to this question may relate to the fact that the operon contains a ribosomal protein gene, as well as the gene for PNPase. It is possible that the promoters are not only critical to the regulation of *pnp* expression, but that they also play and important role in ribosome biogenesis via their regulation of the levels of the *rpsO* transcript. Mutation of the four promoter sequences may provide insight into these possibilities.

Second, what is the significance, if there is any, to the fact that the *S. coelicolor rpsO–pnp* operon produces six transcripts (two *rpsO* transcripts from P*rpsO*A and B, two readthrough transcripts from the same two promoters, and two *pnp* transcripts from P*pnp*A and B)? It should be noted that Northern blot analysis of the transcripts derived from the *S. coelicolor rpsO–pnp* operon did not reveal the presence of six separate transcripts [65]. It is possible that the different transcripts are not sufficiently different in size to have been resolved on the Northern blotting gels. Another intriguing possibility is that the longer transcripts, obtained from the upstream promoter in each case, might be processed at their 5′-ends by RNase J, which possesses 5′–3′-exoribonuclease activity. RNase J has recently been characterized in *S. coelicolor* [66,67].

Third, as described above, PNPase is a cold shock protein in *Streptomyces*. It is relevant to ask whether PNPase responds to other environmental stresses, such as heat, oxidative stress, metal ion stress, etc. It would be of interest, in particular, to examine the effects of various types of stress on the activities of the *rpsO–pnp* promoters. Mutational analyses again might reveal important aspects of promoter function in stress conditions in *Streptomyces*.

Fourth, a number of small effector molecules modulate the activity of *E. coli* PNPase, e.g., ATP, citrate, and cyclic-diGMP [16–19]. It has been proposed that these effectors connect RNA decay to other metabolic pathways in bacterial cells. It would be interesting to determine whether these effectors also affect the activity of *Streptomyces* PNPase. It is noteworthy, in this regard, that in silico molecular docking studies suggest that citrate, which inhibits the activity of *E. coli* PNPase, will bind to PNPase from *S. antibioticus* [18].

Finally, in *E. coli* and other organisms, PNPase is part of a larger macromolecular complex generally referred to as the degradosome ([68,69]. In *E. coli*, the components of the degradosome are organized around a scaffold provided by the single strand specific endoribonuclease, RNase E [70]. RNase E is present in *S. coelicolor*, and has been shown to interact with PNPase in vivo [71]. However, unlike the situation in *E. coli*, the identities of other proteins that might be involved in the degradative machine are unknown in *Streptomyces*.

It is fervently hoped that the foregoing and other important questions related to PNPase structure and function will continue to attract interest and experimentation to provide answers to them.

Acknowledgments: Much of the research described in this report was supported by grants MCB-0133520 and MCB-0817177 from the U.S. National Science Foundation to the author.

References

1. Grunberg-Manago, M.; Ochoa, S. Enzymatic synthesis and breakdown of polynucleotides: Polynucleotide phosphorylase. *J. Am. Chem. Soc.* **1955**, *77*, 3165–3166. [CrossRef]
2. Godefroy-Colburn, T.; Grunberg-Manago, M. Polynucleotide phosphorylase. *Enzymes* **1972**, *7*, 533–574.
3. Littauer, U.Z.; Soreq, H. Polynucleotide phosphorylase. *Enzymes* **1982**, *15*, 517–553.

4.   Lengyel, P.; Speyer, J.F.; Ochoa, S. Synthetic polynucleotides and the amino acid code. *Proc. Natl. Acad. Sci. USA* **1962**, *47*, 1936–1942. [CrossRef]

5.   Matthaei, J.H.; Jones, O.W.; Martin, R.G.; Nirenberg, M. Characteristics and composition of RNA coding units. *Proc. Natl. Acad. Sci. USA* **1962**, *48*, 666–676. [CrossRef] [PubMed]

6.   Zuo, Y.; Deutscher, M. Exoribonuclease superfamilies: Structural analysis and phylogenetic distribution. *Nucleic Acids. Res.* **2001**, *29*, 1017–1026. [CrossRef] [PubMed]

7.   Lin-Chao, S.; Chiou, N.T.; Schuster, G. The PNPase, exosome and RNA helicases as the building components of evolutionarily-conserved RNA degradation machines. *J. Biomed. Sci.* **2007**, *14*, 523–532. [CrossRef] [PubMed]

8.   Donovan, W.P.; Kushner, S.R. Polynucleotide phosphorylase and ribonuclease II are required for cell viability and mRNA turnover in *Escherichia coli* k-12. *Proc. Natl. Acad. Sci. USA* **1986**, *83*, 120–124. [CrossRef] [PubMed]

9.   Clarke, D.J.; Dowds, B.C. The gene coding for polynucleotide phosphorylase in *Photorhabdus* sp. Strain k122 is induced at low temperatures. *J. Bacteriol.* **1994**, *176*, 3775–3784. [CrossRef] [PubMed]

10.   Goverde, R.L.J.; Huis in't Veld, J.H.J.; Kusters, J.G.; Mooi, F.R. The psychrotropic bacterium *Yersinia enterocolitica* requires expression of *pnp*, the gene for polynucleotide phosphorylase, for growth at low termperature (5 °C). *Mol. Microbiol.* **1998**, *28*, 555–569. [CrossRef] [PubMed]

11.   Zangrossi, S.; Briani, F.; Ghisotti, D.; Regonesi, M.E.; Tortora, P.; Deho, G. Transcriptional and post-transcriptional control of polynucleotide phosphorylase during cold acclimation in *Escherichia coli*. *Mol. Microbiol.* **2000**, *36*, 1470–1480. [CrossRef] [PubMed]

12.   Carzaniga, T.; Antoniani, D.; Deho, G.; Briani, F.; Landini, P. The RNA processing enzyme polynucleotide phosphorylase negatively controls biofilm formation by repressing poly-*N*-acetylglucosamine (PNAG) production in *Escherichia coli* C. *BMC Microbiol.* **2012**, *12*, 270. [CrossRef] [PubMed]

13.   Pobre, V.; Arraiano, C.M. Next generation sequencing analysis reveals that the ribonucleases RNAse II, RNAse R and PNPase affect bacterial motility and biofilm formation in *E. coli*. *BMC Genomics* **2015**, *16*, 72. [CrossRef] [PubMed]

14.   Rosenzweig, J.A.; Chopra, A.K. The exoribonuclease polynucleotide phosphorylase influences the virulence and stress responses of *Yersiniae* and many other pathogens. *Front. Cell. Infect. Microbiol.* **2013**, *3*, 81. [CrossRef] [PubMed]

15.   Engman, J.; Negrea, A.; Sigurlasdottir, S.; Georg, M.; Eriksson, J.; Eriksson, O.S.; Kuwae, A.; Sjolinder, H.; Jonsson, A.B. *Neisseria meningitidis* polynucleotide phosphorylase affects aggregation, adhesion, and virulence. *Infect. Immun.* **2016**, *84*, 1501–1513. [CrossRef] [PubMed]

16.   Del Favero, M.; Mazzantini, E.; Briani, F.; Zangrossi, S.; Tortora, P.; Deho, G. Regulation of *Escherichia coli* polynucleotide phosphorylase by ATP. *J. Biol. Chem.* **2008**, *283*, 27355–27359. [CrossRef] [PubMed]

17.   Nurmohamed, S.; Vincent, H.A.; Titman, C.M.; Chandran, V.; Pears, M.R.; Du, D.; Griffin, J.L.; Callaghan, A.J.; Luisi, B.F. Polynucleotide phosphorylase activity may be modulated by metabolites in *Escherichia coli*. *J. Biol. Chem.* **2011**, *286*, 14315–14323. [CrossRef] [PubMed]

18.   Tuckerman, J.R.; Gonzalez, G.; Gilles-Gonzalez, M.A. Cyclic di-GMP activation of polynucleotide phosphorylase signal-dependent RNA processing. *J. Mol. Biol.* **2011**, *407*, 633–639. [CrossRef] [PubMed]

19.   Stone, C.M.; Butt, L.E.; Bufton, J.C.; Lourenco, D.C.; Gowers, D.M.; Pickford, A.R.; Cox, P.A.; Vincent, H.A.; Callaghan, A.J. Inhibition of homologous phosphorolytic ribonucleases by citrate may represent an evolutionarily conserved communicative link between RNA degradation and central metabolism. *Nucleic Acids Res.* **2017**, *45*, 4655–4666. [CrossRef] [PubMed]

20.   Liu, G.; Chater, K.F.; Chandra, G.; Niu, G.; Tan, H. Molecular regulation of antibiotic biosynthesis in *Streptomyces*. *Microbiol. Mol. Biol. Rev.* **2013**, *77*, 112–143. [CrossRef] [PubMed]

21.   Chandra, G.; Chater, K.F. Developmental biology of *Streptomyces* from the perspective of 100 actinobacterial genome sequences. *FEMS Microbiol. Rev.* **2014**, *38*, 345–379. [CrossRef] [PubMed]

22.   Berdy, J. Recent advances in and prospects of antibiotic research. *Process. Biochem.* **1980**, *15*, 28–35.

23.   Littauer, U.Z. From polynucleotide phosphorylase to neurobiology. *J. Biol. Chem.* **2005**, *280*, 38889–38897. [CrossRef] [PubMed]

24.   Briani, F.; Carzaniga, T.; Deho, G. Regulation and functions of bacterial PNPase. *Wiley Interdiscip. Rev. RNA* **2016**, *7*, 241–258. [CrossRef] [PubMed]

25. Régnier, P.; Portier, C. Initiation, attenuation and RNase III processing of transcripts from the *Escherichia coli* operon encoding ribosomal protein S15 and polynucleotide phosphorylase. *J. Mol. Biol.* **1986**, *187*, 23–32. [CrossRef]

26. Luttinger, A.; Hahn, J.; Dubnau, D. Polynucleotide phosphorylase is necessary for competence development in *Bacillus subtilis*. *Mol. Microbiol.* **1996**, *19*, 343–356. [CrossRef] [PubMed]

27. Portier, C.; Regnier, P. Expression of the *rpsO* and *pnp* genes: Structural analysis of a DNA fragment carrying their control regions. *Nucleic Acids Res.* **1984**, *12*, 6091–6102. [CrossRef] [PubMed]

28. Robert-Le Meur, M.; Portier, C. *E. coli* polynucleotide phosphorylase expression is autoregulated through an RNase III-dependent mechanism. *EMBO J.* **1992**, *11*, 2633–2641. [PubMed]

29. Robert-Le Meur, M.; Portier, C. Polynucleotide phosphorylase of *Escherichia coli* induces degradation of its RNase III processed messenger by preventing its translation. *Nucleic Acids Res.* **1994**, *22*, 397–403. [CrossRef] [PubMed]

30. Jarrige, A.-C.; Mathy, N.; Portier, C. Pnpase autocontrols its expression by degrading a double-stranded structure in the *pnp* mRNA leader. *EMBO J.* **2001**, *20*, 6845–6855. [CrossRef] [PubMed]

31. Bralley, P.; Gatewood, M.L.; Jones, G.H. Transcription of the *rpsO-pnp* operon of *Streptomyces coelicolor* involves four temporally regulated, stress responsive promoters. *Gene* **2014**, *536*, 177–185. [CrossRef] [PubMed]

32. Strohl, W.R. Compilation and analysis of DNA sequences associated with apparent streptomycete promoters. *Nucleic Acids Res.* **1992**, *20*, 961–974. [CrossRef] [PubMed]

33. Yamazaki, H.; Ohnishi, Y.; Horinouchi, S. Transcriptional switch on of ssgA by a-factor, which is essential for spore septum formation in *Streptomyces griseus*. *J. Bacteriol.* **2003**, *185*, 1273–1283. [CrossRef] [PubMed]

34. Seghezzi, N.; Amar, P.; Koebmann, B.; Jensen, P.R.; Virolle, M.J. The construction of a library of synthetic promoters revealed some specific features of strong *Streptomyces* promoters. *Appl. Microbiol. Biotechnol.* **2011**, *90*, 615–623. [CrossRef] [PubMed]

35. Jones, G.H. Integrative, *xyle*-based promoter probe vectors for use in *Streptomyces*. *Plasmid* **2011**, *65*, 219–225. [CrossRef] [PubMed]

36. Sun, D.; Liu, C.; Zhu, J.; Liu, W. Connecting metabolic pathways: Sigma factors in *Streptomyces* spp. *Front. Microbiol.* **2017**, *8*, 2546. [CrossRef] [PubMed]

37. Mohanty, B.K.; Kushner, S.R. Bacterial/archaeal/organellar polyadenylation. *Wiley Interdiscip. Rev. RNA* **2011**, *2*, 256–276. [CrossRef] [PubMed]

38. Cao, G.J.; Sarkar, N. Identification of the gene for an *Escherichia coli* poly(A) polymerase. *Proc. Natl. Acad. Sci. USA* **1992**, *89*, 10380–10384. [CrossRef] [PubMed]

39. Cao, G.J.; Kalapos, M.P.; Sarkar, N. Polyadenylated mrna in *Escherichia coli*: Modulation of poly(A) RNA levels by polynucleotide phosphorylase and ribonuclease II. *Biochimie* **1997**, *79*, 211–220. [CrossRef]

40. Mohanty, B.K.; Kushner, S.R. Polynucleotide phosphorylase functions both as a 3′-5′ exonuclease and a poly(A) polymerase in *Escherichia coli*. *Proc. Natl. Acad. Sci. USA* **2000**, *97*, 11966–11971. [CrossRef] [PubMed]

41. Bralley, P.; Jones, G.H. cDNA cloning confirms the polyadenylation of RNA decay intermediates in *Streptomyces coelicolor*. *Microbiology* **2002**, *148*, 1421–1425. [CrossRef] [PubMed]

42. Bralley, P.; Gust, B.; Chang, S.A.; Chater, K.F.; Jones, G.H. RNA 3′-tail synthesis in *streptomyces*: In vitro and in vivo activities of RNase PH, the *SCO3896* gene product and pnpase. *Microbiology* **2006**, *152*, 627–636. [CrossRef] [PubMed]

43. Yehudai-Resheff, S.; Hirsh, M.; Schuster, G. Polynucleotide phosphorylase functions as both an exonuclease and a poly(A) polymerase in spinach chloroplasts. *Mol. Cell Biol.* **2001**, *21*, 5408–5416. [CrossRef] [PubMed]

44. Rott, R.; Zipor, G.; Portnoy, V.; Liveanu, V.; Schuster, G. RNA polyadenylation and degradation in cyanobacteria are similar to the chloroplast but different from *E. coli*. *J. Biol. Chem.* **2003**, *278*, 15771–15777. [CrossRef] [PubMed]

45. Sohlberg, B.; Huang, J.; Cohen, S.N. The *Streptomyces coelicolor* polynucleotide phosphorylase homologue, and not the putative poly(A) polymerase can polyadenylate RNA. *J. Bacteriol.* **2003**, *185*, 7273–7278. [CrossRef] [PubMed]

46. Spickler, C.; Mackie, G.A. Action of RNase II and polynucleotide phosphorylase against RNAs containing stem-loops of defined structure. *J. Bacteriol.* **2000**, *182*, 2422–2427. [CrossRef] [PubMed]

47. Chang, S.A.; Cozad, M.; Mackie, G.A.; Jones, G.H. Kinetics of polynucleotide phosphorylase: Comparison of enzymes from *Streptomyces* and *Escherichia coli* and effects of nucleoside diphosphates. *J. Bacteriol.* **2008**, *190*, 98–106. [CrossRef] [PubMed]

48. Symmons, M.; Jones, G.H.; Luisi, B. A duplicated fold is the structural basis for polynucleotide phosphorylase catalytic activity, processivity and regulation. *Structure* **2000**, *8*, 1215–1226. [CrossRef]

49. Jones, G.H.; Mackie, G.A. *Streptomyces coelicolor* polynucleotide phosphorylase can polymerize nucleoside diphosphates under phosphorolysis conditions, with implications for the degradation of structured rnas. *J. Bacteriol.* **2013**, *195*, 5151–5159. [CrossRef] [PubMed]

50. Potrykus, K.; Cashel, M. (p)ppgpp: Still magical? *Annu. Rev. Microbiol.* **2008**, *62*, 35–51. [CrossRef] [PubMed]

51. Srivatsan, A.; Wang, J.D. Control of bacterial transcription, translation and replication by (p)ppgpp. *Curr. Opin. Microbiol.* **2008**, *11*, 100–105. [CrossRef] [PubMed]

52. Petersen, F.S.; Kjelgaard, N.O. Analysis of the *relA* gene product of *Escherichia coli*. *Eur. J. Biochem.* **1977**, *76*, 91–97. [CrossRef]

53. Chakraburtty, R.; White, J.; Takano, E.; Bibb, M.J. Cloning and characterization and disruption of a (p)ppgpp synthetase gene (*relA*) of *Streptomyces coelicolor* a3(2). *Mol. Microbiol.* **1996**, *19*, 357–368. [CrossRef] [PubMed]

54. Chakraburtty, R.; Bibb, M.J. The ppgpp synthetase gene (*relA*) of *Streptomyces coelicolor* a3(2) plays a conditional role in antibiotic production and morphological differentiation. *J. Bacteriol.* **1997**, *179*, 5854–5864. [CrossRef] [PubMed]

55. Hoyt, S.; Jones, G.H. *RelA* is required for actinomycin production in *Streptomyces antibioticus*. *J. Bacteriol.* **1999**, *181*, 3824–3829. [PubMed]

56. Jin, W.; Ryu, Y.G.; Kang, S.G.; Kim, S.K.; Saito, N.; Ochi, K.; Lee, S.H.; Lee, K.J. Two *relA*/*spoT* homologous genes are involved in the morphological and physiological differentiation of *Streptomyces clavuligerus*. *Microbiology* **2004**, *150*, 1485–1493. [CrossRef] [PubMed]

57. Jones, G.H. Purification and properties of atp:Gtp 3′-pyrophosphotransferase (guanosine pentaphosphate synthetase) from *Streptomyces antibioticus*. *J. Bacteriol.* **1994**, *176*, 1475–1481. [CrossRef] [PubMed]

58. Jones, G.H. Activation of ATP-GTP 3′-pyrophosphotransferase (guanosine pentaphosphate synthetase) in *Streptomyces antibioticus*. *J. Bacteriol.* **1994**, *176*, 1482–1487. [CrossRef] [PubMed]

59. Gatewood, M.L.; Jones, G.H. (p)ppgpp inhibits polynucleotide phosphorylase from *Streptomyces* but not from *Escherichia coli* and increases the stability of bulk mRNA in *Streptomyces coelicolor*. *J. Bacteriol.* **2010**, *192*, 4275–4280. [CrossRef] [PubMed]

60. Jones, G.H. RNA synthesis in *Streptomyces antibioticus*: In vitro effects of actinomycin and transcriptional inhibitors from 48-h cells. *Biochemistry* **1976**, *15*, 3331–3341. [CrossRef] [PubMed]

61. Liras, P.; Villanueva, J.R.; Martin, J.F. Sequential expression of macromolecule biosynthesis and candicidin formation in *Streptomyces griseus*. *J. Gen. Microbiol.* **1977**, *102*, 269–277. [CrossRef] [PubMed]

62. Kelly, K.S.; Ochi, K.; Jones, G.H. Pleiotropic effects of a *relC* mutation in *Streptomyces antibioticus*. *J. Bacteriol.* **1991**, *173*, 2297–2300. [CrossRef] [PubMed]

63. Hesketh, A.; Sun, J.; Bibb, M.J. Induction of ppGpp synthesis in *Streptomyces coelicolor* A3(2) grown under conditions of nutritional sufficiency elicits *actII-ORF4* transcription and actinorhodin biosynthesis. *Mol. Microbiol.* **2001**, *39*, 136–141. [CrossRef] [PubMed]

64. Siculella, L.; Damiano, F.; di Summa, R.; Tredici, S.M.; Alduina, R.; Gnoni, G.V.; Alifano, P. Guanosine 5′-diphosphate 3′-diphosphate (ppgpp) as a negative modulator of polynucleotide phosphorylase activity in a 'rare' actinomycete. *Mol. Microbiol.* **2010**, *77*, 716–729. [CrossRef] [PubMed]

65. Gatewood, M.L.; Bralley, P.; Jones, G.H. RNase III-dependent expression of the *rpsO-pnp* Operon of *Streptomyces coelicolor*. *J. Bacteriol.* **2011**, *193*, 4371–4379. [CrossRef] [PubMed]

66. Bralley, P.; Aseem, M.; Jones, G.H. SCO5745, a bifunctional RNase J Ortholog, affects antibiotic production in *Streptomyces coelicolor*. *J. Bacteriol.* **2014**, *196*, 1197–1205. [CrossRef] [PubMed]

67. Pei, X.Y.; Bralley, P.; Jones, G.H.; Luisi, B.F. Linkage of catalysis and 5′ end recognition in ribonuclease RNase J. *Nucleic Acids Res.* **2015**, *43*, 8066–8076. [CrossRef] [PubMed]

68. Py, B.; Causton, C.F.; Mudd, E.A.; Higgins, C.F. A protein complex that mediates mRNA degradation in *Escherichia coli*. *Mol. Microbiol.* **1994**, *14*, 717–729. [CrossRef] [PubMed]

69. Ait-Bara, S.; Carpousis, A.J. RNA degradosomes in bacteria and chloroplasts: Classification, distribution and evolution of RNase E homologs. *Mol. Microbiol.* **2015**, *97*, 1021–1135. [CrossRef] [PubMed]

70. Vanzo, N.E.; Li, Y.S.; Py, B.; Blum, E.; Higgins, C.F.; Raynal, L.C.; Krisch, H.M.; Carpousis, A.J. Ribonuclease E organizes the protein interactions in the *Escherichia coli* degradosome. *Genes Dev.* **1998**, *12*, 2770–2781. [CrossRef] [PubMed]

71. Lee, K.; Cohen, S.N. A *Streptomyces coelicolor* functional orthologue of *Escherichia coli* RNAse e shows shuffling of catalytic and PNPase-binding domains. *Mol. Microbiol.* **2003**, *48*, 349–360. [CrossRef] [PubMed]

10

Specificity of Induction of Glycopeptide Antibiotic Resistance in the Producing Actinomycetes

Elisa Binda [1,2] ⓘ, **Pamela Cappelletti** [1,2], **Flavia Marinelli** [1,2] **and Giorgia Letizia Marcone** [1,2,*] ⓘ

[1] Department of Biotechnology and Life Sciences, University of Insubria, via J.H. Dunant 3, 21100 Varese, Italy; elisa.binda@uninsubria.it (E.B.); pamela.cappelletti@uninsubria.it (P.C.); flavia.marinelli@uninsubria.it (F.M.)

[2] The Protein Factory Research Center, Politecnico di Milano and University of Insubria, via J.H. Dunant 3, 21100 Varese, Italy

* Correspondence: giorgia.marcone@uninsubria.it

Abstract: Glycopeptide antibiotics are drugs of last resort for treating severe infections caused by Gram-positive pathogens. It is widely believed that glycopeptide-resistance determinants (*van* genes) are ultimately derived from the producing actinomycetes. We hereby investigated the relationship between the antimicrobial activity of vancomycin and teicoplanins and their differential ability to induce *van* gene expression in *Actinoplanes teichomyceticus*—the producer of teicoplanin—and *Nonomuraea gerenzanensis*—the producer of the teicoplanin-like A40926. As a control, we used the well-characterized resistance model *Streptomyces coelicolor*. The enzyme activities of a cytoplasmic-soluble D,D-dipeptidase and of a membrane-associated D,D-carboxypeptidase (corresponding to VanX and VanY respectively) involved in resistant cell wall remodeling were measured in the actinomycetes grown in the presence or absence of subinhibitory concentrations of vancomycin, teicoplanin, and A40926. Results indicated that actinomycetes possess diverse self-resistance mechanisms, and that each of them responds differently to glycopeptide induction. Gene swapping among teicoplanins-producing actinomycetes indicated that cross-talking is possible and provides useful information for predicting the evolution of future resistance gene combinations emerging in pathogens.

Keywords: actinomycetes; glycopeptide antibiotics; teicoplanin; A40926; *van* resistance genes

1. Introduction

Glycopeptide antibiotics (GPAs) are drugs of last resort for treating severe infections caused by Gram-positive pathogens such as *Staphylococcus aureus* (SA), *Enterococcus* spp., and *Clostridioides difficile* [1]. Clinically important GPAs include first-generation vancomycin and teicoplanin—which, although discovered many decades ago, continue to be extensively used in clinical practice—and second-generation telavancin, dalbavancin, and oritavancin, which were recently approved for clinical use for their increased antimicrobial potency and superior pharmacokinetic properties [2–4]. Vancomycin and teicoplanin are natural product GPAs produced by soil-dwelling filamentous actinomycetes. Their common structural motif is a core heptapeptide scaffold containing aromatic amino acids that have undergone extensive oxidative cross-linking and decoration with different moieties, such as sugar residues, chlorine atoms and—in case of teicoplanin—a lipid chain. GPAs inhibit peptidoglycan (PG) synthesis by binding to the D-alanyl-D-alanine (D-Ala-D-Ala) terminus of the peptide stem of PG-precursor lipid II. The binding of GPAs to lipid II by forming five hydrogen bonds locks PG precursors, impeding subsequent cross-linking reactions [5,6]. Second-generation GPAs are semisynthetic derivatives of vancomycin- and teicoplanin-like molecules, where the chemical modifications were introduced outside the D-Ala-D-Ala binding pocket, mainly involving the appendage of hydrophobic aryl or acyl groups that mimic the natural lipid chain of teicoplanin. In fact, the superior antimicrobial potency of teicoplanin-like molecules is due to membrane anchoring of the hydrophobic tail, which strengthens the bond to membrane-localized lipid II [7,8]. Additionally, Dong et al. [9] demonstrated that lipidation is the key functional difference between vancomycin and teicoplanin related to their differing abilities of inducing a GPA resistance response in enterococci. More recently Kwun and Hong [10], using the harmless actinomycete *Streptomyces coelicolor* as a model resistance system, confirmed that teicoplanin-like derivatives are poor inducers of GPA resistance, and a lack of induction accounts for the susceptibility to these molecules.

Many different GPA-resistant phenotypes have been described in enterococci and staphylococci (for an extensive review, see Binda et al., 2014 [2]). In the two most prominent manifestations of resistance (VanA or VanB phenotypes), the GPA-induced expression of *van* genes remodels the bacterial cell wall. The replacement of the dipeptide (D-Ala-D-Ala) terminus of PG precursor with the depsipeptide D-alanyl-D-lactate (D-Ala-D-Lac) reduces by 1000-fold the GPA affinity to their molecular target [11]. Strains displaying this type of resistance are either resistant to both vancomycin and teicoplanin (VanA phenotype), or they are resistant only to vancomycin and susceptible to teicoplanin (VanB phenotype) [12]. Although the proteins directly involved in conferring VanA resistance—i.e., VanH, which converts pyruvate into D-lactate; VanA, a D-Ala-D-Lac ligase; and VanX, a D-Ala-D-Ala dipeptidase—are highly homologous to their counterparts in the VanB phenotype (VanHB, VanB, VanXB), the two-component regulatory systems controlling *van* gene transcription (VanS/VanR in VanA phenotype and VanSB/VanRB in VanB phenotype) are only distantly related [13]. In particular, the membrane-associated sensor domains of VanS and VanSB are unrelated in amino acid sequence, and they respond to GPAs by different mechanisms which account for the difference in induction specificity by vancomycin and teicoplanin and their semi-synthetic derivatives [13–15]. Many efforts [12,14,16,17] have been devoted to identifying the molecular species responsible for differently inducing VanS and VanSB, but their entity and mode of action—i.e., direct binding of the GPAs to the sensor domain or its activation by cell wall intermediates that accumulate as a result of antibiotic action—is still being questioned.

Since it is widely believed that GPA resistance mechanisms are ultimately derived from GPA-producing actinomycetes, which use them to avoid suicide during antibiotic production [2,14], in this paper we investigated the specificity of induction of GPA resistance in teicoplanin- and A40926-producing actinomycetes. Teicoplanin is produced by *Actinoplanes teichomyceticus*, and the teicoplanin-like molecule A40926 [18], which is the natural precursor of the second-generation dalbavancin, is produced by the recently classified *Nonomuraea gerenzanensis* [19,20]. As a control, we used the well-characterized resistance model *S. coelicolor*, which does not synthesize any GPA but does possess a *van* gene cluster conferring inducible resistance to vancomycin but not to teicoplanin, showing the features of the VanB phenotype [10,16,21]. The purpose of this study was to elucidate the relationship between GPA activity and the ability to induce *van* gene expression in the producing actinomycetes, which are considered the evolutionary source of resistance determinants emerging in pathogens, shedding light on the possible evolution of the *van* gene cluster.

2. Results and Discussion

Table 1 reports the minimal inhibitory concentrations (MICs) of vancomycin, teicoplanin, and A40926 against *S. coelicolor*, *A. teichomyceticus*, and *N. gerenzanensis* on solid media. MICs were measured on solid media, since the standard broth dilution method used in unicellular bacteria to determine MICs by turbidity is compromised in mycelial actinomycetes by the formation of multicellular aggregates and by the coexistence of cells in different physiological states (e.g., vegetative mycelium, aerial mycelium, and spores). This is particularly true for difficult-to-cultivate nonstreptomyces actinomycetes such as *Actinoplanes* and *Nonomuraea* strains, which form compact and different-sized clumps when growing in liquid cultures.

Table 1. Minimal inhibitory concentrations (MICs) of glycopeptide antibiotics (GPAs), ramoplanin and bacitracin. The values represent the average of the data from three independent experiments.

Actinomycetes	Vancomycin (μg/mL)	Teicoplanin (μg/mL)	A40926 (μg/mL)	Ramoplanin (μg/mL)	Bacitracin (μg/mL)
S. coelicolor	>100	1.5 ± 0.025	1.5 ± 0.075	0.9 ± 0.045	0.9 ± 0.05
S. coelicolor ΔvanRS	1.25 ± 0.03	1.5 ± 0.02	1.5 ± 0.02	0.9 ± 0.025	0.9 ± 0.035
A. teichomyceticus	90 ± 4.2	20 ± 1.5	32.5 ± 1.5	20 ± 1	20 ± 1.15
N. gerenzanensis	20 ± 1.6	0.9 ± 0.01	4 ± 0.2	20 ± 1.2	20 ± 1.3
N. gerenzanensis pST30	20 ± 1.05	2.75 ± 0.15	17.5 ± 0.875	20 ± 1.1	20 ± 1.2

As expected, *S. coelicolor* was resistant to vancomycin and susceptible to teicoplanin and A40926. Its Δ*vanRS* mutant did not respond to vancomycin, and consequently, it was sensitive to it [10]. For these *Streptomyces* strains, MICs values were slightly higher than those previously reported in a liquid medium [10], which is likely due to the different cultivation method used. Interestingly, *S. coelicolor* and its Δ*vanRS* mutant were equally sensitive to bacitracin and ramoplanin, which are antibiotics structurally unrelated to GPAs that inhibit the late steps of PG synthesis by a diverse mode of action [22,23], evidently not mediated by VanS interaction.

A. teichomyceticus was resistant to all the GPAs tested (Table 1), although its chromosome harbours a canonical *vanHAX* gene cluster including the *vanRS* two component-regulatory system associated with the teicoplanin biosynthetic genes [24]. In this actinomycete, *van* genes are expressed constitutively, even in the absence of the antibiotic, making the cells intrinsically resistant to GPAs [24,25].

In contrast, the A40926-producing strain *N. gerenzanensis* was resistant to vancomycin (less than *A. teichomyceticus* and *S. coelicolor*) but sensitive to teicoplanin and to its own product, albeit at a lower extent. As previously described [26], *N. gerenzanensis* does not possess a *vanHAX* gene cluster, and the only known mechanism of resistance relies on the action of a VanY metallo-D,D-carboxypeptidase (named VanYn) that hydrolyses the C-terminal D-Ala residue of PG pentapeptide precursors. Interestingly, the well-characterized VanA and VanB type enterococci possess, in addition to *vanHAX* genes, an extra *vanY* gene that plays an ancillary unessential role in conferring glycopeptide resistance [27]. Upon vancomycin induction, enterococcal VanX cleaves any residual cytoplasmic D-Ala-D-Ala dipeptide, ensuring that the newly formed PG precursors terminate mostly in D-Ala-D-Lac, whereas VanY just acts on PG precursors that have escaped VanX hydrolysis and converts them into GPA-resistant tetrapeptides [27]. The integration of the pST30 plasmid containing the complete *vanRSHAX* gene cluster from *A. teichomyceticus* [25,28] into the *N. gerenzanensis* chromosome, consistently rendered the host strain more resistant to teicoplanin and A40926 in comparison to the parental strain harbouring only the *vanY* gene (Table 1), confirming the role of *vanHAX* genes in conferring high GPA resistance.

In contrast to *S. coelicolor*, both *A. teichomyceticus* and *N. gerenzanensis* were intrinsically resistant to both bacitracin and ramoplanin. This last result merits further investigation, although it is well-known that PG structure and density, and consequently antibiotic resistance profile, might dramatically vary among different genera of actinomycetes [19,29,30].

To determine the correlation between the antimicrobial activity of the GPAs and their ability to induce the *van* resistance system in actinomycetes, we followed the enzyme activities corresponding to either VanX or VanY peptidases in cells growing in liquid culture in the presence or absence of subinhibitory concentrations of GPAs (Figures 1 and 2). The D,D-dipeptidase activity of VanX (Figure 1) and the D,D-carboxypeptidase activity of VanY (Figure 2) were measured by determining the amount of D-Ala released from the hydrolysis of the D-Ala-D-Ala dipeptide and of the N_ε-acetyl-L-Lys-D-Ala-D-Ala tripeptide, respectively. D-Ala release was measured by using a D-amino acid oxidase coupled to a peroxidase [25,31]. As in the case of enterococci [27], VanX activity was detectable in the cytoplasmic fractions of *S. coelicolor*, *S. coelicolor* Δ*vanRS*, *A. teichomyceticus*, and *N. gerenzanensis* pST30 (Figure 1), and it was specific for the hydrolysis of D,D-dipeptides, being inactive on the ester D-Ala-D-Lac and on dipeptides substituted at the C or N terminus (data not shown). No VanX activity was detectable in *N. gerenzanensis* cytoplasmic fractions (see Table S1 Supplementary Material). Alternatively, VanY activity was detectable only in the membrane fractions of *N. gerenzanensis* and in its recombinant-derived *N. gerenzanensis* pST30 strain (Figure 2), consistent with the predicted VanY N-terminal structure, which contains a hydrophobic domain [31]. No VanY activity was detectable in *S. coelicolor*, *S. coelicolor* Δ*vanRS*, and *A. teichomyceticus* (see Table S1 Supplementary Material).

In *S. coelicolor* and *S. coelicolor* Δ*vanRS*, basal VanX activity (without any GPA addition) reached the maximum value within the 24 h of growth. When *S. coelicolor* parental strain was grown in the presence of subinhibitory concentrations of vancomycin (10 µg/mL), teicoplanin (0.75 µg/mL), and A40926 (0.75 µg/mL), only vancomycin induced an increase in VanX activity, and the level of enzyme activity doubled within the first 24 h from the induction (Figure 1). The addition of ramoplanin and bacitracin (both added at 0.45 µg/mL) did not show any effect on VanX activity (data not shown), thus indicating the specificity of vancomycin induction. Moreover, the addition of subinhibitory concentrations of vancomycin (in this case 0.6 µg /mL), teicoplanin (0.75 µg/mL), A40926 (0.75 µg/mL), and ramoplanin and bacitracin (both added at 0.45 µg/mL) to *S. coelicolor* Δ*vanRS* did not induce any increase in VanX activity, confirming the role of VanS in responding to vancomycin induction (Figure 1).

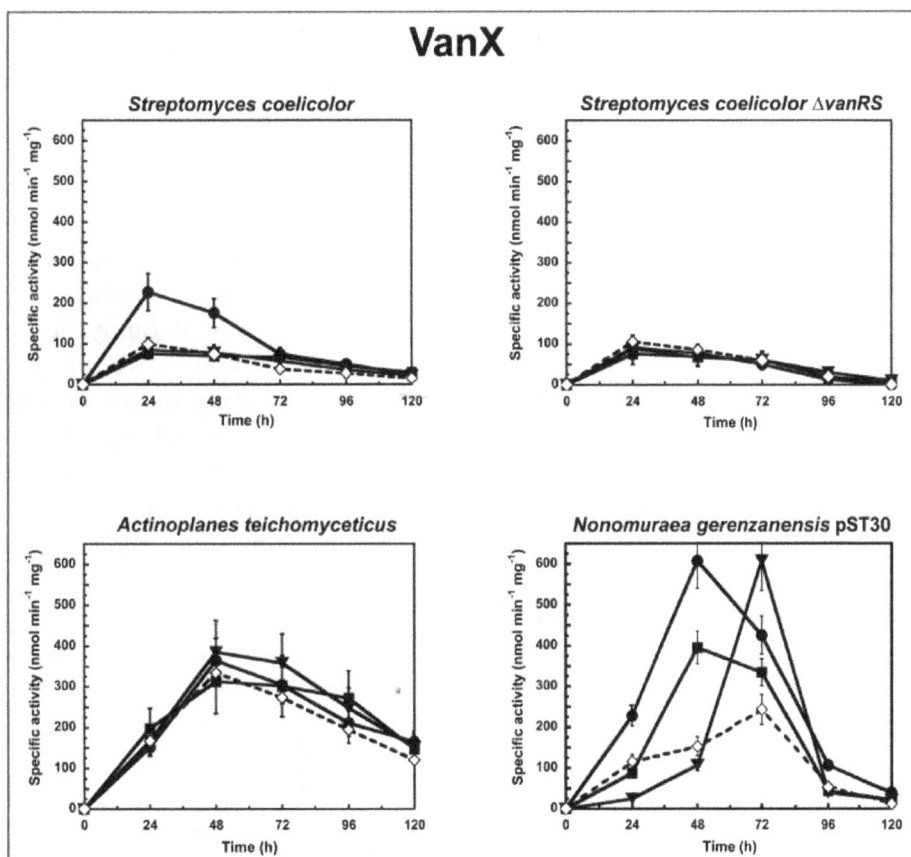

Figure 1. VanX activity in *S. coelicolor*, *S. coelicolor* Δ*vanRS*, *A. teichomyceticus*, and *N. gerenzanensis* pST30 grown in the absence (dotted line) or in the presence (continuous line) of subinhibitory concentrations of GPAs added at the moment of inoculum (see material and methods). VanX-specific activity is defined as the number of nanomoles of D-Ala released by the hydrolysis of D-Ala-D-Ala dipeptide at 37 °C per minute per milligram of protein contained in cytoplasmic fractions. Symbols represent non-induction (◇), induction with vancomycin (●), or teicoplanin (■), or A40926 (▼). The values represent the averages from three independent experiments, with a standard deviation of <5%.

In *A. teichomyceticus*, basal VanX activity (without any GPA addition) reached the maximum value after 48 h of growth. No significant variation in VanX activity was detectable following the addition of 45 µg/mL of vancomycin, of 10 µg/mL of teicoplanin, or of 15 µg/mL of A40926 (Figure 1). As expected, the MICs of GPAs measured on *A. teichomyceticus* after 48 and 72 h of growth in the presence of teicoplanin were the same as reported in Table 1 (see Table S2 in Supplementary Material). These results are in agreement with the constitutive expression of *vanHAX* genes that, according to Beltrametti et al. [24], is due to an impaired phosphatase function of the mutated VanS, which is consequently locked in the "on" state in this organism [14]. The addition of ramoplanin and bacitracin did not exert any specific effect on the VanX activity in *A. teichomyceticus* (data not shown).

Interesting is what occurred in the recombinant strain *N. gerenzanensis* pST30 that, in addition to *vanYn*, also harbours the heterologous *vanX* from *A. teichomyceticus*. In this strain, the basal D,D-dipeptidase activity of VanX reached the maximum value after 72 h of growth. VanX activity was induced by 10 µg/mL of vancomycin, by 1.75 µg/mL of teicoplanin, and by 10 µg/mL of A40926, albeit with different kinetics and intensity (Figure 1). When the *A. teichomyceticus vanRSHAX* genes were integrated into the host genome, VanX activity was not longer under the control of the parental *vanRS* but became inducible by GPAs, undergoing regulation by a still-unknown circuit present in *N. gerenzanensis*, which responds to subinhibitory concentrations of vancomycin (within the 48 h of growth), A40926 (within the 72 h), and, albeit to less extent, teicoplanin (within the 48 h) (Figure 1).

To shed light on the specificity of induction of GPA resistance in *N. gerenzanensis*, we compared the VanY activity in *N. gerenzanensis* and in its recombinant strain *N. gerenzanensis* pST30 when grown in the absence or presence of GPAs (Figure 2). In both the strains, basal VanY activity reached its maximum activity after 72 h of growth. Upon induction with 10 µg/mL of vancomycin, 0.45 µg/mL of teicoplanin, or 2 µg/mL of A40926, VanY activity in the parental strain increased within the first 24 h (Figure 2), suggesting that VanY-based resistance was induced by the exposure to the three GPAs. As expected, MICs of GPAs measured on *N. gerenzanensis* after 48 and 72 h of growth in the presence of A40926 increased, as reported in Table S2 of Supplementary Material. Again, the addition of ramoplanin and bacitracin did not influence the activity profile (data not shown). Surprisingly, the membrane-associated VanY activity in *N. gerenzanensis* pST30 was significantly induced only by vancomycin, and its detection was delayed in comparison to the parental strain, reaching its maximum value after 96 h of growth (Figure 2). In the presence of A40926 and teicoplanin, the VanY activity was comparable to the basal level previously observed in the noninduced recombinant strain (Figure 2). Intriguingly, these data suggest that swapping heterologous *A. teichomyceticus* genes in *N. gerenzanensis* pST30 did alter the specificity of induction of the homologous VanY activity, although the heterologous VanX activity responded to induction by the three GPAs as the VanY activity did in the parental strain. It seems that in the presence of the heterologous VanX dipeptidase, homologous VanY carboxyesterase tends to play an auxiliary role as it occurs in VanA and VanB enterococci [21]. Irrespective of this finding, further investigations on the still-unknown regulatory genes controlling GPA resistance in *N. gerenzanensis* are needed to better explain these diverse responses to GPA induction. In a previous 'van genes' swapping experiment conducted by Hutchings et al., 2006, introducing the *Streptomyces toyocaensis* VanRS signal transduction system into *S. coelicolor* Δ*vanRS* switched inducer specificity to that of *S. toyocaensis*, whose resistant genes are induced by A47934 but not by vancomycin [21]. The authors concluded that the inducer specificity was determined by the origin of VanS/VanR [21]. More recently, Kilian et al. reported that the VanRS homologous two-component system VnlRS of *Amycolatopsis balhimycina* (which produces the vancomycin-type balhimycin) activated the transcription of the *vanHAX* genes in *S. coelicolor*, but not in *A. balhimycina* [32]. Surprisingly, the introduction of VnlRS from *A. balhimycina* into *S. coelicolor* induced teicoplanin resistance, most likely by activating further unknown genes required for teicoplanin resistance [32]. Although two members of a putative VanRS-like two-component signal transduction system were previously identified in the A40926 biosynthetic cluster in *N. gerenzanensis* [33], their role in controlling the VanY-based self-resistance mechanism and in responding to GPA induction is still unveiled and merit further investigations.

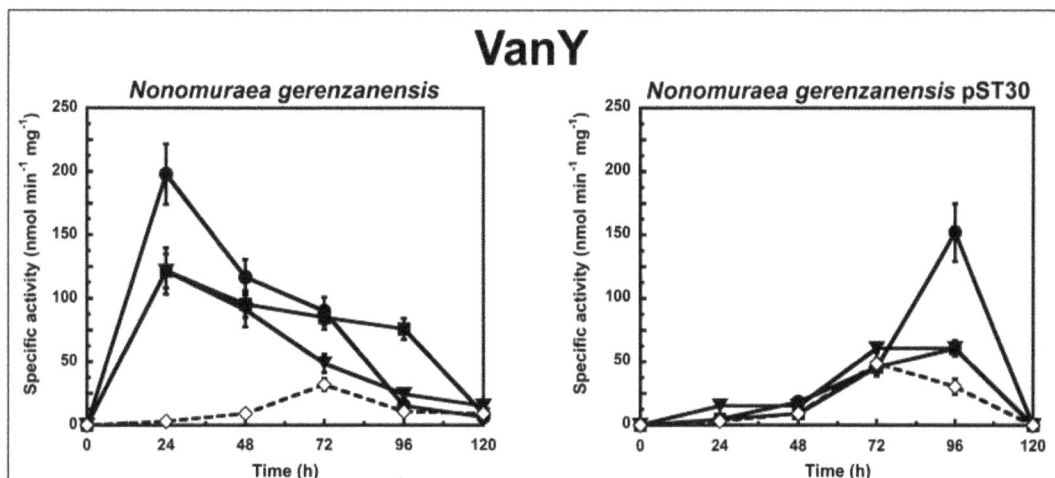

Figure 2. VanY activity in *N. gerenzanensis* and *N. gerenzanensis* pST30 grown in the absence (dotted line) or in the presence (continuous line) of subinhibitory concentrations of GPAs added at the moment of inoculum (see material and methods). VanY-specific activity is defined as the number of nanomoles of D-Ala released by the hydrolysis of N_ε-acetyl-L-Lys-D-Ala-D-Ala tripeptide at 37 °C per minute per milligram of protein contained in membrane extracts. Symbols represent non-induction (◇), induction with vancomycin (●), or teicoplanin (■), or A40926 (▼). The values represent the averages from three independent experiments, with a standard deviation of <5%.

3. Materials and Methods

3.1. Strains and Media

S. coelicolor A3(2) was a gift from Mervyn Bibb, John Innes Institute, Norwich, UK [34]. The ΔvanRS mutant of S. coelicolor was generously donated by Hee-Jeon Hong, University of Cambridge, UK [21]. Streptomyces spp. strains were maintained as spores in 10% (v/v) glycerol and propagated in MS agar media [34]. Liquid media for streptomycetes were YEME [34] and BTSB (Difco). Colonies were picked up from agar plates and inoculated into 300 mL Erlenmeyer flasks containing 50 mL of YEME. Flask cultures were incubated on a rotary shaker at 200 rpm and 28 °C.

N. gerenzanensis ATCC 39727 [19], its recombinant strain N. gerenzanensis pST30 [25], and A. teichomyceticus ATCC 31121 [35] were maintained as lyophilized master cell banks (MCBs). The mycelium from the MCBs was streaked on slants of a salt medium (SM) [34] solidified with agar (15 g/liter). After its growth, the mycelium from a slant was homogenized in 10 mL of 0.9% (w/v) NaCl, inoculated into liquid SM, grown for 96 h at 28 °C with aeration, and stored as a working cell bank (WCB) in 1.5 mL cryovials at −80 °C. One vial was used to inoculate each 300 mL Erlenmeyer flask containing 50 mL VSP medium [26], and the flasks were incubated at 28 °C, with shaking at 200 rpm. Previous HPLC data showed that no A40926 or teicoplanin production occurred in this vegetative medium [26,35]. In the case of N. gerenzanensis pST30, the VSP medium was added with 50 μg/mL apramycin to maintain plasmid selection. Surface cultures were grown on V0.1 agar [26]. All medium components were from Sigma-Aldrich (St. Louis, MO, USA) unless otherwise stated.

3.2. Induction Experiments

S. coelicolor A3(2), its ΔvanRS mutant, A. teichomyceticus ATCC 31121, N. gerenzanensis ATCC 39727, and N. gerenzanensis pST30 were grown as described above. Vancomycin, teicoplanin, A40926, bacitracin, and ramoplanin (all from Sigma-Aldrich) were dissolved in MilliQ water and sterilized by filtration using 0.22 μm filters. Antibiotics were added to the cultures at the moment of inoculation using concentrations calculated as the half-point of MICs (see below and Table 1), except for vancomycin (10 µg/mL) in *S. coelicolor* A3(2), as reported by Kwun et al. [10]. At these concentrations, growth curves of noninduced and induced strains were overlapping.

3.3. MIC Determination

Cryovials of WCBs were thawed at room temperature and used to inoculate a VSP medium for *Nonomuraea* spp. and *Actinoplanes* spp. or YEME for *Streptomyces* spp. in the presence or the absence of GPAs. The strains were grown to exponential phase (approximately 72 h) at 28 °C with shaking. The mycelium was harvested by centrifugation, suspended in 0.9% (*w/v*) NaCl, and fragmented by sonication with a Vibracell Albra sonicator 400 W [26]. A suspension of sonicated hyphae (corresponding to 10^7 CFU) was seeded onto V0.1 (*Nonomuraea* spp. and *Actinoplanes* spp.) or MS (*Streptomyces* spp.) agar plates supplemented with increasing concentrations of the following antibiotics: 0 to 100 µg/mL vancomycin in 10-µg/mL increments; 0 to 2 µg/mL teicoplanin in 0.1-µg/mL increments or 0 to 40 µg/mL teicoplanin in 10-µg/mL increments depending on the strain; and 0 to 5 µg/mL or 5 to 50 µg/mL A40926, depending on the strain, in 0.5-µg/mL or 2.5-µg/mL increments. The plates were dried and then incubated at 28 °C. MIC values were determined as the lowest antibiotic concentrations that inhibited visible growth after 10 days of incubation.

3.4. D,D-dipeptidase and D,D-carboxypeptidase Assays

Cells were harvested by centrifugation at 3600× *g* for 20 min at 4 °C, and then they were suspended in 2 mL of 0.9% (*w/v*) NaCl per gram of cells (wet weight). All of the following manipulations were conducted at 0 to 4 °C. The mycelium was fragmented by sonication with a Sonics Vibracell VCX 130. Sonication was carried out for 5 min on ice, with cycles of 30 s with an amplitude of 90% (90% of 60 Hz), with breaks of 10 s. The samples were then centrifuged at 39,000× *g* for 15 min, and the supernatants (cytoplasmic fractions) were collected. An alkaline extraction of the pellets (cell debris and membrane fractions) was carried out by adapting a protocol developed previously for extracting membrane-bound proteins [25,36]. The sedimented pellets were resuspended in ice-cold distilled water containing proteinase inhibitors (0.19 mg/mL phenylmethanesulfonyl fluoride and 0.7 µg/mL pepstatin, both purchased from Sigma-Aldrich), and then, immediately before centrifugation (28,000× *g* for 15 min at 4 °C), the pH was adjusted to 12 by adding an appropriate volume of 2.5 N NaOH. Immediately after centrifugation, the supernatants were neutralized to pH 7 by adding 0.5 M sodium acetate (pH 5.4). Enzymatic activities in the supernatant (cytoplasmic fractions) and in the resuspended insoluble fractions (membranes) were assayed as reported previously [36] by measuring the release of D-Ala from commercially available dipeptide (D-Ala-D-Ala, 10 mM; Sigma-Aldrich) and tripeptide (N$_\varepsilon$-acetyl-L-Lys-D-Ala-D-Ala, 10 mM; Sigma-Aldrich). D,D-carboxypeptidase activity was confirmed using 10 mM UDP-MurNAc-L-Ala-D-Glu-*meso*-Dap-D-Ala-D-Ala (UK-BaCWAN, University of Warwick) as a substrate. The release of D-Ala was followed spectrophotometrically at 510 nm with a D-amino acid oxidase–peroxidase coupled reaction. Reaction mixtures contained 5 mM of the peroxidase colorimetric substrate 4-aminoantipyrine (Sigma-Aldrich), 3 U/mL D-amino acid oxidase (Sigma-Aldrich), 7.5 U/mL horseradish peroxidase (Sigma-Aldrich), and 6 mM phenol in 50 mM 1,3-bis[tris(hydroxymethyl)methylamino]propane (pH 7.4) in a final volume of 1 mL, as described in detail in [36]. To compare the D,D-dipeptidase and D,D-carboxypeptidase activities in the cytoplasmic and membrane extracts, the activity was expressed as the number of nanomoles of D-Ala released from the dipeptide or tripeptide per min per mg of protein in the extract.

4. Conclusions

By comparing the specificity of induction of VanX and VanY peptidases in three different soil-dwelling actinomycetes, we confirm that *S. coelicolor* has a VanB-phenotype responding to vancomycin but not to teicoplanin or to teicoplanin-like A40926. *S. coelicolor* does not produce any GPA but possessing resistance genes confers it a selective advantage since it shares the ecological niche (soil) with many other GPAs-producing actinomycetes. Interestingly, by a culture-independent approach using molecular probes, it has been recently estimated that the frequency of encountering a vancomycin-type producer in soil is from 2.5 to 5 times higher than for a teicoplanin-like producing actinomycete [37]. In contrast, the teicoplanin producer *A. teichomyceticus* is highly and constitutively resistant to all the GPAs, including its own product. On the contrary, lower resistance in *N. gerenzanensis* is induced either by vancomycin or teicoplanins, and is based on the action of a VanY carboxypeptidase, which in many enterococci and staphylococci plays an unessential and ancillary role in the presence of VanHAX system [27]. Evidently, although producing structurally similar GPAs, *A. teichomyceticus* and *N. gerenzanensis* do not share the same self-resistant mechanism. Previous comparative analyses of their biosynthetic GPA clusters indicated that many A40926 biosynthetic genes are more related to vancomycin-type genes than to their teicoplanin homologs [38]. The production of A40926 and teicoplanin are most likely the result of a convergent evolution rather than originating from the same common ancestor. Although the identity and the role of the putative VanRS-like two-component signal transduction system in *N. gerenzanensis* needs to be investigated, the results of gene swapping between *A. teichomyceticus* and *N. gerenzanensis* indicate that cross-talking of the two-component systems is possible, as previously demonstrated in other actinomycetes [21,32]. Determining the sequences and the protein structures of the putative VanRS two-component system in *N. gerenzanensis* may help to confirm that the inducer specificity is determined by the origin of VanRS proteins and may provide additional evidence on the role of GPAs as VanS effector ligands. Additionally, since the genes involved in GPAs resistance in pathogens have been recruited from the different antibiotic-producing actinomycetes, gene swapping among different GPA-producing actinomycetes is proving to be useful for unveiling the specificity of regulation and predicting the evolution of future resistance gene combinations emerging in pathogens.

Supplementary Materials:
Table S1: Maximum VanX and VanY activities during the growth (in the absence of GPAs) of *S. coelicolor*, *S. coelicolor* Δ*vanRS*, *A. teichomyceticus*, *N. gerenzanensis* and *N. gerenzanensis* pST30. The values represent the average of the data from three independent experiments, Table S2: MICs of GPAs in noninduced and teicoplanins-induced actinomycetes. The values represent the average of the data from three independent experiments.

Author Contributions: E.B., F.M. and G.L.M. conceived and designed the experiments; E.B. and P.C. performed the experiments; E.B., P.C. and G.L.M. analyzed the data; E.B., F.M. and G.L.M. wrote the paper.

Acknowledgments: This work was supported by public grants "Fondo di Ateneo per la Ricerca" 2015, 2016, 2017 to F. Marinelli and G.L. Marcone and by Federation of European Microbiological Societies (FEMS) Research Fellowship 2015 to E. Binda.

References

1. European Centre for Disease Prevention and Control. Available online: https://ecdc.europa.eu/en/about-us/partnerships-and-networks/disease-and-laboratoy-networks/ears-net (accessed on 16 January 2018).

2. Binda, E.; Marinelli, F.; Marcone, G.L. Old and new glycopeptide antibiotics: Action and resistance. *Antibiotics* **2014**, *3*, 572–594. [CrossRef] [PubMed]

3. Marcone, G.L.; Binda, E.; Berini, F.; Marinelli, F. Old and new glycopeptide antibiotics: From product to gene and back in the post-genomic era. *Biotechnol. Adv.* **2018**, *36*, 534–554. [CrossRef] [PubMed]

4. Van Bambeke, F. Lipoglycopeptide antibacterial agents in Gram-positive infections: A comparative review. *Drugs* **2015**, *18*, 2073–2095. [CrossRef] [PubMed]

5. Cooper, M.A.; Williams, D.H. Binding of glycopeptide antibiotics to a model of a vancomycin-resistant bacterium. *Chem. Biol.* **1999**, *6*, 891–899. [CrossRef]

6. Perkins, H.R.; Nieto, M. The chemical basis for the action of the vancomycin group of antibiotics. *Ann. N. Y. Acad. Sci.* **1974**, *235*, 348–363. [CrossRef] [PubMed]

7. Allen, N.E.; Nicas, T.I. Mechanism of action of oritavancin and related glycopeptide antibiotics. *FEMS Microbiol. Rev.* **2003**, *26*, 511–532. [CrossRef] [PubMed]

8. Treviño, J.; Bayón, C.; Ardá, A.; Marinelli, F.; Gandolfi, R.; Molinari, F.; Jimenez-Barbero, J.; Hernáiz, M.J. New insights into glycopeptide antibiotic binding to cell wall precursors using SPR and NMR spectroscopy. *Chemistry* **2014**, *20*, 7363–7372. [CrossRef] [PubMed]

9. Dong, S.D.; Oberthür, M.; Losey, H.C.; Anderson, J.W.; Eggert, U.S.; Peczuh, M.W.; Walsh, C.T.; Kahne, D. The structural basis for induction of VanB resistance. *J. Am. Chem. Soc.* **2002**, *124*, 9064–9065. [CrossRef] [PubMed]

10. Kwun, M.J.; Hong, H.J. The activity of glycopeptide antibiotics against resistant bacteria correlates with their ability to induce the resistance system. *Antimicrob. Agents Chemother.* **2014**, *58*, 6306–6310. [CrossRef] [PubMed]

11. Bugg, T.D.; Wright, G.D.; Dutka-Malen, S.; Arthur, M.; Courvalin, P.; Walsh, C.T. Molecular basis for vancomycin resistance in *Enterococcus faecium* BM4147: Biosynthesis of a depsipeptide peptidoglycan precursor by vancomycin resistance proteins VanH and VanA. *Biochemistry* **1991**, *30*, 10408–10415. [CrossRef] [PubMed]

12. Arthur, M.; Quintiliani, R. Regulation of VanA- and VanB-type glycopeptide resistance in enterococci. *Antimicrob. Agents Chemother.* **2001**, *45*, 375–381. [CrossRef] [PubMed]

13. Evers, S.; Courvalin, P. Regulation of VanB-type vancomycin resistance gene expression by the VanS(B)-VanR(B) two-component regulatory system in *Enterococcus faecalis* V583. *J. Bacteriol.* **1996**, *178*, 1302–1309. [CrossRef] [PubMed]

14. Hong, H.J.; Hutchings, M.I.; Buttner, M.J. Vancomycin resistance VanS/VanR two-component systems. *Adv. Exp. Med. Biol.* **2008**, *631*, 200–213. [CrossRef] [PubMed]

15. Depardieu, F.; Podglajen, I.; Leclercq, R.; Collatz, E.; Courvalin, P. Modes and modulations of antibiotic resistance gene expression. *Clin. Microbiol. Rev.* **2007**, *20*, 79–114. [CrossRef] [PubMed]

16. Kwun, M.J.; Novotna, G.; Hesketh, A.R.; Hill, L.; Hong, H.J. In vivo studies suggest that induction of VanS-dependent vancomycin resistance requires binding of the drug to D-Ala-D-Ala termini in the peptidoglycan cell wall. *Antimicrob. Agents Chemother.* **2013**, *57*, 4470–4480. [CrossRef] [PubMed]

17. Koteva, K.; Hong, H.J.; Wang, X.D.; Nazi, I.; Hughes, D.; Naldrett, M.J.; Buttner, M.J.; Wright, G.D. A vancomycin photoprobe identifies the histidine kinase VanSsc as a vancomycin receptor. *Nat. Chem. Biol.* **2010**, *6*, 327–329. [CrossRef] [PubMed]

18. Goldstein, B.P.; Selva, E.; Gastaldo, L.; Berti, M.; Pallanza, R.; Ripamonti, F.; Ferrari, P.; Denaro, M.; Arioli, V.; Cassani, G. A40926, a new glycopeptide antibiotic with anti-*Neisseria* activity. *Antimicrob. Agents Chemother.* **1987**, *31*, 1961–1966. [CrossRef] [PubMed]

19. Dalmastri, C.; Gastaldo, L.; Marcone, G.L.; Binda, E.; Congiu, T.; Marinelli, F. Classification of *Nonomuraea* sp. ATCC 39727, an actinomycete that produces the glycopeptide antibiotic A40926, as *Nonomuraea gerenzanensis* sp. nov. *Int. J. Syst. Evol. Microbiol.* **2016**, *66*, 912–921. [CrossRef] [PubMed]

20. D'Argenio, V.; Petrillo, M.; Pasanisi, D.; Pagliarulo, C.; Colicchio, R.; Talà, A.; de Biase, M.S.; Zanfardino, M.; Scolamiero, E.; Pagliuca, C.; et al. The complete 12 Mb genome and transcriptome of *Nonomuraea gerenzanensis* with new insights into its duplicated "Magic" RNA polymerase. *Sci. Rep.* **2016**, *6*, 18. [CrossRef] [PubMed]

21. Hutchings, M.I.; Hong, H.J.; Buttner, M.J. The vancomycin resistance VanRS two-component signal transduction system of *Streptomyces coelicolor*. *Mol. Microbiol.* **2006**, *59*, 923–935. [CrossRef] [PubMed]

22. Siewert, G.; Strominger, J.L. Bacitracin: An inhibitor of the dephosphorylation of lipid pyrophosphate, an intermediate in the biosynthesis of the peptidoglycan of bacterial cell walls. *Proc. Natl. Acad. Sci. USA* **1967**, *57*, 767–773. [CrossRef] [PubMed]

23. Hamburger, J.B.; Hoertz, A.J.; Lee, A.; Senturia, R.J.; McCafferty, D.G.; Loll, P.J. A crystal structure of a dimer of the antibiotic ramoplanin illustrates membrane positioning and a potential lipid II docking interface. *Proc. Natl. Acad. Sci. USA* **2009**, *106*, 13759–13764. [CrossRef] [PubMed]

24. Beltrametti, F.; Consolandi, A.; Carrano, L.; Bagatin, F.; Rossi, R.; Leoni, L.; Zennaro, E.; Selva, E.; Marinelli, F. Resistance to glycopeptide antibiotics in the teicoplanin producer is mediated by *van* gene homologue expression directing the synthesis of a modified cell wall peptidoglycan. *Antimicrob. Agents Chemother.* **2007**, *51*, 1135–1141. [CrossRef] [PubMed]

25. Marcone, G.L.; Binda, E.; Carrano, L.; Bibb, M.; Marinelli, F. Relationship between glycopeptide production and resistance in the actinomycete *Nonomuraea* sp. ATCC 39727. *Antimicrob. Agents Chemother.* **2014**, *58*, 5191–5201. [CrossRef] [PubMed]

26. Marcone, G.L.; Beltrametti, F.; Binda, E.; Carrano, L.; Foulston, L.; Hesketh, A.; Bibb, M.; Marinelli, F. Novel mechanism of glycopeptide resistance in the A40926 producer *Nonomuraea* sp. ATCC 39727. *Antimicrob. Agents Chemother.* **2010**, *54*, 2465–2472. [CrossRef] [PubMed]

27. Arthur, M.; Depardieu, F.; Cabanié, L.; Reynolds, P.; Courvalin, P. Requirement of the VanY and VanX D,D-peptidases for glycopeptide resistance in enterococci. *Mol. Microbiol.* **1998**, *30*, 819–830. [CrossRef] [PubMed]

28. Serina, S.; Radice, F.; Maffioli, S.; Donadio, S.; Sosio, M. Glycopeptide resistance determinants from the teicoplanin producer *Actinoplanes teichomyceticus*. *FEMS Microbiol. Lett.* **2004**, *240*, 69–74. [CrossRef] [PubMed]

29. Marcone, G.L.; Carrano, L.; Marinelli, F.; Beltrametti, F. Protoplast preparation and reversion to the normal filamentous growth in antibiotic-producing uncommon actinomycetes. *J. Antibiot.* **2010**, *63*, 83–88. [CrossRef] [PubMed]

30. Marcone, G.L.; Binda, E.; Reguzzoni, M.; Gastaldo, L.; Dalmastri, C.; Marinelli, F. Classification of *Actinoplanes* sp. ATCC 33076, an actinomycete that produces the glycolipodepsipeptide antibiotic ramoplanin, as *Actinoplanes ramoplaninifer* sp. nov. *Int. J. Syst. Evol. Microbiol.* **2017**, *67*, 4181–4188. [CrossRef] [PubMed]

31. Binda, E.; Marcone, G.L.; Pollegioni, L.; Marinelli, F. Characterization of VanYn, a novel D,D-peptidase/D,D-carboxypeptidase involved in glycopeptide antibiotic resistance in *Nonomuraea* sp. ATCC 39727. *FEBS J.* **2012**, *279*, 3203–3213. [CrossRef] [PubMed]

32. Kilian, R.; Frasch, H.J.; Kulik, A.; Wohlleben, W.; Stegmann, E. The VanRS homologous two-component system VnlRSAb of the glycopeptide producer *Amycolatopsis balhimycina* activates transcription of the *vanHAXSc* genes in *Streptomyces coelicolor*, but not in *A. balhimycina*. *Microb. Drug Resist.* **2016**, *22*, 499–509. [CrossRef] [PubMed]

33. Sosio, M.; Stinchi, S.; Beltrametti, F.; Lazzarini, A.; Donadio, S. The gene cluster for the biosynthesis of the glycopeptide antibiotic A40926 by *Nonomuraea* species. *Chem. Biol.* **2003**, *10*, 541–549. [CrossRef]

34. Kieser, T.; Bibb, M.J.; Buttner, M.J.; Chater, K.F.; Hopwood, D.A. *Practical Streptomyces Genetics*; The John Innes Foundation: Norwich, UK, 2000; ISBN 0-7084-0623-8.

35. Taurino, C.; Frattini, L.; Marcone, G.L.; Gastaldo, L.; Marinelli, F. *Actinoplanes teichomyceticus* ATCC 31121 as a cell factory for producing teicoplanin. *Microb. Cell Fact.* **2011**, *10*, 82–94. [CrossRef] [PubMed]

36. Binda, E.; Marcone, G.L.; Berini, F.; Pollegioni, L.; Marinelli, F. *Streptomyces* spp. as efficient expression system for a D,D-peptidase/D,D-carboxypeptidase involved in glycopeptide antibiotic resistance. *BMC Biotechnol.* **2013**, *13*, 24. [CrossRef] [PubMed]

37. Thaker, M.N.; Wang, W.; Spanogiannopoulos, P.; Waglechner, N.; King, A.M.; Medina, R.; Wright, G.D. Identifying producers of antibacterial compounds by screening for antibiotic resistance. *Nat. Biotechnol.* **2013**, *31*, 922–927. [CrossRef] [PubMed]

38. Donadio, S.; Sosio, M.; Stegmann, E.; Weber, T.; Wohlleben, W. Comparative analysis and insights into the evolution of gene clusters for glycopeptide antibiotic biosynthesis. *Mol. Genet. Genom.* **2005**, *274*, 40–50. [CrossRef] [PubMed]

11

Toxicological Assessment of a Lignin Core Nanoparticle Doped with Silver as an Alternative to Conventional Silver Core Nanoparticles

Cassandra E. Nix [1], Bryan J. Harper [1], Cathryn G. Conner [2], Alexander P. Richter [2], Orlin D. Velev [2] and Stacey L. Harper [1,3,4,*]

[1] Department of Environmental & Molecular Toxicology, Oregon State University, Corvallis, OR 97331, USA; nixc@oregonstate.edu (C.E.N.); Bryan.Harper@oregonstate.edu (B.J.H.)

[2] Department of Chemical and Biomolecular Engineering, North Carolina State University, Raleigh, NC 27606, USA; cgconner@ncsu.edu (C.G.C.); aprichte@ncsu.edu (A.P.R.); odvelev@ncsu.edu (O.D.V.)

[3] Oregon Nanoscience and Microtechnologies Institute, Corvallis, OR 97330, USA

[4] School of Chemical, Biological and Environmental Engineering, Oregon State University, Corvallis, OR 97331, USA

* Correspondence: stacey.harper@oregonstate.edu

Abstract: Elevated levels of silver in the environment are anticipated with an increase in silver nanoparticle (AgNP) production and use in consumer products. To potentially reduce the burden of silver ion release from conventional solid core AgNPs, a lignin-core particle doped with silver ions and surface-stabilized with a polycationic electrolyte layer was engineered. Our objective was to determine whether any of the formulation components elicit toxicological responses using embryonic zebrafish. Ionic silver and free surface stabilizer were the most toxic constituents, although when associated separately or together with the lignin core particles, the toxicity of the formulations decreased significantly. The overall toxicity of lignin formulations containing silver was similar to other studies on a silver mass basis, and led to a significantly higher prevalence of uninflated swim bladder and yolk sac edema. Comparative analysis of dialyzed samples which had leached their loosely bound Ag^+, showed a significant increase in mortality immediately after dialysis, in addition to eliciting significant increases in types of sublethal responses relative to the freshly prepared non-dialyzed samples. ICP-OES/MS analysis indicated that silver ion release from the particle into solution was continuous, and the rate of release differed when the surface stabilizer was not present. Overall, our study indicates that the lignin core is an effective alternative to conventional solid core AgNPs for potentially reducing the burden of silver released into the environment from a variety of consumer products.

Keywords: nanotechnology; environmentally-friendly; pesticide; antimicrobial; zebrafish

1. Introduction

Silver nanoparticles (AgNPs) are an effective antimicrobial agent and the most widely commercialized engineered nanomaterial, incorporated into half of all reported consumer and medical products in the Nanotechnology Consumer Products Inventory [1]. Prominent examples include cosmetics, clothing, shoes, detergents, water filters, phones, laptops, and toys [2–4]. AgNP use has risen steadily in the past decade (~52 new consumer products per year), and global production is estimated based on surveys of European producers to be between 12–1216 tons per year by 2020, assuming the number of products on the market continues to increase at the current rate [5,6]. With the increasing production and use of AgNPs, the fate and the subsequent release of silver in nanomaterial and ionic form into the environment are of concern.

Research indicates that AgNPs can enter aqueous environments from discharges at the point of production, by erosion from household products, and from disposal of silver-containing products [7–11]. These studies have prompted the investigation of AgNP interactions in the environment [12], particularly aquatic systems, to determine which general intrinsic and extrinsic properties are important in determining fate [9,13–15]. Extrinsic properties include environmental factors and processes that can impact the fate of the particles in aquatic systems, such as pH, temperature, ionic strength of the water, and natural organic matter, as well as processes like sedimentation, deposition, dissolution, agglomeration, and/or particle sulfidation [16–19]. Intrinsic factors address inherent particle characteristics, such as size, shape, chemical composition, surface structure, and surface charge [12,20–23]. Extrinsic factors can interact with intrinsic features of nanoparticles to alter particle behavior with concomitant effects on properties, such as the bioavailability of AgNPs to living organisms; thus, a more comprehensive understanding is needed [13,24].

AgNPs are known to be toxic to many aquatic organisms, including algae, bacteria, invertebrates, and fish [2]. Several mechanisms of action have been proposed, mainly attributing the toxicity of AgNPs to silver ions released from the nanoparticle. However, nanoparticle-specific mechanisms are also being investigated, with data suggesting that mechanistic differences exist compared to dissolved silver [5,25]. Silver ion specific mechanisms include interactions with thiols and electron donor groups, which can impact enzymes and DNA, which makes them unavailable for cellular processes [26–28], denaturing of DNA and RNA, which ultimately affects protein synthesis [29,30], and production of superoxide radicals and other reactive oxygen species via reactions with oxygen [29]. Particle-specific mechanisms have been suggested that focus on the ability of AgNPs to cause cell membrane damage, leading to disruption in the ion efflux system in cells [31,32], as well as by intracellular ion release elicited by the acidic conditions of the lysosomal cellular compartment where particles are internalized (Trojan horse effect) [33]. Since multiple aquatic organisms may be at risk due to an increased prevalence of silver in the environment, it is important to consider ways to reduce the environmental silver burden related to AgNP production and use.

By applying the principles of green chemistry during nanomaterial design and synthesis, harmful effects to the environment can be limited while maintaining the desired antimicrobial activity [34]. In order to reduce silver ion release into the environment, a silver-doped lignin nanoparticle was engineered, which is anticipated to have lower environmental impacts upon release into the environment [35]. During the synthesis of these particles, we replaced the silver core with lignin, which was chosen as it is a natural biodegradable biopolymer [36]. Similar synthesized lignin nanoparticles have been shown to have no impact on algae and yeast survival, suggesting they have a high level of biocompatibility [37]. The lignin is easily precipitated into nanosized particles using environmentally-friendly solvents, and the resulting nanoparticles can be infused with up to ten times lower (Ag^+) than silver core nanoparticles, and still maintain the same antimicrobial efficacy [35]. The particles are then surface-functionalized with a polycationic electrolyte layer to stabilize the particle, as well as to provide additional antimicrobial impact. The lignin nanoparticles exhibit both high and low affinity binding regions for silver ions, and these differing affinities, as well as the electrostatic barrier provided by the surface stabilizer, impact the rate of silver ion release to the surrounding solution [35,36]. It is expected that the low affinity binding sites will primarily release the majority of the weakly bound silver in the first 24 h [35]; however, we also wanted to investigate the long-term release from the high affinity binding sites, so two of the formulated samples were dialyzed to remove the weakly bound silver. When compared to their non-dialyzed counterparts, this allowed us to determine whether there are any differences in toxicological responses after the release of the loosely bound silver ions to quantify the potential environmental risks of these particles.

Our aim was to elucidate which aspects of the formulation contribute most to the toxicity of the formulation, and to discover whether these nanoparticles exhibit any toxicity after dialysis, which intended to simulate post-consumer use. We hypothesized that (1) released silver ions from the lignin particle and the surface stabilizer are the main contributors to the aquatic toxicity of these nanoparticles; and (2) once the particles have been dialyzed to remove the ionic silver from the low affinity lignin-binding sites, there would be a reduction in toxicity of the formulated particles. To test these hypotheses, we utilized the embryonic zebrafish assay, which is a widely-used model for toxicity testing as it provides a suite of developmental endpoints that are critical to the survival of the organism [38,39]. Zebrafish also develop quickly and are optically transparent, which allows for easy observations of phenotypic responses [38]. Additionally, they share similar homology to humans, so observed effects of chemical stressors from this assay can potentially be extrapolated to human physiological responses [40].

2. Materials and Methods

2.1. Materials and Characterization

Reference component solutions of silver nitrate ($AgNO_3$) salt (CAS# 7761-88-8, Fisher Scientific, Hampton, NH, USA) at 50 mg/L of Ag^+ dissolved in ultrapure water and poly (diallyldimethylammonium chloride) (PDAC, MW 100,000–200,000, CAS# 26062-79-3, Sigma Aldrich, St. Louis, MO, USA) at 200 mg/L in ultrapure water were prepared and refrigerated at 4 °C until use. The lignin (Indulin AT) for the nanoparticle core was extracted from biomass as a by-product of kraft pulping processes [36,41]. The Indulin AT lignin powder (lot MB05) and supporting documentation were obtained from MeadWestVaco, SC. The size range of the particles after synthesis with the pH-drop flash precipitation method (Figure S1c) was 84 ± 5 nm in ultrapure water [35]. PDAC was chosen to provide a cationic surface charge to the particles, such that they would be attracted to the negatively charged bacterial cell membranes. Stock nanomaterial suspensions of the lignin nanoparticle (NP), the silver functionalized lignin nanoparticle (NP + Ag), the silver functionalized particle with the cationic PDAC surface (NP + Ag + PDAC), and the lignin nanoparticle with PDAC alone (NP + PDAC) were prepared as previously described, and tested for antimicrobial efficacy, as is reported in previous publications [35,36]. Stock concentrations of each component were as follows: 500 mg/L lignin nanoparticle, 5 mg/L Ag^+, and 200 mg/L PDAC. All stock materials were stored in distilled water at 4 °C until use. Seven-fold dilutions of stock nanomaterial suspensions were performed with fishwater to prepare the varied exposure solutions. Fishwater was prepared by dissolving 260 mg/L Instant Ocean salts (Aquatic Ecosystems, Apopka, FL, USA) in reverse osmosis water and adjusting pH to 7.2 ± 0.2 using ~0.1 g sodium bicarbonate (conductivity 480–600 µS/cm) [39]. Experimental materials were stored under the same conditions as the reference materials. The NP + Ag and NP + PDAC formulations were solely used for comparative purposes, whereas the NP + Ag + PDAC is the proposed complete product formulation.

The samples to be dialyzed (NP + Ag and NP + Ag + PDAC) were placed in deionized water for 24 h which included a Slide-A-Lyzer MINI Dialysis Device (Thermo Scientific, Waltham, MA, USA) with a 10 K molecular weight cutoff membrane to remove dissolved silver from solution prior to dilution and testing. A second sample of NP + Ag was also dialyzed and allowed to age for 5 months prior to testing. Thus, the dialyzed samples included NP + Ag Aged, NP + Ag Fresh, and NP + Ag + PDAC Fresh, with the "Fresh" and "Aged" designations referring to when the sample was tested relative to when it was dialyzed.

The hydrodynamic diameter (HDD) and the zeta potential of each formulation that contained particles were measured in triplicate using a Zetasizer Nano ZS (Malvern Instruments Ltd., Worcestershire, UK) at 26.8 °C after dilution with fishwater to 50 mg/L. Aliquots (1 mL) were stored in an incubator under the same conditions as the embryonic zebrafish, until ready for analysis. Measurements were made over a five-day period, which also included an initial measurement (Day 0) which correlates with the exposure time of the experiment. Metadata associated with the zeta potential measurements can be found in Table S1.

2.2. Embryonic Zebrafish Assay

Exposure solutions of reference and nanomaterial suspensions were dispensed into 96-well plates, with each row having 12 wells of a given concentration of test material. Each well was filled with 200 µL of test solution and one of the eight rows on the plate was reserved for fishwater alone as a control. Adult zebrafish (*Danio rerio*) were maintained at the Sinnhuber Aquatic Research Laboratory (SARL) at Oregon State University, Corvallis, OR, USA. Embryos received from SARL were approximately 6–8 h post-fertilization (hpf) and were inspected under a dissecting microscope to ensure viability and developmental stage, then placed individually into wells of a 96-well plate. The chorionic membrane surrounding the zebrafish was preserved. Two replicate exposures were conducted over two weeks for each material, which allowed us to have a total sample size of 24 fish per concentration, per material. After plating, the exposure wells were covered with Parafilm to reduce evaporation, and embryos were incubated at 26.8 °C under a 14:10 light/dark photoperiod.

2.3. Toxicological Evaluations of Embryonic Zebrafish

Fish were observed at 24 hpf and 120 hpf for mortality, as well as a suite of developmental, morphological, and physiological abnormalities. At 24 hpf, embryos were evaluated for mortality, presence of spontaneous movement, delayed developmental progression, and notochord malformations. At 120 hpf, mortality was evaluated in conjunction with malformations of the snout, brain, pectoral and caudal fin, eye, jaw, otic structures, axis, trunk, somites, swim bladder, and body pigmentation. In addition, physiological and behavioral endpoints evaluated at 120 hpf include the presence of pericardial or yolk sac edema, impaired circulation and active touch response [39]. Hatching success was measured between 48 and 120 hpf, with embryos that hatched between 48 and 72 hpf being considered normal, and any individuals hatching after 72 hpf were considered delayed [42]. All endpoints were reported as either absent or present. Representative images of control fish and any individuals that displayed developmental abnormalities at 24 and 120 hpf were taken with an Olympus SZX10 microscope (Tokyo, Japan) fitted with an Olympus SC100 high resolution digital color camera (Olympus Corporation, Center Valley, PA, USA), and representative images are included in the Supplementary Materials (Figure S1). All experiments were performed in compliance with national care and use guidelines, and approved by the Institutional Animal Care and Use Committee (IACUC) at Oregon State University (ACUP #4764).

2.4. Measurement of Dissolved Silver and Particle-Associated Silver

Both the concentration of dissolved silver released from the nanoparticles and the silver associated with the particle itself were quantified by inductively coupled plasma-optical emission spectroscopy or mass spectrometry (ICP-OES or ICP-MS). To quantify silver content in solution, acid digestion of particles was performed using established methods [18,43]. Triplicate 0.5 mL samples of stock suspensions were centrifuged at $13,000 \times g$ for 10 min in a 3 kDa centrifugal filter (VWR, Radnor, PA, USA) with a polyethersulfone (PES) membrane, to separate the lignin particles from the filtrate. A total of 0.45 mL of filtrate sample was collected, diluted 10-fold with ultrapure water, and adjusted with 70% trace-metal grade HNO_3 to a final concentration of 3% HNO_3. For the lignin particle digestion, 0.1 mL of stock solution was digested in the same manner as the filtrate samples, without the centrifugation step. All samples were digested in Teflon tubes at 200 °C with 3 mL 70% trace-metal grade HNO_3. The acid was allowed to completely evaporate, and the process was repeated three times. Final digested samples were dissolved in 5 mL of 3% HNO_3 prior to ICP-OES/MS analysis. The silver ICP standard was purchased from RICCA Chemical Company (Ricca Chemical Company, Arlington, TX, USA) and diluted to six concentrations spanning the expected concentrations. All samples, including standards, were analyzed in triplicate with ICP-OES

(Teledyne Leeman Labs, Hudson, NH, USA) for silver content, except the filtrate from the NP + Ag + PDAC sample, which was analyzed by ICP-MS (Thermo-Fisher, Waltham, MA, USA) to provide a lower level of detection ($\geq$5 µg/L).

2.5. Statistical Analyses

All statistical analyses were conducted with SigmaPlot version 13.0 (Systat Software, San Jose, CA, USA), unless otherwise noted, and all differences were considered significant at $p \leq 0.05$. For measurements of zeta potential and HDD, significant differences were determined with repeated measures analysis of variance (ANOVA) and Tukey's post hoc analysis. Two-way ANOVA was conducted to ensure that there was no significant difference in mortality between replicate exposure plates prior to pooling of the data. Concentration–response curves were generated with the Environmental Protection Agency's Toxicity Relationship Analysis Program (EPA TRAP v. 1.30, March 2015). EPA TRAP was also used to calculate the concentration at which fifty percent of exposed zebrafish perished (LC_{50}) for each material, and the Litchfield/Wilcoxon formula was utilized for LC_{50} comparisons between treatments [44]. Significant sublethal endpoints were determined by Fisher's Exact Test, by comparing the control (fishwater alone) response to each concentration response tested. To determine whether there were significant differences in the concentration of silver associated with the particle versus the filtrate in the ICP analysis, a paired *t*-test was utilized.

3. Results and Discussion

3.1. Particle Characterization

Average zeta potential and HDD for the formulated particles in fishwater were measured over a five-day period. As expected, the zeta potential of the formulated particles varied with the presence of the surface stabilizer with the lignin NP alone, and the NP + Ag, both having negative zeta potentials in fishwater (−24.6 and −29.0 mV, respectively), while the particles with the cationic surface stabilizer had positive zeta potentials with and without silver ions present (28.1 and 25.5 mV respectively. Over the five day incubation in fishwater, only relatively minor changes in particle zeta potential were identified (Figure S2a). Zeta potentials for the dialyzed particles in fishwater were similarly consistent over time, and correlated well with their non-dialyzed counterparts (Figure S2b).

The initial HDD of the various particle formulations in fishwater were similar to the 84 nm primary particle size ranging from 80 to 95 nm, depending on the particle type (Figure S2c). Most of the formulated particles had consistent HDDs over time, however, the NP + Ag sample had the largest increase in size, reaching 124 nm by the end of the five day incubation. The dialyzed NP + Ag samples (both freshly dialyzed and aged dialyzed samples) had much more consistent HDD than the non-dialyzed counterparts (Figure S2d). These data suggest that the rapid loss of silver ions from the non-dialyzed components to the solution can lead to some particle swelling, however, the surface stabilizer effectively stabilized the particles from agglomeration.

3.2. Analysis of Dissolved Silver and Particle-Associated Silver

The concentration of silver in solution and the silver associated with the particles was quantified for the five nanoparticle samples that included silver. Figure 1 shows the concentration of silver present in the particle and in the solution which, when combined, matches the nominal concentration provided for each material. In all cases, the silver associated with the particle was greater than the silver present in solution (1.62 to 132 times greater. The full formulation (NP + Ag + PDAC) contains approximately 11 times more silver associated with the particle than the dialyzed full formulation (NP + Ag + PDAC Fresh). Additionally, the age of the NP + Ag sample played a role in silver distribution, as the older formulation contained approximately 10 times more silver in the filtrate than the particle.

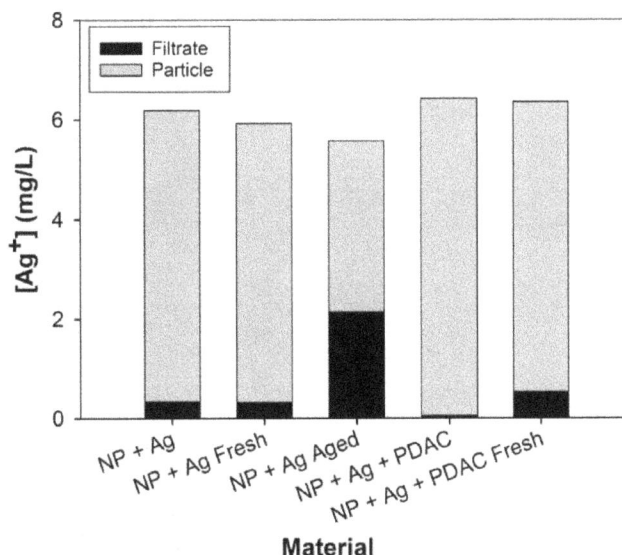

Figure 1. Concentration of silver associated with the filtrate and the particle as determined by ICP analysis. "Fresh" and "Aged" designations relate to the amount of time since the samples were dialyzed. All samples were analyzed via ICP-OES, except for the filtrate in the NP + Ag + PDAC sample, which was analyzed with ICP-MS.

Previous analyses of similar particles by Richter and colleagues [35] found that the concentration of silver associated with the particle after dialysis was approximately 18%; however, in this study, we found much higher concentrations associated with the particle (61.7–99.2%). This may have been due to variance between batches of the lignin nanoparticle stock solutions, as well as the differences in digestion techniques. Although the dialysis process is effective at releasing the loosely bound silver from the particles, the electrostatic barrier in the samples that contained PDAC may have impacted the rate at which silver was released. The full formulation had the lowest release of dissolved silver, although there was significantly more silver released from the freshly dialyzed full formulation sample, suggesting that PDAC may retard the release of ionic silver by repulsive electrostatic interactions. Additionally, through previous characterization of the lignin particle functional groups by Richter and colleagues [35,36], there is a higher proportion of organically-bound sulfur compared to other lignin types (nine times that of high-purity lignin), which would likely provide strong binding sites for dissolved silver [45].

3.3. Comparative Analysis of Formulation Toxicity

No significant differences were found between replicate exposure plates; therefore, replicates were pooled to increase the sample size to 24 fish per concentration, per material. To encompass all possible comparisons, but for clarity in interpreting the data, two groupings were made, which parallel our hypotheses. These two groupings are formulation comparisons and dialyzed sample comparisons. Concentration-response curves for the two groupings are illustrated in the SI (Figure S3). Additionally, a modeled concentration-response curve was generated for the reference material silver nitrate, which is included in the SI (Figure S4).

3.3.1. Formulation Components

As represented in Figure 2a, the lignin core nanoparticle (NP) itself was the least toxic component (LC_{50} = 323 mg/L), and when the NP was combined with the other aspects of the formulation, LC_{50} values decreased significantly in all cases (NP + Ag LC_{50} = 164 mg/L, NP + PDAC LC_{50} = 33 mg/L, NP + Ag + PDAC LC_{50} = 32 mg/L). The presence of silver in the full formulation (NP + Ag + PDAC) did not change the overall toxicity relative to NP + PDAC. Additionally, when PDAC was present in the formulation (NP + PDAC or NP + Ag + PDAC), a significant increase in mortality events occurred. PDAC and Ag$^+$ alone were the two most toxic constituents, with LC$_{50}$'s of 5.39 mg/L and 1.53 mg/L, respectively.

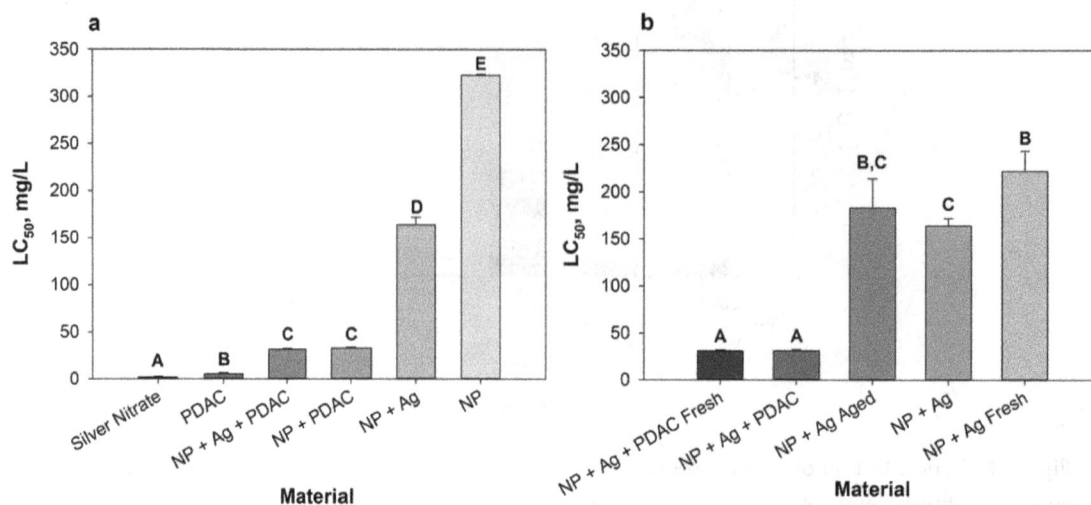

Figure 2. LC$_{50}$'s for nanoparticles and components (**a**) and dialyzed samples (**b**) with standard error of two experimental replicates with 12 embryos exposed at each concentration in each replicate test (24 embryos per concentration total). Significant differences between LC$_{50}$ values are indicated with a change in letter above the bar.

The estimated LC$_{50}$ for Ag$^+$ is greater than many published literature values for zebrafish [46–50], however, exposure time and conditions differ in these studies, which may explain the observed differences in toxicity. Our zebrafish embryos were exposed at 8 hpf with the chorion intact, whereas some of the referenced studies did not expose the fish until after hatching, or even as adults. Th chorionic membrane can modulate silver toxicity by sequestering ions to prevent them from entering the perivitelline fluid [51], and removing the chorion has been shown to increase toxic responses [40,51]. It is likely that the presence of the chorion may have played a large role in modulating silver toxicity, but the exposure media may have also played a role as well.

The hardness of our prepared fishwater may have altered the toxicity of silver nitrate, as well as nanoparticle-containing formulations to the embryonic zebrafish. Based on dissolved magnesium and calcium concentrations, our fishwater is categorized as soft water (<60 mg/L CaCO$_3$), whereas many of the above studies utilize moderately hard to hard water when exposing their zebrafish (up to 148 mg/L CaCO$_3$). It has been reported that LC$_{50}$'s tend to be higher in the presence of dissolved organic matter, which has the greatest effect on silver toxicity, followed by Cl$^-$, Na$^+$, and Ca^{2+} [52]. This is based on the coalescence effect, which leads to complexation and/or formation of nanoparticle agglomerates and/or aggregates, which can decrease apparent toxicity by minimizing particle uptake by the organism [53]. As our fishwater was categorized as soft water (low concentrations of Na$^+$ and Ca^{2+}), we then determined the concentration of chloride ions present, as silver ion bioavailability can be impacted due to complexation and subsequent precipitation of silver chloride [24,47].

In the Instant Ocean salt formulation used to make the fishwater, the majority of the cations are paired with chloride, and we determined the chloride concentration in our fishwater to be 142 mg/L, which is approximately 55% of the dissolved ion content. It is possible that when the fishwater was used to dilute the silver-containing treatments, the silver complexed with the chloride and precipitated out of solution, which may have led to a greater LC$_{50}$ value. To determine whether precipitation was a significant factor, we utilized Visual MINTEQ (v.3.1) for each silver-containing formulation. We used the filtrate concentrations from the ICP data for each of the formulations that contained silver, and determined that nearly all of the dissolved silver (98.2–99.8%) would complex with the chloride present in the fishwater to form a precipitate of silver chloride, except the NP + Ag + PDAC sample, as the concentration of Ag^+ in solution was very low. However, as the exposures occurred over a five day period, and the movement of silver from the particle to the surrounding solution is a dynamic process, dissolved silver could have still been bioavailable to the zebrafish.

Considering our nanoparticle and silver combination formulations, comparisons to published LC_{50} values for conventional silver core AgNPs differ significantly. Reported AgNP LC_{50}'s for fish generally range between 0.05 and 20 mg/L [2,54]. Variations in reported LC_{50} values may relate to differences in the type of exposure, exposure time, age of the fish, the presence of the chorionic membrane, the use of bare or coated nanoparticles, and/or differences in exposure media. A study completed by Bar-Ilan and colleagues [55] matched our exposure conditions most consistently, and had reported LC_{50}'s within the range above, although the LC_{50}'s differed from our findings. They exposed embryonic zebrafish to different sizes of colloidal AgNPs (3–100 nm), and found a range of LC_{50}'s, from 10.1 to 14.7 mg/L. Although the sizes of the particles, length and timing of the exposure, and retention of the chorionic membrane is consistent with our experiment, our LC_{50}'s were an order of magnitude less toxic based on total particle mass (for example, the measured LC_{50} for the NP + Ag formulation was 164 mg/L). Thus, the silver doped lignin nanoparticles have a lower mass-based toxicity than solid core AgNPs, while maintaining a similar antimicrobial efficacy [35]. The difference may be due to the use of the lignin particle, which was shown via ICP-OES/MS analysis to retain bound silver, probably due to the higher binding affinity sites (Figure 1). It should be noted that there was a 100:1 ratio of lignin to Ag^+ in the nanoparticles, so the amount of silver in each particle was only a hundredth of the mass of the total particle, making our LC_{50} values, based on silver content alone, similar to those measured for solid core AgNPs reported in other studies. Therefore, potential exposure to silver ions would be reduced in the presence of the lignin particles, leading to an apparent increase in the LC_{50}. This suggests that by replacing the silver core typical of conventional AgNPs, the concentration of silver released to the environment may be reduced, which was one of the goals of formulating the nanoparticle with a lignin core.

PDAC alone was the second most toxic component tested, and formulations that contained PDAC were significantly more toxic than formulations that did not contain PDAC (Figure 2a). Although PDAC is a high charge density cationic polymer commonly used as a flocculant/coagulant in wastewater treatment, it is also cited as a cytotoxin that interacts with cell membranes to elicit cell damage, and eventually necrosis [56,57]. Our results correspond with this literature finding, as embryos that were exposed to PDAC alone progressively blackened and disintegrated, starting at 5.75 mg/L. Other formulations that contained PDAC did not elicit this response, perhaps because the PDAC is electrostatically associated with the lignin particle, or was "complexed". Free, or "non-complexed" PDAC, can interact with blood components, such as erythrocytes and plasma proteins, cell membranes, and extracellular matrix proteins, leading to undesired side effects not seen with complexed polycations [58]. Our experimental observations support this, as we see that the uncomplexed PDAC sample is indeed more toxic than any formulation that contains a nanoparticle–PDAC complex (Figure 2a). Additionally, research suggests polycationic polymers like PDAC can disrupt the lipid bilayer, with larger polymers leading to the formation of holes in the lipid membrane that increased membrane permeability [59,60]. Given that information, it is possible that PDAC made the fish more susceptible to both dissolved and particle-bound silver as a result of changes in membrane permeability. The positively charged PDAC-coated particles (SI, Figure S2) may have also been attracted to the negatively-charged membranes of the zebrafish, which could have increased the exposure to silver associated with the particle.

3.3.2. Dialyzed Formulations

The purpose of dialyzing the samples was to simulate post-consumer use of the nanoparticle by purging the surrounding solution of excess silver ions. In the LC_{50} comparisons of dialyzed materials, two results can be observed (Figure 2b). First, there was no difference in LC_{50} between the dialyzed complete formulation (NP + Ag + PDAC Fresh) and its non-dialyzed counterpart (NP + Ag + PDAC). This may be due to similar nominal concentrations of silver, as calculated by adding the silver associated with the particle and silver present in the filtrate (Figure 1). Second, the NP + Ag samples showed a significant decrease in toxicity post-dialysis, with LC_{50} values increasing immediately after dialysis (NP + Ag Fresh, LC_{50} = 222 mg/L), however, the dialyzed aged sample had a similar toxicity to the non-dialyzed sample (NP + Ag LC_{50} = 164 mg/L and NP + Ag Aged LC_{50} = 184 mg/L). Perhaps over time, the higher affinity binding sites on the lignin release more silver into solution compared to the freshly dialyzed sample, leading to the slight decrease in the aged LC_{50} (Figure 1).

3.4. Analysis of Sublethal Endpoints

There were several endpoints that were significant ($p \leq 0.05$), which included morphological abnormalities, including uninflated swim bladder and snout malformations, developmental endpoints, such as delay in hatching and delayed developmental progression, and physiological anomalies, such as impaired circulation, yolk sac edema, and pericardial edema (Figure 3a–f). Exposure to the silver nitrate at concentrations similar to the amount of silver in the NPs did not cause any significant malformations in the embryos. Overall, there was a significant increase in the types of sublethal responses observed in the dialyzed samples compared to the non-dialyzed samples. The dialyzed samples, particularly the aged sample, had proportionally less silver associated with the particle than the non-dialyzed samples (Figure 1), which could explain the increase in sublethal impacts, as well as the lack of sublethal endpoints for NP + Ag + PDAC (Figure 3).

Swim bladder malformations occurred when silver or PDAC were included in the particle formulation; however, this did not occur when silver and PDAC were both present in the particle formulation (NP + Ag + PDAC), except when freshly dialyzed (Figure 3e). Exposure to silver ions during embryonic zebrafish development has been described as impacting cholinergic signaling, which is important in swim bladder formation [61]. Swim bladder malformations were not significant in the NP + Ag + PDAC sample, likely due to high ratio of silver associated with the particle as compared to the filtrate (Figure 1).

Malformations of the snout were only significant in the freshly dialyzed full formulation (Figure 3e). Although others have reported silver nanoparticles causing snout malformations [54], we do not see this malformation in silver nitrate (Figure S5) or any other formulation containing silver, suggesting some other mechanisms of malformation may be involved. Perhaps the presence of all three formulation components may have contributed to the prevalence of snout malformations, in addition to the increased concentration of silver in the filtrate, as it exceeded the other treatments by a factor of six (Figure 1), except for the aged dialyzed particle (NP + Ag Aged).

Yolk sac edema was present in all fish exposed to formulations containing silver, and impaired circulation was significant in both freshly dialyzed formulations (Figure 3d,e). Significant pericardial edema responses were only noted in the NP + Ag and NP + Ag + PDAC Fresh formulations. Similarly, several other studies have reported that as a result of silver nanoparticle exposure, pericardial edema, yolk sac edema, and impaired circulation are prevalent in the early developmental stages of zebrafish [62–65]. As the development of the circulatory system and the formation of the heart typically occur between 21 and 24 hpf in zebrafish embryos [42,64], it is likely that the release of dissolved silver from the nanoparticles resulted in these endpoints being prevalent, however, particle-specific responses cannot be ruled out. The chorion has been reported to modulate metal toxicity [51], but there has been recent evidence that nanoparticles (30–72 nm) can move through the chorionic membrane pores and distribute to numerous parts of the fish, including the brain, heart, yolk, and blood [66]. Should the distribution of silver include the yolk and heart, edemas would be expected to occur due to disturbances in osmoregulation [55,62,63,67]. Once these developmental pathways are disturbed during early development, normal embryogenesis can be impacted, resulting in numerous defects [68]. In addition, silver nanoparticles may agglomerate in exposure media, which can alter oxygen exchange through chorionic pores, affecting oxygen tension and osmotic balance, which could then result in edemas similar to those observed in our study [66].

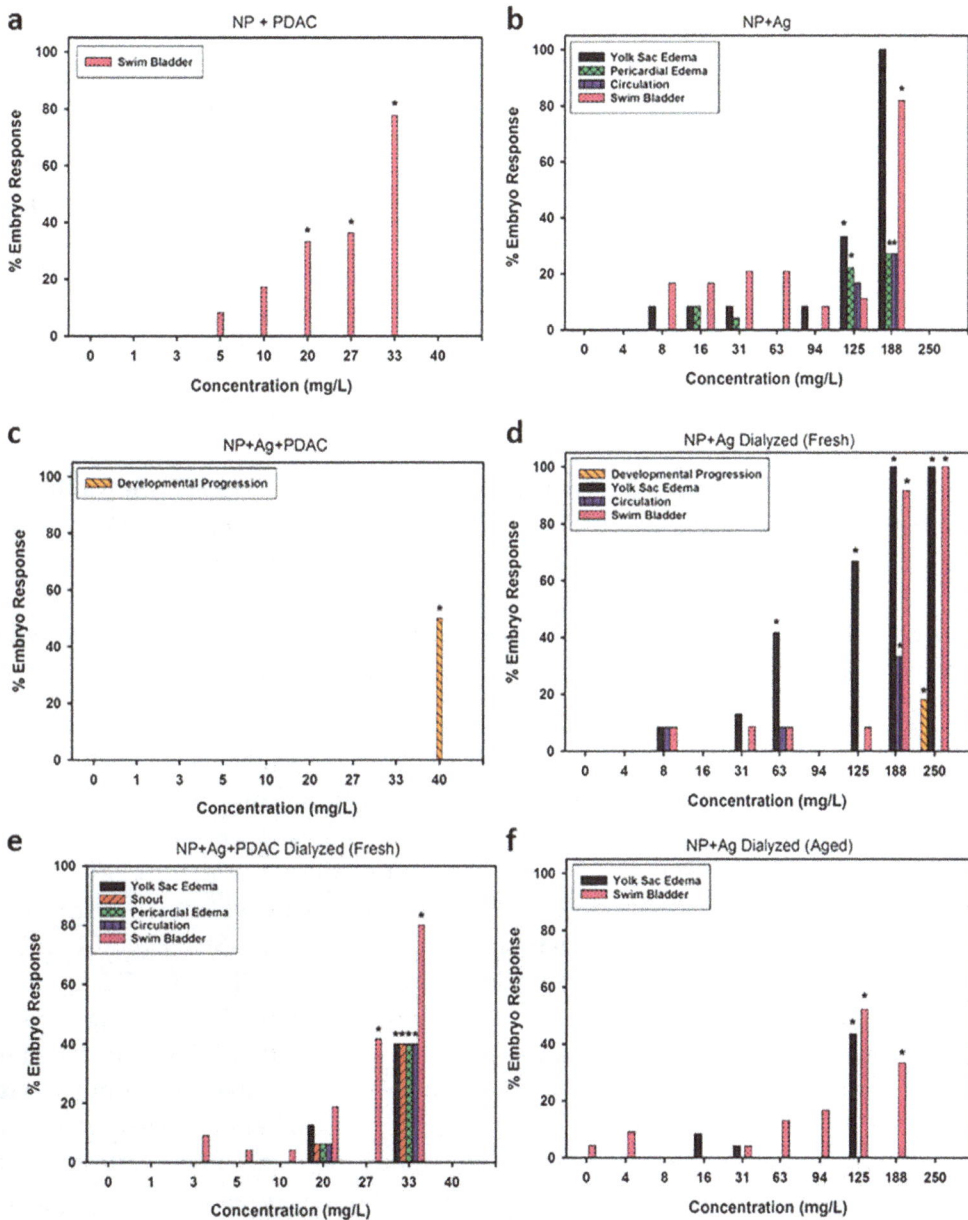

Figure 3. Types of developmental and morphological abnormalities observed in 120 hpf zebrafish embryos exposed to various formulations of the nanoparticles including (**a**) NP + PDAC; (**b**) NP + Ag; (**c**) NP + Ag + PDAC; (**d**) NP + Ag Dialyzed (Fresh); (**e**) NP + Ag + PDAC Dialyzed (Fresh) and (**f**) NP + Ag Dialyzed (Aged). Asterisk represents significant increase relative to unexposed (control) fish embryos at $p \leq 0.05$.

Pericardial edema coupled with impaired circulation following AgNP exposure has been shown to be concentration dependent [63], with an increase in prevalence from 10–100 mg/L. This was the trend we observed in our study, although our study saw increases up to 125 mg/L with a maximum of 17% responding. The most reasonable explanation for the slight difference in observations may be due to differences between solid silver nanoparticles with surface stabilizers, and the lignin-coated particles with specific silver binding sites on the particle core. Polyvinyl alcohol was used as the surface coating in Asharani and colleagues [63], which may have altered the dynamics of silver ion release relative to our samples. Our samples contained PDAC as a surface stabilizer, which provides an electrostatic barrier that could impede silver ion release, which we did see in our samples (Figure 1); however, when freshly dialyzed, PDAC had limited impact on silver ion release, suggesting solution equilibrium may be controlled by PDAC. Additionally, although there was silver present in the filtrate of the freshly dialyzed samples, the lignin core bound the majority of the silver, probably due to the higher affinity silver ion binding sites being utilized.

Significant delay in hatching and delayed developmental progression were the two developmental abnormalities observed in our study following exposure to silver salts (Figure S5) and high concentrations of the bare lignin nanoparticles (Figure S6), respectively. As delayed developmental progression was found following exposure to relatively high concentrations of the bare lignin nanoparticle and no other samples, the bare particle may interact with necessary ions in the solution, making them limited for supporting embryo development at concentrations of 350 mg/L and higher (Figure S6). This is further supported by the finding that this process does not occur when the particle is functionalized with silver, PDAC, or both, as the binding sites on the lignin particle are already occupied. Silver nitrate was the only material tested that led to a delay in hatching. A delay in hatching is primarily caused by deactivation of the ZHE1 enzyme, which prevents chorionic degradation [69]. Lin and colleagues have shown that dissolved metals can interfere with ZHE1, and although silver was included in their assay, it did not lead to a significant decrease in ZHE1 activity [69]. Asharani and colleagues exposed zebrafish to Ag^+ at 2.14 mg/L, and observed a delay in hatching at 4% compared to controls, but this was not significant [62]. Approximately 50% of our surviving fish exhibited a delay in hatching compared to controls following exposure to silver salts, however, this was not seen in lignin nanoparticle formulations containing silver.

4. Conclusions

The results of this study provide several insights into a nanoparticle engineered to be an environmentally friendly alternative to solid silver core nanoparticles. Our data shows that the use of lignin as the nanoparticle core could be a viable alternative, as it did not pose a significant toxicological hazard to our test organism. Since our reported toxicity was similar to other findings when compared on the basis of silver content, the toxicity of silver-enabled nanoparticles may be predictable, based on the silver concentration of the particle. Ionic silver and PDAC alone were the most toxic components of the formulation, which may be attributed to their higher diffusivity and propensity to interact with cell membranes relative to silver and/or PDAC associated with the particle. The inclusion of PDAC not only adds antimicrobial activity to the particle, but also seems to delay the release of silver ions, so in situations where time release of antimicrobial agents is desired, stabilizing the particles with PDAC may be warranted. This data also encourages further development of similar nanomaterials to minimize their impact on the environment, as well as testing the current particle under environmentally relevant conditions to evaluate toxicity. One way of reducing the environmental impact of these engineered nanomaterials is to design them in a way to minimize the release of soluble components, or to replace these components with less toxic ingredients. We are presently investigating the use of an alternative nanoparticle coating which is biologically derived, that may have the potential to be less toxic in comparison to PDAC.

5. Associated Content

Supplemental Information Is Available for This Publication

Representative images of zebrafish with and without significant developmental impacts; Average zeta potential and hydrodynamic diameter measurements for particle-containing formulations over a five day period; Metadata associated with zeta potential measurements; Concentration-response curves for formulation components and dialyzed materials based on zebrafish mortality at 120 hpf;

Modeled concentration-response curve for the reference material silver nitrate based on zebrafish mortality at 120 hpf; Visual MINTEQ output for all silver-containing formulations.

Supplementary Materials:
Figure S1: Representative images of zebrafish with and without significant developmental impacts, Figure S2: Average zeta potential and hydrodynamic diameter (HDD) of particle formulations over a five day period in fishwater. Figure S1a,b are average zeta potential measurements for the formulation components (a) and the dialyzed formulations (b), and Figure S1c,d are the average HDD measurements for the formulation components (c) and the dialyzed formulations (d), Figure S3: Concentration–response comparisons for formulation components (a) and dialyzed materials (b) based on zebrafish mortality at 120 hpf (a) Significant differences ($p \leq 0.05$) existed between materials in the formulation component treatments. The lignin particle exhibited the lowest toxicity, followed by silver, and PDAC. (b) No significant differences ($p > 0.05$) existed in the dialyzed sample treatments. Comparisons included the two full formulations (NP + Ag + PDAC) and the three NP + Ag formulations, Figure S4: Concentration–response curve for silver nitrate based on zebrafish mortality at 120 hpf, Figure S5: Frequency of delayed hatching in zebrafish embryos exposed to Ag^+ as silver nitrate in fishwater. Asterisk represents significant increase ($p \leq 0.05$) relative to unexposed (control) fish embryos, Figure S6: Frequency of delayed developmental progression in zebrafish embryos exposed to lignin nanoparticles in fishwater. Asterisk represents significant increase ($p \leq 0.05$) relative to unexposed (control), Table S1: Metadata associated with zeta potential measurements.

Author Contributions: Alexander P. Richter and Orlin D. Velev conceived the materials, Cathryn G. Conner synthesized and provided the materials, Bryan J. Harper and Stacey L. Harper designed the experiments and contributed to the analysis of the data and Cassandra E. Nix performed the toxicological experiments, contributed to the data analysis and wrote the paper.

Acknowledgments: We would like to thank Alicea Meredith, Lindsay Denluck and Teresa Peterson for their assistance on the project and the Sinnhuber Aquatic Research Laboratory (Grant #P30 ES000210) for providing the zebrafish embryos. This work was supported by the United States Department of Agriculture National Institute of Food and Agriculture (USDA-NIFA), Grant 2013-67021-21181, partially supported by an Oregon State University Agricultural Research Foundation Grant (ARF8301A), as well as a grant from the National Institute of Environmental and Health Sciences (Grant # R01ES017552) to Stacey Harper. Alexander P. Richter thanks the Lemelson Foundation and the Lemelson-MIT program for support. We also acknowledge the support provided to Cathryn G. Conner by the Molecular Biotechnology Training Program (MBTP) sponsored by the National Institutes of Health and the Graduate School at North Carolina State University (5 T32 GM008776-15).

References

1. Vance, M.E.; Kuiken, T.; Vejerano, E.P.; McGinnis, S.P.; Hochella, M.F.; Rejeski, D.; Hull, M.S. Nanotechnology in the real world: Redeveloping the nanomaterial consumer products inventory. *Beilstein J. Nanotechnol.* **2015**, *6*, 1769–1780. [CrossRef] [PubMed]

2. Bondarenko, O.; Juganson, K.; Ivask, A.; Kasemets, K.; Mortimer, M.; Kahru, A. Toxicity of ag, cuo and zno nanoparticles to selected environmentally relevant test organisms and mammalian cells in vitro: A critical review. *Arch. Toxicol.* **2013**, *87*, 1181–1200. [CrossRef] [PubMed]

3. Bystrzejewska-Piotrowska, G.; Golimowski, J.; Urban, P.L. Nanoparticles: Their potential toxicity, waste and environmental management. *Waste Manag.* **2009**, *29*, 2587–2595. [CrossRef] [PubMed]

4. Marambio-Jones, C.; Hoek, E.M.V. A review of the antibacterial effects of silver nanomaterials and potential implications for human health and the environment. *J. Nanopart. Res.* **2010**, *12*, 1531–1551. [CrossRef]

5. Massarsky, A.; Trudeau, V.L.; Moon, T.W. Predicting the environmental impact of nanosilver. *Environ. Toxicol. Pharmacol.* **2014**, *38*, 861–873. [CrossRef] [PubMed]

6. Piccinno, F.; Gottschalk, F.; Seeger, S.; Nowack, B. Industrial production quantities and uses of ten engineered nanomaterials in europe and the world. *J. Nanopart. Res.* **2012**, *14*, 1109. [CrossRef]

7. Benn, T.; Cavanagh, B.; Hristovski, K.; Posner, J.D.; Westerhoff, P. The release of nanosilver from consumer products used in the home. *J. Environ. Qual.* **2010**, *39*, 1875–1882. [CrossRef] [PubMed]

8. Benn, T.M.; Westerhoff, P. Nanoparticle silver released into water from commercially available sock fabrics. *Environ. Sci. Technol.* **2008**, *42*, 4133–4139. [CrossRef] [PubMed]

9. Gottschalk, F.; Sun, T.; Nowack, B. Environmental concentrations of engineered nanomaterials: Review of modeling and analytical studies. *Environ. Pollut.* **2013**, *181*, 287–300. [CrossRef] [PubMed]

10. Kaegi, R.; Sinnet, B.; Zuleeg, S.; Hagendorfer, H.; Mueller, E.; Vonbank, R.; Boller, M.; Burkhardt, M. Release of silver nanoparticles from outdoor facades. *Environ. Pollut.* **2010**, *158*, 2900–2905. [CrossRef] [PubMed]

11. Mackevica, A.; Olsson, M.E.; Hansen, S.F. The release of silver nanoparticles from commercial toothbrushes. *J. Hazard. Mater.* **2016**, *322*, 270–275. [CrossRef] [PubMed]

12. Dobias, J.; Bernier-Latmani, R. Silver release from silver nanoparticles in natural waters. *Environ. Sci. Technol.* **2013**, *47*, 4140–4146. [CrossRef] [PubMed]

13. Handy, R.D.; Owen, R.; Valsami-Jones, E. The ecotoxicology of nanoparticles and nanomaterials: Current status, knowledge gaps, challenges, and future needs. *Ecotoxicology* **2008**, *17*, 315–325. [CrossRef] [PubMed]

14. Maurer-Jones, M.A.; Gunsolus, I.L.; Murphy, C.J.; Haynes, C.L. Toxicity of engineered nanoparticles in the environment. *Anal. Chem.* **2013**, *85*, 3036–3049. [CrossRef] [PubMed]

15. Selck, H.; Handy, R.D.; Fernandes, T.F.; Klaine, S.J.; Petersen, E.J. Nanomaterials in the aquatic environment: A european union-united states perspective on the status of ecotoxicity testing, research priorities, and challenges ahead: Nanomaterials in the aquatic environment. *Environ. Toxicol. Chem.* **2016**, *35*, 1055–1067. [CrossRef] [PubMed]

16. Furtado, L.M.; Bundschuh, M.; Metcalfe, C.D. Monitoring the fate and transformation of silver nanoparticles in natural waters. *Bull. Environ. Contam. Toxicol.* **2016**, *97*, 445–449. [CrossRef] [PubMed]

17. Furtado, L.M.; Norman, B.C.; Xenopoulos, M.A.; Frost, P.C.; Metcalfe, C.D.; Hintelmann, H. Environmental fate of silver nanoparticles in boreal lake ecosystems. *Environ. Sci. Technol.* **2015**, *49*, 8441–8450. [CrossRef] [PubMed]

18. Kim, K.-T.; Truong, L.; Wehmas, L.; Tanguay, R.L. Silver nanoparticle toxicity in the embryonic zebrafish is governed by particle dispersion and ionic environment. *Nanotechnology* **2013**, *24*, 115101. [CrossRef] [PubMed]

19. Peijnenburg, W.J.G.M.; Baalousha, M.; Chen, J.; Chaudry, Q.; Von der kammer, F.; Kuhlbusch, T.A.J.; Lead, J.; Nickel, C.; Quik, J.T.K.; Renker, M.; et al. A review of the properties and processes determining the fate of engineered nanomaterials in the aquatic environment. *Crit. Rev. Environ. Sci. Technol.* **2015**, *45*, 2084–2134. [CrossRef]

20. Lacave, J.M.; Retuerto, A.; Vicario-Parés, U.; Gilliland, D.; Oron, M.; Cajaraville, M.P.; Orbea, A. Effects of metal-bearing nanoparticles (Ag, Au, CdS, ZnO, SiO$_2$) on developing zebrafish embryos. *Nanotechnology* **2016**, *27*, 325102. [CrossRef] [PubMed]

21. Nel, A.; Xia, T.; Mädler, L.; Li, N. Toxic potential of materials at the nanolevel. *Science* **2006**, *311*, 622–627. [CrossRef] [PubMed]

22. Sharma, V.K.; Siskova, K.M.; Zboril, R.; Gardea-Torresdey, J.L. Organic-coated silver nanoparticles in biological and environmental conditions: Fate, stability and toxicity. *Adv. Colloid Interface Sci.* **2014**, *204*, 15–34. [CrossRef] [PubMed]

23. Shin, S.; Song, I.; Um, S. Role of physicochemical properties in nanoparticle toxicity. *Nanomaterials* **2015**, *5*, 1351–1365. [CrossRef] [PubMed]

24. Groh, K.J.; Dalkvist, T.; Piccapietra, F.; Behra, R.; Suter, M.J.F.; Schirmer, K. Critical influence of chloride ions on silver ion-mediated acute toxicity of silver nanoparticles to zebrafish embryos. *Nanotoxicology* **2015**, *9*, 81–91. [CrossRef] [PubMed]

25. Ivask, A.; ElBadawy, A.; Kaweeteerawat, C.; Boren, D.; Fischer, H.; Ji, Z.; Chang, C.H.; Liu, R.; Tolaymat, T.; Telesca, D.; et al. Toxicity mechanisms in escherichia coli vary for silver nanoparticles and differ from ionic silver. *ACS Nano* **2014**, *8*, 374–386. [CrossRef] [PubMed]

26. Clement, J.; Jarrett, P. Antibacterial silver. *Met. Based Drugs* **1994**, *1*, 467–482. [CrossRef] [PubMed]

27. Gordon, O.; Vig Slenters, T.; Brunetto, P.S.; Villaruz, A.E.; Sturdevant, D.E.; Otto, M.; Landmann, R.; Fromm, K.M. Silver coordination polymers for prevention of implant infection: Thiol interaction, impact on respiratory chain enzymes, and hydroxyl radical induction. *Antimicrob. Agents Chemother.* **2010**, *54*, 4208–4218. [CrossRef] [PubMed]

28. Morones, J.R.; Elechiguerra, J.L.; Camacho, A.; Holt, K.; Kouri, J.B.; Ramírez, J.T.; Yacaman, M.J. The bactericidal effect of silver nanoparticles. *Nanotechnology* **2005**, *16*, 2346–2353. [CrossRef] [PubMed]

29. Feng, Q.L.; Wu, J.; Chen, G.Q.; Cui, F.Z.; Kim, T.N.; Kim, J.O. A mechanistic study of the antibacterial effect of silver ions on escherichia coli and staphylococcus aureus. *J. Biomed. Mater. Res.* **2000**, *52*, 662–668. [CrossRef]

30. Fong, J.; Wood, F. Nanocrystalline silver dressings in wound management: A review. *Int. J. Nanomed.* **2006**, *1*, 441–449. [CrossRef]

31. Hwang, E.T.; Lee, J.H.; Chae, Y.J.; Kim, Y.S.; Kim, B.C.; Sang, B.-I.; Gu, M.B. Analysis of the toxic mode of action of silver nanoparticles using stress-specific bioluminescent bacteria. *Small* **2008**, *4*, 746–750. [CrossRef] [PubMed]

32. Sharma, V.K.; Yngard, R.A.; Lin, Y. Silver nanoparticles: Green synthesis and their antimicrobial activities. *Adv. Colloid Interface Sci.* **2009**, *145*, 83–96. [CrossRef] [PubMed]

33. Sabella, S.; Carney, R.P.; Brunetti, V.; Malvindi, M.A.; Al-Juffali, N.; Vecchio, G.; Janes, S.M.; Bakr, O.M.; Cingolani, R.; Stellacci, F.; et al. A general mechanism for intracellular toxicity of metal-containing nanoparticles. *Nanoscale* **2014**, *6*, 7052–7061. [CrossRef] [PubMed]

34. Anastas, P.; Eghbali, N. Green chemistry: Principles and practice. *Chem. Soc. Rev.* **2010**, *39*, 301–312. [CrossRef] [PubMed]

35. Richter, A.P.; Brown, J.S.; Bharti, B.; Wang, A.; Gangwal, S.; Houck, K.; Cohen Hubal, E.A.; Paunov, V.N.; Stoyanov, S.D.; Velev, O.D. An environmentally benign antimicrobial nanoparticle based on a silver-infused lignin core. *Nat. Nanotechnol.* **2015**, *10*, 817–823. [CrossRef] [PubMed]

36. Richter, A.P.; Bharti, B.; Armstrong, H.B.; Brown, J.S.; Plemmons, D.; Paunov, V.N.; Stoyanov, S.D.; Velev, O.D. Synthesis and characterization of biodegradable lignin nanoparticles with tunable surface properties. *Langmuir* **2016**, *32*, 6468–6477. [CrossRef] [PubMed]

37. Frangville, C.; Rutkevičius, M.; Richter, A.P.; Velev, O.D.; Stoyanov, S.D.; Paunov, V.N. Fabrication of environmentally biodegradable lignin nanoparticles. *ChemPhysChem* **2012**, *13*, 4235–4243. [CrossRef] [PubMed]

38. Hill, A.J. Zebrafish as a model vertebrate for investigating chemical toxicity. *Toxicol. Sci.* **2005**, *86*, 6–19. [CrossRef] [PubMed]

39. Truong, L.; Harper, S.; Tanguay, R. Evaluation of embryotoxicity using the zebrafish model. In *Drug Safety Evaluation: Methods and Protocols*; Humana Press: New York, NY, USA, 2011; pp. 271–279.

40. Kim, K.-T.; Tanguay, R.L. The role of chorion on toxicity of silver nanoparticles in the embryonic zebrafish assay. *Environ. Health Toxicol.* **2014**, *29*, e2014021. [CrossRef] [PubMed]

41. Duval, A.; Lawoko, M. A review on lignin-based polymeric, micro- and nano-structured materials. *React. Funct. Polym.* **2014**, *85*, 78–96. [CrossRef]

42. Kimmel, C.B.; Ballard, W.W.; Kimmel, S.R.; Ullmann, B.; Schilling, T.F. Stages of embryonic development of the zebrafish. *Dev. Dyn.* **1995**, *203*, 253–310. [CrossRef] [PubMed]

43. Wu, F.; Harper, B.J.; Harper, S.L. Differential dissolution and toxicity of surface functionalized silver nanoparticles in small-scale microcosms: Impacts of community complexity. *Environ. Sci. Nano* **2017**, *4*, 359–372. [CrossRef]

44. Sprague, J.; Fogels, A. *Watch the y in Bioassay*; EPS-5-AR-77-1; Procedural 3rd Aquatic Toxicology Workshop: Halifax, NS, Canada, 1977; pp. 107–118.

45. Bielmyer, G.K.; Grosell, M.; Paquin, P.R.; Mathews, R.; Wu, K.B.; Santore, R.C.; Brix, K.V. Validation study of the acute biotic ligand model for silver. *Environ. Toxicol. Chem.* **2007**, *26*, 2241–2246. [CrossRef] [PubMed]

46. Alsop, D.; Wood, C.M. Metal uptake and acute toxicity in zebrafish: Common mechanisms across multiple metals. *Aquat. Toxicol.* **2011**, *105*, 385–393. [CrossRef] [PubMed]

47. Bielmyer, G.; Brix, K.; Grosell, M. Is Cl^- protection against silver toxicity due to chemical speciation? *Aquat. Toxicol.* **2008**, *87*, 81–87. [CrossRef] [PubMed]

48. Bilberg, K.; Hovgaard, M.B.; Besenbacher, F.; Baatrup, E. In vivo toxicity of silver nanoparticles and silver ions in zebrafish (*Danio rerio*). *J. Toxicol.* **2012**, *2012*, 1–9. [CrossRef] [PubMed]

49. Powers, C.M.; Slotkin, T.A.; Seidler, F.J.; Badireddy, A.R.; Padilla, S. Silver nanoparticles alter zebrafish development and larval behavior: Distinct roles for particle size, coating and composition. *Neurotox. Teratol.* **2011**, *33*, 708–714. [CrossRef] [PubMed]

50. Powers, C.M.; Yen, J.; Linney, E.A.; Seidler, F.J.; Slotkin, T.A. Silver exposure in developing zebrafish (*danio rerio*): Persistent effects on larval behavior and survival. *Neurotoxicol. Teratol.* **2010**, *32*, 391–397. [CrossRef] [PubMed]

51. Rombough, P. The influence of zona radiata on the toxicities of zinc, lead, mercury, copper and silver ions to embryos of steelhead trout salmo gairdneri. *Comp. Biochem. Physiol.* **1985**, *82*, 115–117. [CrossRef]

52. McGeer, J.C.; Playle, R.C.; Wood, C.M.; Galvez, F. A physiologically based biotic ligand model for predicting the acute toxicity of waterborne silver to rainbow trout in freshwaters. *Environ. Sci. Technol.* **2000**, *34*, 4199–4207. [CrossRef]

53. Lapresta-Fernández, A.; Fernández, A.; Blasco, J. Nanoecotoxicity effects of engineered silver and gold nanoparticles in aquatic organisms. *TrAC Trends Anal. Chem.* **2012**, *32*, 40–59. [CrossRef]

54. Reidy, B.; Haase, A.; Luch, A.; Dawson, K.; Lynch, I. Mechanisms of silver nanoparticle release, transformation and toxicity: A critical review of current knowledge and recommendations for future studies and applications. *Materials* **2013**, *6*, 2295–2350. [CrossRef] [PubMed]

55. Bar-Ilan, O.; Albrecht, R.M.; Fako, V.E.; Furgeson, D.Y. Toxicity assessments of multisized gold and silver nanoparticles in zebrafish embryos. *Small* **2009**, *5*, 1897–1910. [CrossRef] [PubMed]

56. Fischer, D.; Li, Y.; Ahlemeyer, B.; Krieglstein, J.; Kissel, T. In vitro cytotoxicity testing of polycations: Influence of polymer structure on cell viability and hemolysis. *Biomaterials* **2003**, *24*, 1121–1131. [CrossRef]

57. Wandrey, C.; Hernandez-Barajas, J.; Hunkeler, D. Diallyldimethylammonium chloride and its polymers. *Adv. Polym. Sci.* **1999**, *145*, 123–177.

58. Kircheis, R.; Wightman, L.; Wagner, E. Design and gene delivery activity of modified polyethylenimines. *Adv. Drug Del. Rev.* **2001**, *53*, 341–358. [CrossRef]

59. Hong, S.; Leroueil, P.R.; Janus, E.K.; Peters, J.L.; Kober, M.-M.; Islam, M.T.; Orr, B.G.; Baker, J.R.; Banaszak Holl, M.M. Interaction of polycationic polymers with supported lipid bilayers and cells: Nanoscale hole formation and enhanced membrane permeability. *Bioconjug. Chem.* **2006**, *17*, 728–734. [CrossRef] [PubMed]

60. Mecke, A.; Majoros, I.J.; Patri, A.K.; Baker, J.R.; Banaszak Holl, M.M.; Orr, B.G. Lipid bilayer disruption by polycationic polymers: The roles of size and chemical functional group. *Langmuir* **2005**, *21*, 10348–10354. [CrossRef] [PubMed]

61. Robertson, G.N.; McGee, C.A.S.; Dumbarton, T.C.; Croll, R.P.; Smith, F.M. Development of the swimbladder and its innervation in the zebrafish,danio rerio. *J. Morphol.* **2007**, *268*, 967–985. [CrossRef] [PubMed]

62. Asharani, P.V.; Lian Wu, Y.; Gong, Z.; Valiyaveettil, S. Toxicity of silver nanoparticles in zebrafish models. *Nanotechnology* **2008**, *19*, 255102. [CrossRef] [PubMed]

63. Asharani, P.V.; Lian Wu, Y.; Gong, Z.; Valiyaveettil, S. Comparison of the toxicity of silver, gold and platinum nanoparticles in developing zebrafish embryos. *Nanotoxicology* **2011**, *5*, 43–54. [CrossRef] [PubMed]

64. Lee, K.J.; Browning, L.M.; Nallathamby, P.D.; Osgood, C.J.; Xu, X.-H.N. Silver nanoparticles induce developmental stage-specific embryonic phenotypes in zebrafish. *Nanoscale* **2013**, *5*, 11625–11636. [CrossRef] [PubMed]

65. Osborne, O.J.; Johnston, B.D.; Moger, J.; Balousha, M.; Lead, J.R.; Kudoh, T.; Tyler, C.R. Effects of particle size and coating on nanoscale ag and tio2 exposure in zebrafish (*danio rerio*) embryos. *Nanotoxicology* **2013**, *7*, 1315–1324. [CrossRef] [PubMed]

66. Liu, W.; Long, Y.; Yin, N.; Zhao, X.; Sun, C.; Zhou, Q.; Jiang, G. Toxicity of engineered nanoparticles to fish. In *Engineered Nanoparticles and the Environment: Biophysicochemical Processes and Toxicity*; John Wiley & Sons: Hoboken, NJ, USA, 2016; Volume 4.

67. Lee, K.J.; Nallathamby, P.D.; Browning, L.M.; Osgood, C.J.; Xu, X.-H.N. In vivo imaging of transport and biocompatibility of single silver nanoparticles in early development of zebrafish embryos. *ACS Nano* **2007**, *1*, 133–143. [CrossRef] [PubMed]

68. Kiener, T.K.; Selptsova-Friedrich, I.; Hunziker, W. TJP3/ZO-3 is critical for epidermal barrier function in zebrafish embryos. *Dev. Biol.* **2008**, *316*, 36–49. [CrossRef] [PubMed]

69. Lin, S.; Zhao, Y.; Ji, Z.; Ear, J.; Chang, C.H.; Zhang, H.; Low-Kam, C.; Yamada, K.; Meng, H.; Wang, X.; et al. Zebrafish high-throughput screening to study the impact of dissolvable metal oxide nanoparticles on the hatching enzyme, ZHE1. *Small* **2013**, *9*, 1776–1785. [CrossRef] [PubMed]

12

Antimicrobial Potential and Cytotoxicity of Silver Nanoparticles Phytosynthesized by Pomegranate Peel Extract

Renan Aparecido Fernandes [1,2], Andresa Aparecida Berretta [3], Elina Cassia Torres [3], Andrei Felipe Moreira Buszinski [3], Gabriela Lopes Fernandes [2], Carla Corrêa Mendes-Gouvêa [2], Francisco Nunes de Souza-Neto [4], Luiz Fernando Gorup [4,5], Emerson Rodrigues de Camargo [4] and Debora Barros Barbosa [2,*]

[1] Department of Dentistry, University Center of Adamantina (UNIFAI), Adamantina 17800-000, São Paulo, Brazil; renanfernandes@fai.com.br

[2] Department of Dental Materials and Prosthodontics, São Paulo State University (UNESP), School of Dentistry, Araçatuba 16015-050, São Paulo, Brazil; fernandesgabriela@hotmail.com (G.L.F.); carla_cmendes@hotmail.com (C.C.M.-G.)

[3] Laboratory of Research, Development & Innovation, Apis Flora Industrial e Comercial Ltda., Ribeirão Preto 14020-670, São Paulo, Brazil; andresa.berretta@apisflora.com.br (A.A.B.); elinacassia@hotmail.com (E.C.T.); andrei.buszinski@apisflora.com.br (A.F.M.B.)

[4] Department of Chemistry, Federal University of São Carlos, São Carlos 13565-905, São Paulo, Brazil; francisconsn29@gmail.com (F.N.S.-N.); lfgorup@gmail.com (L.F.G.); camargo@ufscar.br (E.R.C.)

[5] FACET-Department of Chemistry, Federal University of Grande Dourados, Dourados 79804-970, Mato Grosso do Sul, Brazil

* Correspondence: debora@foa.unesp.br

Abstract: The phytosynthesis of metal nanoparticles is nowadays attracting the increased attention of researchers and is much needed given the worldwide matter related to environmental contamination. The antimicrobial activity of colloidal and spray formulation of silver nanoparticles (AgNPs) synthesized by pomegranate peel extract against *Candida albicans* and *Staphylococcus aureus*, and their cytotoxicity in mammalian cells were tested in the present study. Dry matter, pH, total phenolics, and ellagic acid in the extract were determined. Then, AgNPs were phytosynthesized and characterized by X-ray diffraction, electron transmission microscopy, dynamic light scattering, zeta potential, and Ag^+ dosage. Spray formulations and respective chemical-AgNP controls were prepared and tested. The peel extract reduced more than 99% of Ag^+, and produced nanoparticles with irregular forms and an 89-nm mean size. All AgNP presented antimicrobial activity, and the spray formulation of green-AgNP increased by 255 and 4 times the effectiveness against *S. aureus* and *C. albicans*, respectively. The cytotoxicity of colloidal and spray green-AgNP was expressively lower than the respective chemical controls. Pomegranate peel extract produced stable AgNP with antimicrobial action and low cytotoxicity, stimulating its use in the biomedical field.

Keywords: silver; nanoparticles; *Candida albicans*; *Staphylococcus aureus*; herbal medicine; Punicaceae

1. Introduction

Recently, a state of alert on a topic that affects people globally, antimicrobial resistance, has received much attention. This has led to the deaths of more than 700,000 people a year worldwide and this number has risen every year [1]. It is estimated that there will be a reduction in the world population of 11–444 million people in 2050 if antimicrobial resistance is not bypassed [1].

As an alternative against antimicrobial resistance, one approach gaining in strength is the use of inorganic particles at the nanoscale. The most prominent metals in the group of inorganic nanoparticles are copper, zinc, titanium, magnesium, gold, and silver [2–4]. In this context, silver nanoparticles have been the most exploited as they have a wide range of toxicity against several microorganisms such as *Staphylococcus aureus, Escherichia coli, Candida albicans*, and others [5].

The incorporation and use of silver nanoparticles has been observed in sundry sectors, for instance, in the food industry as an attempt to produce packaging with antimicrobial activity [6]. Its use in the area of cosmetics has also received prominence, as has its use in housecleaning, antiseptics, sunscreens, soap, and shampoo [7–9] as well as in textile manufacturing [10].

Considering the synthesis of silver nanoparticles, many routes have been presented such as electrochemical [11], radiation [12], photochemistry [13], and by biological methods [14]. Phytochemical synthesis has been noteworthy since the use of chemical compounds may result in undesirable toxic effects not only for the human organism but also for the environment. Its effectiveness in the production of silver nanoparticles has been demonstrated by the use of compounds of different plants in the ion reduction, being characterized as rapid, low cost, and environmentally friendly synthesis [15]. Furthermore, green-silver nanoparticles are usually less cytotoxic when compared to those reduced by conventional chemical agents [16]. It is believed that silver nanoparticles reduced by plant extracts do not carry on their surface chemical compounds used for the reduction and stabilization of chemically produced silver nanoparticles that are toxic to human cells. It is still believed that the phytochemicals present in the extracts are carried on the surface of the silver nanoparticles, reducing their cytotoxic effect, aside from presenting different forms of chemically produced silver nanoparticles [16]. Important aspects in green-synthesis should be taken into account including the choice of plant to be used, being the plants which grow in different regions of the world more eligible for this [16]. The previously known potential of the plant including antioxidant, anti-inflammatory, and antimicrobial such as the case of *Punica granatum* (pomegranate) should also be considered [17–19]. Some studies have also used *Punica granatum* to reduce silver ions to silver nanoparticles [19–21]. Silver nanoparticles were green-synthesized and showed significantly lower cytotoxicity when compared to the silver nanoparticles synthesized by a chemical pathway. This fact has stimulated the search for the use of reduced silver nanoparticles by means of plant extracts for biological purposes such as the treatment of contagious infectious diseases, especially those in need of topical treatment.

Thus, taking together the benefits of pomegranate and the antimicrobial applicability of silver nanoparticles, the present study aimed to synthesize silver nanoparticles using pomegranate peel extract, and to produce spray formulations containing the previously green-synthesized silver nanoparticles. Their antimicrobial activity against *Staphylococcus aureus* and *Candida albicans*, and their cytotoxicity effect on fibroblast cells were investigated.

2. Results

2.1. Characterization of Peel Extract, Silver Nanoparticles and Formulations

The pH and the dry matter of the peel extract obtained by maceration followed by percolation were 3.13 and 86.39 ($\pm$0.96) % *w/w*, and the total phenolics expressed in gallic acid and the ellagic acid were 392.0 ($\pm$9) and 3.64 ($\pm$0.03) mg/g, respectively.

The formation of silver nanoparticles was confirmed by comparing the XRD patterns and the corresponding standard patterns of cubic of silver nanoparticles (Figure 1), according to the diffraction standard (JCPDS file No. 04-0783). The reflection peak (2 2 2) is characteristic of the substrate (Si), where silver particles were deposited as a thin film. TEM images (Figure 2) showed different forms and sizes of silver nanoparticles produced by green and conventional chemical routes as well as in their respective formulations. In general, green-synthesis produced particles with a larger size than those obtained by conventional synthesis. Dynamic Laser Scanning (DLS) analyses of the formulations prepared with green or conventional silver nanoparticles demonstrated different particle sizes, being the mean values of 89 ± 21 and 19 ± 4 nm for the green and conventional formulation, respectively. The values of zeta potential of green and conventional silver nanoparticles were lower than -30 mV (-46.2 ± 6.06 mV green, and -67.5 ± 3.69 mV conventional), indicating the stability of both colloidal silver nanoparticles.

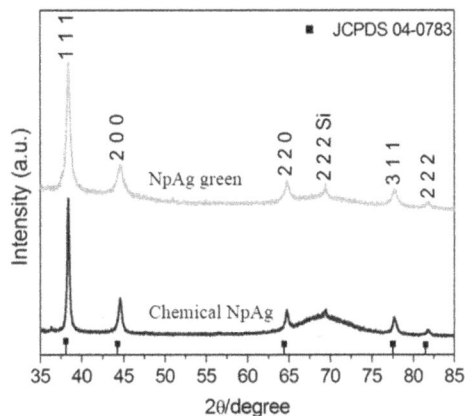

Figure 1. X-ray diffraction (XRD) of the green and chemical silver nanoparticles.

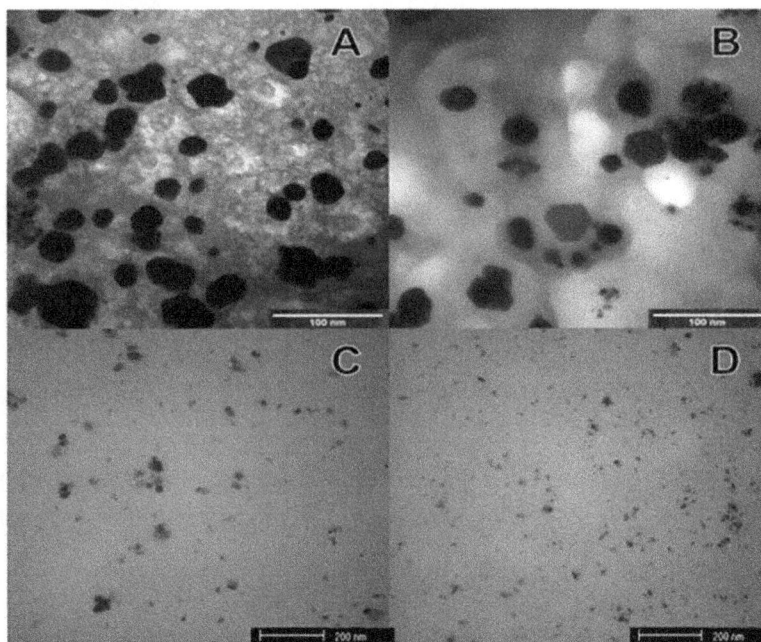

Figure 2. Images of transmission electron microscopy (TEM): (A) Green silver nanoparticles; (B) Silver nanoparticles green formulation; (C) Chemical silver nanoparticles; (D) Silver nanoparticles chemical formulation.

Almost 100% of the Ag^+ ions coming from $AgNO_3$ were reduced by the pomegranate peel extract (99.89%) and sodium citrate (99.51%). However, in the spray formulation containing chemical-silver nanoparticles, the percentage of reduction was diminished to 68.18% although the formulation maintained stable regarding Ag^+ ions concentration for 28 days (Table 1). Zeta potential data confirmed the stability of the spray formulations regardless of the method used to obtain the silver nanoparticles (Table 2). The total phenolics in the spray formulations with or without silver nanoparticles were quantified at 0, 7, 14, and 28 days after having been prepared (Figure 3), and it has been significantly reduced in the green-synthesized silver nanoparticle formulation after 14 days with values ranging from 0.405 to 0.295 mg/g.

Table 1. Values of the silver ionic reduction and zeta potential for green and chemical silver nanoparticle formulations in different periods.

Time	Silver Nanoparticles Green Formulation			Silver Nanoparticles Chemical Formulation		
	$\mu g Ag^+/mL$	% of Reduction	Zeta Potential	$\mu g Ag^+/mL$	% of Reduction	Zeta Potential
T0	0.249	99.93%	-73.7 ± 6.49	1.769	68.15%	-78.2 ± 3.06
T7	0.178	99.95%	-68.3 ± 4.92	1.927	65.31%	-72.9 ± 3.10
T14	0.220	99.94%	-72.8 ± 6.49	1.543	72.22%	-85.5 ± 3.36
T28	0.186	99.95%	-68.6 ± 5.62	1.846	66.77%	-76.5 ± 4.05

Table 2. Silver ion concentration ($\mu g Ag^+/mL$) and percentage of silver ions reduction after the reactions, AgNP percentage, and values of minimum inhibitory concentration (MIC) of silver nanoparticles and pomegranate peel extract found for *Staphylococcus aureus* and *Candida albicans*.

Samples	Silver Ions Concentration	Silver Ions Remaining %	Ag NP %	MIC ($\mu g/mL$)	
				S. aureus	*C. albicans*
Control *	10,303.26	95.52	4.48	4.13	4.59
Pomegranate peel extract	-	-	-	391	781
Silver nanoparticles green	10.89	0.11	99.89	67.50	68.75
Silver nanoparticles chemical	130.40	1.21	98.79	0.50	0.25
Pomegranate peel extract formulation	-	-	-	0.37	0.18
Silver nanoparticles green formulation	0.249	0.01	99.99	0.26	16.87
Silver nanoparticles chemical formulation	1.769	31.85	68.15	0.56	1.12

* Control = Carboxymethylcellulose, propylene glycol, silver nitrate.

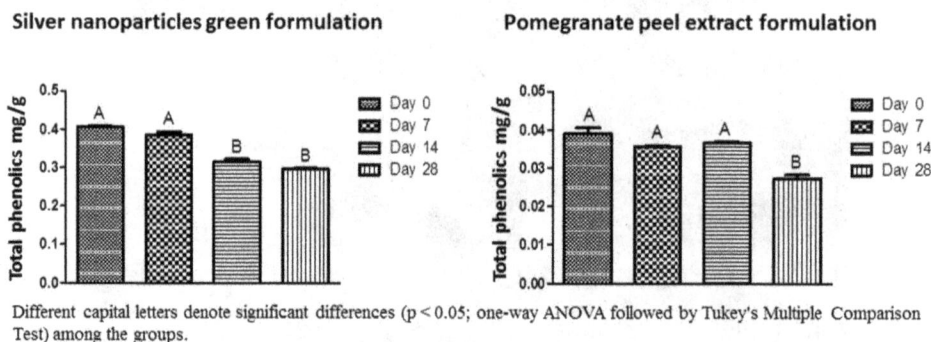

Different capital letters denote significant differences ($p < 0.05$; one-way ANOVA followed by Tukey's Multiple Comparison Test) among the groups.

Figure 3. Total phenolics concentration for the silver nanoparticles green formulation and pomegranate peel extract formulation in different periods. Different capital letters denote significant difference ($p < 0.05$; one-way ANOVA followed by Tukey's multiple comparison test) among the groups.

2.2. Antimicrobial Activity

The antimicrobial activity expressed as MIC values of silver nanoparticles and pomegranate peel extract ($\mu g/mL$) (Table 1) was, in general, considerably lower for the spray formulations than the active inputs regardless of the microorganisms tested. MIC values against *C. albicans* for active inputs and spray formulations were 781 and 0.18 for the peel extract, 68.75 and 16.87 for the green-, and 0.25 and 1.12 for the chemical-silver nanoparticles. While for *S. aureus*, the values were 391 and 0.37, 67.5, and 0.26, and 0.5 and 0.56 for pomegranate peel extract, green-, and chemical-silver nanoparticles in the active inputs and spray formulations, respectively. In addition, different conditions of humidity and temperature did not affect the effectiveness of the spray formulations against both microorganisms.

2.3. Cytotoxicity

Figure 4 shows the fibroblast L929 cells viability in view of different concentrations of silver nanoparticles (green and conventional route). Green silver nanoparticles presented lower cytotoxicity than conventional ones. A dosage of 50 $\mu g/mL$ was necessary to initiate the toxicity, but the cell viability was nearly 80%, while conventional-silver nanoparticles were quite toxic at very low concentration (6.25 μg/mL) and was similar to the negative control (DMSO) with viability lower than 20%. Furthermore, the addition of the reagents to prepare the formulations did not interfere in the toxicity of the conventional-silver nanoparticles, whereas the cytotoxicity for the green-silver nanoparticles formulation as well as for the extract formulation was considerably increased.

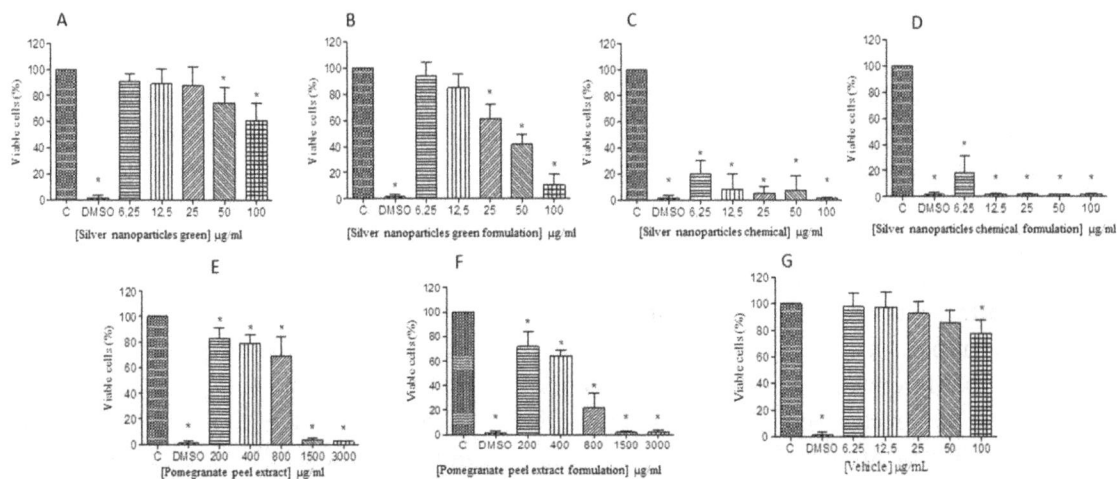

*p<0.05 Significant statistical difference compared to the control group (C) 100% viable cells, using one-way ANOVA, followed by the Bonferroni test.

Figure 4. Cytotoxicity evaluation of respective active input (green and chemical silver nanoparticles and pomegranate peel extract), their respective formulations, and the vehicle (compounds of spray-formulation without the active inputs). (**A**) Silver nanoparticles green; (**B**) Silver nanoparticles green formulation; (**C**) Silver nanoparticles chemical; (**D**) Silver nanoparticles chemical formulation; (**E**) Pomegranate peel extract; (**F**) Pomegranate peel extract formulation and (**G**) Vehicle.

3. Discussion

For future reproducibility of the experiment, the extract obtained by maceration followed by percolation was duly characterized in relation to dry matter, total phenolics content, ellagic acid, and pH. Total phenolics were determined only in samples that contained the pomegranate peel extract, and then the chemical formulation did not present any phenolic content in its composition. Polyphenols are effective hydrogen donors and are correlated to the number and position of hydroxyl groups and conjugations as well as the presence of donor electrons in the aromatic ring B, because of the ability of this aromatic ring to withstand the electron depletion located in the π electron system [22]. The antimicrobial activity of various polyphenols and plant extracts have been evaluated in pharmaceutical and food studies [23,24]. Some phenolic compounds present in sage, rosemary, thyme, hops, coriander, tea, cloves, and basil are known to exhibit antimicrobial effects against foodborne pathogens. Their mechanisms of action need to be further elucidated, and might be due to a plethora of phenolic compounds present in a very single plant extract. Furthermore, as the bioactive compounds in the extract presented antioxidant and anti-inflammatory activities, the antimicrobial potential of the pomegranate peel extract in the in vivo trials could show better results, and should be strongly stimulated in further studies. Regarding the multi conceptual nature of the term antioxidant and bringing it into the context of this study, some polyphenols present in low concentrations could prevent or reduce the extent of oxidative damage in mammalian cells. Taken together, these natural biomolecules could indirectly protect the cells and reduce the cytotoxicity of silver nanoparticles.

The correct selection of the plant and the standardization of the methods to obtain the extracts to be used as reducing or capping agent in the nanosynthesis of metal particles should be preponderant when the green process is elected for the production of products in large scale. Additionally, a plethora of plants used in the phytosynthesis of metal nanoparticles [25–27] and the lack of information of the extraction techniques used in the articles has hindered the comparison of the present results with those found in the literature. For instance, different values and methods of total phenolics quantification can be observed in the literature as described by Kalaycioglu et al. (2017) [28]. Similarly, other factors can interfere in the evaluation and comparisons of the extracts such as the chemical and genotypic composition of the plant, the variety and the soil type, the place of the plant origin, the harvest season, maturation method, aside from the solvent and the process used for the obtention of the pomegranate extract, among others [29].

Scanning electron microscopy (SEM) and transmission electron microscopy (TEM) images showed the smallest particles obtained by conventional chemical synthesis, and DLS data confirmed these findings with mean sizes of 89 and 19 nm for green and chemical nanoparticles, respectively. The fission of colloidal particles of different sizes and shapes may be related to additives (salts, polymers), solvent properties (boiling temperature, affinity with created surfaces), the addition of nucleation, among others [30]. The reagents used in the chemical synthesis would produce particles with more predictable characteristics than the several substances and compounds present in the plant extract and used in the phytosynthesis route, which would interfere with the size and form of the nanoparticles and make phytosynthesis a challenge in controlling the reaction process and the morphological aspects of the particles. Moreover, the presence of different bioactive substances in the extract would reduce only a fraction of the silver ions present in the solution. The remaining silver ions would form other nuclei and further the growth of the previously formed silver nanoparticles [31]. This process is called Ostwald Ripening, where the largest particles consume the smaller ones and grow larger, where the dissolution of the smaller ones and deposition of ions on the surface of larger ones occur [32].

Almost 100% of ions reduction was observed for both synthesis routes. However, when the chemical silver nanoparticles were added to the formulation, a dissociation of ions from nearly 30% was observed when compared to chemical silver nanoparticles alone. This fact could be due to the presence of the components as carboxymethylcellulose and propylene glycol in the spray formulation which possibly favored the silver ion dissociation into the system [33]. The presence of oxygen or ligands for Ag^+ in the formulations may increase the dissolution rate of AgNP and lead to increased dissolution through the formation of Ag^+ complexes [34]. Ag^+ in solution will interact with various ions and molecules that are present in aqueous media. Important ligands to be considered for Ag^+ are sulfide and organic ligands such as the carboxylic acids group which are used as Ag coatings (e.g., citrate, lactate). Carboxyl ligands such as carboxymethylcellulose strongly bind Ag^+, which may affect the dissolution of AgNP and the bioavailability of Ag^+ [35].

Furthermore, the size of the Ag in the NP affects the extent and kinetics of the AgNP dissolution as the smallest nanoparticles dissolve faster and to a greater extent [36]. This would explain the difference in the dissolution of the nanoparticles in the formulations. Their dissolution is of high relevance for the possible toxic effects of AgNP as Ag^+ appears in many cases to determine their toxicity [37]. This fact was not observed when green-synthesis was carried out. This could be related to several compounds present in the extract which would readily react with the released silver ions, or the encapsulation of the silver nanoparticles promoted by those phytocompounds may have avoided the silver ions dissociation from the silver nanoparticles and its release to the solution.

Zeta potential test demonstrated the stability of the silver nanoparticles, most notedly in the spray formulations. Electrical charges on the surface of the nanoparticles prevent agglomeration, and thus afford the stability of the nanoparticles [38,39]. Indeed, silver nanoparticles and spray formulations presented a mean of 70 mV, which indicates their high stability of silver nanoparticles [40].

Antimicrobial results are also promising for the silver nanoparticles as well as the pomegranate extract obtained. The formulations notably showed better results when compared with the input active only. This fact could be explained for the proper dispersion of the active inputs (silver nanoparticles and pomegranate peel extract) in the spray formulation. Additionally, a synergistic effect could have occurred between those active inputs and the methylparaben present in the formulation. In the literature, studies with an antimicrobial effect of pomegranate extract were conducted against

Staphylococcus aureus, Enterobacter aerogene, Salmonella typhi, and *Klebsiella pneumonia* [41]. The MIC values obtained in this study for pomegranate extract were in accordance with Bakkiyaraj et al. (2013) [42] for both the microorganisms studied, and a difference was observed in *C. albicans,* but this fact may be explained by the difference between the *C. albicans* strains used in the studies.

Chemical-silver nanoparticles, in formulation or not, produced MIC values against *S. aureus* about 10-fold lower than those produced by Prema et al. (2017) [33] (60 μg/mL), who also produced silver nanoparticles stabilized with CMC. Indeed, the antimicrobial activity of chemical silver nanoparticles was also determined by Monteiro et al. (2011) [43] with MIC values for *C. albicans* (0.5 μg/mL) in accordance with this present study.

Noteworthy is the difference found in the present study in respect of cytotoxicity between the chemical and green routes to obtain silver nanoparticles. Studies have shown that silver nanoparticles produced with *Protium serratum* and *Nyctanthes arbortristis* extracts were biocompatible when tested in L929 fibroblasts [44,45]. It is believed that what makes the silver nanoparticle toxic to human cells is the type of reducing agent used such as sodium citrate or sodium borohydride [46]. Even in conventional syntheses of silver nanoparticles, reagents are used that prevent the aggregation of these nanoparticles [47], which may further favor their cytotoxicity.

In the case of phytosynthesis of metal nanoparticles, plant extracts, aside from acting as reducing agents, would act to stabilize the particles against dissolution, hence reducing the toxicity of the silver nanoparticles solution. Furthermore, it is possible that some compounds in the extracts may have a synergistic effect with the silver nanoparticles [48], making them less toxic to human cells. Furthermore, extracts of *Punica granatum* have exhibited antioxidant [49] and anti-inflammatory [50] activity, and may have contributed to reducing the cytotoxicity of green- in comparison with chemical-silver nanoparticles.

In general, the stability assay (silver ions dosage, zeta potential, and antimicrobial activity) showed a high stabilizing capacity of the formulations. However, the spray formulations of green silver nanoparticles and pomegranate peel extract showed a significant reduction in the content of total phenolics in 14 and 28 days. The decrease in the content of total phenolics may have occurred due to the temperature variations inherent in the stability test, as occurred in the study of [51] where the temperature affected the total phenolics content in the roselle-mango juice blends. Moreover, in formulations containing green-silver nanoparticles, the components of the extract may have been degraded or associated with the nanoparticles, explaining the faster decrease of the total phenolics content when compared to the pomegranate extract formulation. Interestingly, ion dosage, zeta potential, and antimicrobial activity were not affected by different conditions of temperature, time, and humidity of the stability test.

Altogether, the reported results suggest that the plant extract mediated syntheses of AgNP showed a pronounced lower cytotoxic effect in mouse fibroblast cells (L929) than the syntheses of AgNP by the chemical method. Of note is the implication that different sizes between the green- chemical-AgNP as well as the expected impurities sedimented on both obtained nanoparticles could have had on their toxicity. Although it is quite tricky to obtain AgNP with a well-defined form and size and prevent the particles aggregation [52], it is of importance to complement and support our findings, then strongly recommend an eco-friendly approach to producing green-AgNP and prototype wound-care sprays containing these particles.

4. Materials and Methods

4.1. Plant Material and Preparation of Pomegranate Peel Extract

Pomegranate samples were collected from a crop cultivated in Eixo (21°08′01″ S, 51°06′06″ W), Mirandópolis, São Paulo, Brazil, during May 2015. Pomegranate peels were separated and stove-dried at 50 °C, ground, and sieved to a granulometry lower than 2 mm. Peels were submitted to alcohol extraction using 70% ethanol by maceration, followed by the percolation process [53]. The extract was characterized in relation to pH, dry matter, and total phenolics expressed as gallic acid. The chemical marker of pomegranate, ellagic acid, was also identified and quantified.

4.1.1. Determination of Total Phenolics, pH, and Dry Matter

To determine the total phenolics, an analytical curve of gallic acid (Sigma-Aldrich Chemical Co., St. Louis, MO, USA) was carried out [54]. All extracts obtained and the standard solution of gallic acid were prepared in 50 mL volumetric flasks using water as the solvent. The samples were homogenized and, the flasks were brought to the ultrasonic bath for 30 min. A 0.5 mL aliquot was transferred to another 50 mL flask where 2.5 mL of Folin-Denis reagent (Qhemis-High Purity, Hexis, São Paulo, Brazil) and 5.0 mL of 29% sodium carbonate (Cinética, São Paulo, Brazil) were added. The samples were protected from light and the readings were performed after 30 min in a UV-Vis spectrophotometer at 760 nm [53]. The pH was measured direct from a solution of 1% extract, using a pH kit (Merck KGaA, Darmstadt, Germany) and dry matter was calculated after drying on a sample stove at 105 °C and was expressed in percentage w/w. All data were analyzed in triplicate.

4.1.2. Determination of the Ellagic Acid Content

A Shimadzu liquid chromatograph and a Shimpack ODS C18 (Shimadzu Corporation, Kyoto, Japan) reverse phase column (100 mm × 2.6 mm) were used to determine the ellagic acid content by high performance liquid chromatography (HPLC). Analytical conditions were optimized based on de Sousa et al. (2007) [55] with modifications. As the mobile phase, HPLC grade methanol and a 2% aqueous acetic acid solution with gradient elution (0–7 min, 20–72.5% v/v methanol, 7–7.5 min, 72.5–95% v/v methanol, 7.5–8.5 min 95% v/v methanol, 8.5–9 min 95–20% v/v methanol, 9–10 min 20% v/v methanol) were used. The flow rate was 1.0 mL/min, and the separation was achieved at 25 °C. The injection volume was 5 μL and the wavelength used was 254 nm. Peaks were determined by comparison with an authenticated ellagic acid standard. Briefly, the sample was transferred to a 20 mL volumetric flask which was diluted with HPLC grade methanol. Extraction was undertaken using a vortex for 5 min and ultrasonic bath for 1 h. For the extracts, samples were transferred to volumetric flasks of 10 mL, using methanol HPLC as the solvent. All samples were vortexed for 5 min and sonicated for 30 min. Samples were filtered through 0.45 μm filter. All samples were prepared in triplicate.

4.2. Synthesis of Green-Silver Nanoparticles

The protocols described by Gorup et al. (2011) [56] and Das et al. 2015 [57] with modifications were used to produce silver nanoparticles. Briefly, 3.5% of carboxymethylcellulose (CMC) (Labsynth, Diadema, Brazil), 20% of propylene glycol (PG) (Labsynth, Diadema, Brazil), 100 mM of silver nitrate (SN) (Merck KGaA, Darmstadt, Germany), pomegranate peel extract at 30 mg/mL, and water to make up 100% of the samples were used. Silver nanoparticles were not purified relative to the excess reagents. The reaction was carried out at 50 °C for 12 min, and it was selected based on previous results.

4.3. Synthesis of Chemical-Silver Nanoparticles

Chemical-silver nanoparticles were produced according to Gorup et al. [53]. $AgNO_3$ (Merck KGaA, Darmstadt, Hesse, Germany) was dissolved in water, and brought to boiling at 90 °C. After 2 min of boiling, an aqueous solution of sodium citrate ($Na_3C_6H_5O_7$) (Merck KGaA, Darmstadt, Hesse, Germany) was added, and kept boiling for another 6 min until the solution reached a yellow amber color. The stoichiometric ratio was 1:3, respectively for $AgNO_3$ and $Na_3C_6H_5O_7$. Silver nanoparticles were not purified relative to the excess reagents.

4.4. Preparation of the Spray Formulations

The reagents used were CMC (Labsynth, Diadema, Brazil), PG (Labsynth, Diadema, Brazil), and methylparaben (Labsynth, Diadema, Brazil) in a proportion of 0.1%, 7%, and 0.1%, respectively. The active inputs (green- or chemical-silver nanoparticles and pomegranate peel extract) concentrations were based on the minimum inhibitory concentration and cytotoxicity. Therefore, the final concentrations of active inputs in the spray formulations were: 337.5 µg/mL of green-silver nanoparticles, 5.55 µg/mL chemical-silver nanoparticles, and 94 µg/mL of crude peel extract dry matter.

4.5. Characterization of the Silver Nanoparticles and the Spray Formulations

4.5.1. X-ray Diffraction (XRD), Dynamic Light Scattering (DLS), and Zeta Potential Analysis

A Shimadzu XRD diffractometer with a Cu Kα radiation operating at 30 kV and 30 mA and 2θ range from 35° to 85° with step scan of 0.02° and scan speed 0.2°·min^{-1} was used to perform XRD analysis. To collect silver nanoparticles patterns, the nanoparticles were deposited on the surface of a silicon substrate (Si) by dripping the aqueous colloidal dispersion on the substrate at room temperature until the solvent had evaporated.

DLS experiments were performed at room temperature and at a fixed angle of 173° on a Zetasizer Nano ZS (Malvern Instruments Ltd., Malvern, UK) equipped with 50 mW 533 nm laser and a digital auto correlator. The number-average values obtained were compared to the size distributions of the silver nanoparticles. For the zeta potential test a Zetasizer (Malvern instruments, Malvern, UK) with an MPT-2 titrator was used. Aliquots from each test suspension were obtained to conduct zeta potential, and mean values were obtained from three independent measurements.

4.5.2. TEM Analyzes

The nanocompounds morphology was characterized by TEM images in a Jeol JEM-100 CXII (JEOL USA Inc., Peabody, St. Louis, MO, USA) microscope equipped with Hamamatsu ORCA-HR digital camera.

4.6. Silver Ions Dosage

The dosages of free silver ions (Ag$^+$) present in the compounds and spray formulations were performed to observe if the total amount of Ag added in the synthesis reaction was successfully reduced. A specific electrode 9616 BNWP (Thermo Scientific, Beverly, MA, USA) coupled to an ion analyzer (Orion 720 A$^+$, Thermo Scientific, Beverly, MA, USA) was used. A 1000 µg Ag/mL standard was prepared by adding 1.57 g of AgNO3 to 1 L of deionized water. The combined electrode was calibrated with standards containing 6.25 to 100 µg Ag/mL to achieve equivalent silver concentrations in the compounds. A silver ionic strength adjuster solution (ISA, Cat. No. 940011) that provided a constant background ionic strength was used (1 mL of each sample/standard: 0.02 mL ISA).

4.7. Stability Test of the Spray Formulations

The spray formulations were submitted to a stability test with controlled conditions of temperature and time. This test was based on Anvisa protocols (Cosmetics stability guide ISBN 85-88233-15-0; Copyright$^©$ Anvisa, 2005) and the guide to stability studies (Ordinance No. 593 of 25 August 2000). Briefly, samples of each spray formulation were submitted to alternating cycles of temperature daily ranging from 40 to −5 °C for 28 days. The tests selected to evaluate the stability of the samples were ion dosage, total phenolics content, zeta potential, and minimal inhibitory concentration (MIC). All tests were done in the same conditions as described before, and were carried out at 0, 7, 14, and 28 days.

4.8. Antimicrobial Activity of the Silver Nanoparticles and the Spray Formulations

Minimal inhibitory concentration of the silver nanoparticles samples were determined following the instructions of the Clinical Laboratory Standards Institute with some modifications. The samples were first diluted in water and subsequently in culture medium specific for each microorganism, Mueller Hinton broth (BD Difco, Franklin Lakes, USA) for *Staphylococcus aureus* (ATCC 25923), and RPMI (Sigma-Aldrich, St. Louis, MO, USA) for *Candida albicans* SC 5314) [58]. The microorganisms were adjusted to 5×10^5 cells/mL for *S. aureus* and 5×10^3 cells/mL for *C. albicans*, and the plates were incubated for 24 h and 48 h in aerobiosis at 37 °C for *S. aureus* and *C. albicans*, respectively. After incubation, the plates were visually read. The assays were performed in triplicate.

4.9. Cytotoxicity Analysis

For the evaluation of cytotoxicity, fibroblast cells of the L929 lineage were used. Cells were cultured in DMEM culture supplemented with 10% fetal bovine serum (FBS), penicillin G (100 U/mL) (Gibco®, Carlsbad, USA), streptomycin (100 µg/mL), amphotericin B (25 µg/mL) and incubated in a stove at 37 °C with 5% CO_2. Cells were subcultured (5–7 days), using 0.9% saline to wash them and 0.25% trypsin to disintegrate them from the vial. After disruption, these cells were centrifuged at 1000 rpm for 10 min at 10 °C, resuspended in complete DMEM medium (supplemented with FBS), and cell counted in a Neubauer's chamber.

The sub-cultured third to eighth passage fibroblasts were inoculated into 96-well microplates at a density of 0.5×10^5 cells/well. They were then incubated at 37 °C with 5% CO_2. After 24 h, 20 µL of different dilutions of each sample were added to the wells of the plate containing the cells in medium not supplemented with SBF (incomplete medium) and incubated. Twenty-four hours post-treatment, the medium was withdrawn, cells were washed with saline and 20 µL of resazurin (Sigma-Aldrich) 0.01% *w/v* in deionized H_2O was added to each well containing 180 µL of DMEM medium supplemented with 10% Of SFB. The plates were then incubated for 4 h at 37 °C and fluorescence was measured at 540 and 590 nm for excitation and emission, respectively [59]. Cell viability was expressed as a percentage of viable cells when compared to the control group without treatment.

4.10. Statistical Analysis

GraphPad Prism software (GraphPad Software, Inc., La Jolla, CA, USA) was employed for the statistical analysis with a confidence level of 95%. Parametric statistical analyses were conducted with one-way ANOVA followed by Tukey's multiple comparison test for total phenols and zeta potential. For the ion test the statistical analyses was Dunn's multiple comparison test.

5. Conclusions

In light of the results obtained and the limitations of the present study, it was concluded that the use of pomegranate peel extract showed it to be an efficient reducing agent for the production of silver nanoparticles. Moreover, the antimicrobial potential and the low cytotoxicity demonstrated by green-silver nanoparticles have stimulated the search for improvements in the bio-nanotechnology field. Furthermore, the anti-inflammatory and antioxidant properties of pomegranate have encouraged further studies to use nanosystems with future application in prophylaxis or treatment of biofilm-dependent diseases.

Author Contributions: R.A.F., D.B.B., and A.A.B. conceived and designed the experiments; R.A.F., E.C.T., A.F.M.B., G.L.F., and C.C.M.-G. performed the experiments; R.A.F., D.B.B., and A.A.B. analyzed the data; F.N. d.S.-N., L.F.G., and E.R.d.C. contributed reagents/materials/analysis tools; R.A.F. and D.B.B. wrote the paper.

Funding: This study was supported by São Paulo Research Foundation (FAPESP), Brazil, (Process n° 2016/04230-9).

Acknowledgments: The authors would like to thank the company Apis Flora Indl. Coml. Ltda. for the facilities and for the production of the spray formulations containing pomegranate peel extract, and the Laboratory of photochemioprotection of the Faculty of Pharmaceutical Sciences of Ribeirão Preto for the facilities in performing some of the laboratory assays. We thank the Brazilian Agricultural Research Corporation (EMBRAPA) to allow for some tests on the research on its premises and also the Federal University of São Carlos for disposal of its dependencies and technologies. This research work was supported by the São Paulo Research Foundation (FAPESP), Brazil, (Process n° 2016/04230-9).

References

1. Raut, S.; Adhikari, B. The need to focus China's national plan to combat antimicrobial resistance. *Lancet Infect. Dis.* **2017**, *17*, 137–138. [CrossRef]

2. Guzman, M.; Dille, J.; Godet, S. Synthesis and antibacterial activity of silver nanoparticles against gram-positive and gram-negative bacteria. *Nanomed. Nanotechnol. Biol. Med.* **2012**, *8*, 37–45. [CrossRef] [PubMed]

3. He, G.; Qiao, M.; Li, W.; Lu, Y.; Zhao, T.; Zou, R.; Li, B.; Darr, J.A.; Hu, J.; Titirici, M.M.; et al. S, N-Co-Doped Graphene-Nickel Cobalt Sulfide Aerogel: Improved Energy Storage and Electrocatalytic Performance. *Adv. Sci.* **2017**, *4*, 1600214. [CrossRef] [PubMed]

4. Jankun, J.; Landeta, P.; Pretorius, E.; Skrzypczak-Jankun, E.; Lipinski, B. Unusual clotting dynamics of plasma supplemented with iron(III). *Int. J. Mol. Med.* **2014**, *33*, 367–372. [CrossRef] [PubMed]

5. Hebeish, A.; El-Rafie, M.H.; El-Sheikh, M.A.; Seleem, A.A.; El-Naggar, M.E. Antimicrobial wound dressing and anti-inflammatory efficacy of silver nanoparticles. *Int. J. Biol. Macromol.* **2014**, *65*, 509–515. [CrossRef] [PubMed]

6. Kuorwel, K.K.; Cran, M.J.; Sonneveld, K.; Miltz, J.; Bigger, S.W. Antimicrobial activity of biodegradable polysaccharide and protein-based films containing active agents. *J. Food Sci.* **2011**, *76*, R90–R102. [CrossRef] [PubMed]

7. Bansod, S.D.; Bawaskar, M.S.; Gade, A.K.; Rai, M.K. Development of shampoo, soap and ointment formulated by green-synthesised silver nanoparticles functionalised with antimicrobial plants oils in veterinary dermatology: Treatment and prevention strategies. *IET Nanobiotechnol.* **2015**, *9*, 165–171. [CrossRef] [PubMed]

8. Tulve, N.S.; Stefaniak, A.B.; Vance, M.E.; Rogers, K.; Mwilu, S.; LeBouf, R.F.; Schwegler-Berry, D.; Willis, R.; Thomas, T.A.; Marr, L.C. Characterization of silver nanoparticles in selected consumer products and its relevance for predicting children's potential exposures. *Int. J. Hyg. Environ. Health* **2015**, *218*, 345–357. [CrossRef] [PubMed]

9. Benn, T.; Cavanagh, B.; Hristovski, K.; Posner, J.D.; Westerhoff, P. The release of nanosilver from consumer products used in the home. *J. Environ. Qual.* **2010**, *39*, 1875–1882. [CrossRef] [PubMed]

10. Velazquez-Velazquez, J.L.; Santos-Flores, A.; Araujo-Melendez, J.; Sánchez-Sánchezc, R.; Velasquilloc, C.; Gonzálezd, C.; Martínez-Castañone, G.; Martinez-Gutierreza, F. Anti-biofilm and cytotoxicity activity of impregnated dressings with silver nanoparticles. *Mater. Sci. Eng. C Mater. Biol. Appl.* **2015**, *49*, 604–611. [CrossRef] [PubMed]

11. Treshchalov, A.; Erikson, H.; Puust, L.; Tsarenko, S.; Saar, R.; Vanetsev, A.; Tammeveski, K.; Sildos, I. Stabilizer-free silver nanoparticles as efficient catalysts for electrochemical reduction of oxygen. *J. Colloid Interface Sci.* **2017**, *491*, 358–366. [CrossRef] [PubMed]

12. Malkar, V.V.; Mukherjee, T.; Kapoor, S. Synthesis of silver nanoparticles in aqueous aminopolycarboxylic acid solutions via gamma-irradiation and hydrogen reduction. *Mater. Sci. Eng. C Mater. Biol. Appl.* **2014**, *44*, 87–91. [CrossRef] [PubMed]

13. Lombardo, P.C.; Poli, A.L.; Castro, L.F.; Perussi, J.R.; Schmitt, C.C. Photochemical Deposition of Silver Nanoparticles on Clays and Exploring Their Antibacterial Activity. *ACS Appl. Mater. Interfaces* **2016**, *8*, 21640–21647. [CrossRef] [PubMed]

14. Rafique, M.; Sadaf, I.; Rafique, M.S.; Tahir, M.B. A review on green-synthesis of silver nanoparticles and their applications. *Artif. Cells Nanomed. Biotechnol.* **2016**, *8*, 1–20. [CrossRef]

15. Roy, N.; Gaur, A.; Jain, A.; Bhattacharya, S.; Rani, V. Green-synthesis of silver nanoparticles: An approach to overcome toxicity. *Environ. Toxicol. Pharmacol.* **2013**, *36*, 807–812. [CrossRef] [PubMed]

16. Das, R.K.; Brar, S.K. Plant mediated green-synthesis: Modified approaches. *Nanoscale* **2013**, *5*, 10155–101562. [CrossRef] [PubMed]

17. Lansky, E.P.; Newman, R.A. *Punica granatum* (pomegranate) and its potential for prevention and treatment of inflammation and cancer. *J. Ethnopharmacol.* **2007**, *109*, 177–206. [CrossRef] [PubMed]

18. Pande, G.; Akoh, C.C. Antioxidant capacity and lipid characterization of six Georgia-grown pomegranate cultivars. *J. Agric. Food Chem.* **2009**, *57*, 9427–9436. [CrossRef] [PubMed]

19. Edison, T.J.; Sethuraman, M.G. Biogenic robust synthesis of silver nanoparticles using *Punica granatum* peel and its application as a green catalyst for the reduction of an anthropogenic pollutant 4-nitrophenol. *Spectrochim. Acta Part A Mol. Biomol. Spectrosc.* **2013**, *104*, 262–264. [CrossRef] [PubMed]

20. Ahmad, N.S.; Rai, R. Rapid green-synthesis of silver and gold nanoparticles using peels of *Punica granatum*. *Adv. Mater. Lett.* **2012**, *3*, 376–380. [CrossRef]

21. Naik, S.K.; Chand, P.K. Silver nitrate and aminoethoxyvinylglycine promote in vitro adventitious shoot regeneration of pomegranate (*Punica granatum* L.). *J. Plant Physiol.* **2003**, *160*, 423–430. [CrossRef] [PubMed]

22. Ramirez-Tortoza, C.; Andersen, O.M.; Gardner, P.T.; Morrice, P.C.; Wood, S.G.; Duthie, S.J.; Collins, A.R.; Duthie, G.G. Anthocyanin-rich extract decreases indices of lipid peroxidation and DNA damage in vitamin E depleted rats. *Free Radic. Biol. Med.* **2001**, *46*, 1033–1037. [CrossRef]

23. Taguri, T.; Takashi, T.; Kouno, I. Antibacterial spectrum of plant polyphenols and extracts depending upon hydroxyphenyl structure. *Biol. Pharm. Bull.* **2006**, *29*, 2226–2235. [CrossRef] [PubMed]

24. Ahn, J.; Grun, I.U.; Mustapha, A. Effects of plant extracts on microbial growth, color change, and lipid oxidation in cooked beef. *Food Microbiol.* **2007**, *24*, 7–14. [CrossRef] [PubMed]

25. Elemike, E.E.; Onwudiwe, D.C.; Ekennia, A.C.; Ehiri, R.C.; Nnaji, N.J. Phytosynthesis of silver nanoparticles using aqueous leaf extracts of *Lippia citriodora*: Antimicrobial, larvicidal and photocatalytic evaluations. *Mater. Sci. Eng. C Mater. Biol. Appl.* **2017**, *75*, 980–989. [CrossRef] [PubMed]

26. Ovais, M.; Khalil, A.T.; Raza, A.; Khan, M.A.; Ahmad, I.; Islam, N.U.; Saravanan, M.; Ubaid, M.F.; Ali, M.; Shinwari, Z.K. Green-synthesis of silver nanoparticles via plant extracts: Beginning a new era in cancer theranostics. *Nanomedicine* **2016**, *11*, 3157–3177. [CrossRef] [PubMed]

27. Soman, S.; Ray, J.G. Silver nanoparticles synthesized using aqueous leaf extract of *Ziziphus oenoplia* (L.) Mill: Characterization and assessment of antibacterial activity. *J. Photochem. Photobiol. B Biol.* **2016**, *163*, 391–402. [CrossRef] [PubMed]

28. Kalaycioglu, Z.; Erim, F.B. Total phenolic contents, antioxidant activities, and bioactive ingredients of juices from pomegranate cultivars worldwide. *Food Chem.* **2017**, *221*, 496–507. [CrossRef] [PubMed]

29. Li, Y.; Yang, F.; Zheng, W.; Hu, M.; Wang, J.; Ma, S.; Deng, Y.; Luo, Y.; Ye, T.; Yin, W. *Punica granatum* (pomegranate) leaves extract induces apoptosis through mitochondrial intrinsic pathway and inhibits migration and invasion in non-small cell lung cancer in vitro. *Biomed. Pharmacother. Biomed. Pharmacother.* **2016**, *80*, 227–235. [CrossRef] [PubMed]

30. Martins, M.A.; Trindade, T. Os nanomateriais e a descoberta de novos mundos na bancada do químico. *Quím. Nova* **2012**, *35*, 1434–1446. [CrossRef]

31. Agnihotri, S.; Mukerji, S.; Mukerji, S. Size-controlled silver nanoparticles synthesized over the range 5–100 nm using the same protocol and their antibacterial efficacy. *RSC Adv.* **2014**, *4*, 3974–3983. [CrossRef]

32. Houk, L.R.; Challa, S.R.; Grayson, B.; Fanson, P.; Datye, A.K. The definition of "critical radius" for a collection of nanoparticles undergoing Ostwald ripening. *Langmuir* **2009**, *25*, 11225–11227. [CrossRef] [PubMed]

33. Prema, P.; Thangapandiyan, S.; Immanuel, G. CMC stabilized nano silver synthesis, characterization and its antibacterial and synergistic effect with broad spectrum antibiotics. *Carbohydr. Polym.* **2017**, *158*, 141–148. [CrossRef] [PubMed]

34. Gondikas, A.P.; Morris, A.; Reinsch, B.C.; Marinakos, S.M.; Lowry, G.V.; Hsu-Kim, H. Cysteine-induced modifications of zero-valent silver nanomaterials: Implications for particle surface chemistry, aggregation, dissolution, and silver speciation. *Environ. Sci. Technol.* **2012**, *46*, 7037–7045. [CrossRef] [PubMed]

35. Solomon, M.M.; Gerengi, H.; Umoren, S.A. Carboxymethyl Cellulose/Silver Nanoparticles Composite: Synthesis, characterization and Application as a Benign Corrosion Inhibitor for St37 Steel in 15% H_2SO_4 Medium. *ACS Appl. Mater. Interfaces* **2017**, *9*, 6376–6389. [CrossRef] [PubMed]

36. Liu, J.; Sonshine, D.A.; Shervani, S.; Hurt, R.H. Controlled release of biologically active silver from nanosilver surfaces. *ACS Nano* **2010**, *4*, 6903–6913. [CrossRef] [PubMed]

37. El Badawy, A.M.; Luxton, T.P.; Silva, R.G.; Scheckel, K.G.; Suidan, M.T.; Tolaymat, T.M. 2010. Impact of environmental conditions (pH, ionic strength, and electrolyte type) on the surface charge and aggregation of silver nanoparticles suspensions. *Environ. Sci. Technol.* **2010**, *44*, 1260–1266. [CrossRef] [PubMed]

38. Sadowski, Z.; Maliszewska, I.H.; Grochowalska, B.; Polowczyk, I.; Koźlecki, T. Synthesis of silver nanoparticles using microorganisms. *Mater. Sci.* **2008**, *26*, 419–424.

39. Salem, H.F.; Eid, K.A.M.; Saraf, M.A. Formulation and evaluation of silver nanoparticles as antibacterial and antifungal agents with a minimal cytotoxic effect. *Int. J. Drug Deliv.* **2011**, *3*, 293–304.

40. Leite, E.R.; Ribeiro, C. *Crystallization and Growth of Colloidal Nanocrystals*; Springer: New York, NY, USA, 2012; ISBN 978-1-4614-1308-0.

41. Malviya, S.; Jha, A.; Hettiarachchy, N. Antioxidant and antibacterial potential of pomegranate peel extracts. *J. Food Sci. Technol.* **2014**, *51*, 4132–4137. [CrossRef] [PubMed]

42. Bakkiyaraj, D.; Nandhini, J.R.; Malathy, B.; Pandian, S.K. The anti-biofilm potential of pomegranate (*Punica granatum* L.) extract against human bacterial and fungal pathogens. *Biofouling* **2013**, *29*, 929–937. [CrossRef] [PubMed]

43. Monteiro, D.R.; Gorup, L.F.; Silva, S.; Negri, M.; de Camargo, E.R.; Oliveira, R.; Barbosa, D.B.; Henriques, M. Silver colloidal nanoparticles: Antifungal effect against adhered cells and biofilms of *Candida albicans* and *Candida glabrata*. *Biofouling* **2011**, *27*, 711–719. [CrossRef] [PubMed]

44. Gogoi, N.; Babu, P.J.; Mahanta, C.; Bora, U. Green-synthesis and characterization of silver nanoparticles using alcoholic flower extract of *Nyctanthes arbortristis* and in vitro investigation of their antibacterial and cytotoxic activities. *Mater. Sci. Eng. C Mater. Biol. Appl.* **2015**, *46*, 463–469. [CrossRef] [PubMed]

45. Mohanta, Y.K.; Panda, S.K.; Bastia, A.K.; Mohanta, T.K. Biosynthesis of Silver Nanoparticles from *Protium serratum* and Investigation of their Potential Impacts on Food Safety and Control. *Front. Microbiol.* **2017**, *8*, 626. [CrossRef] [PubMed]

46. Asharani, P.V.; Lian Wu, Y.; Gong, Z.; Valiyaveettil, S. Toxicity of silver nanoparticles in zebrafish models. *Nanotechnology* **2008**, *19*, 255102. [CrossRef] [PubMed]

47. Ren, M.; Jin, Y.; Chen, W.; Huang, W. Rich capping ligand—Ag colloid interactions. *J. Phys. Chem. C* **2015**, *119*, 27588–27593. [CrossRef]

48. Gengan, R.M.; Anand, K.; Phulukdaree, A.; Chuturgoon, A. A549 lung cell line activity of biosynthesized silver nanoparticles using *Albizia adianthifolia* leaf. *Colloids Surf. B Biointerfaces* **2013**, *105*, 87–91. [CrossRef] [PubMed]

49. Delgado, N.T.; Rouver, W.D.; Freitas-Lima, L.C.; de Paula, T.D.; Duarte, A.; Silva, J.F.; Lemos, V.S.; Santos, A.M.; Mauad, H.; Santos, R.L.; et al. Pomegranate Extract Enhances Endothelium-Dependent Coronary Relaxation in Isolated Perfused Hearts from Spontaneously Hypertensive Ovariectomized Rats. *Front. Pharmacol.* **2016**, *7*, 522. [CrossRef] [PubMed]

50. Houston, D.M.; Bugert, J.; Denyer, S.P.; Heard, C.M. Anti-inflammatory activity of *Punica granatum* L. (Pomegranate) rind extracts applied topically to ex vivo skin. *Eur. J. Pharm. Biopharma.* **2017**, *112*, 30–37. [CrossRef] [PubMed]

51. Mgaya-Kilima, B.; Remberg, S.F.; Chove, B.E.; Wicklund, T. Physiochemical and antioxidant properties of roselle-mango juice blends; effects of packaging material, storage temperature and time. *Food Sci. Nutr.* **2015**, *3*, 100–109. [CrossRef] [PubMed]

52. Zhang, X.F.; Liu, Z.G.; Shen, W.; Gurunathan, S. Silver Nanoparticles: Synthesis, Characterization, Properties, Applications, and Therapeutic Approaches. *Int. J. Mol. Sci.* **2016**, *17*. [CrossRef] [PubMed]

53. De Oliveira, J.R.; de Castro, V.C.; das Gracas Figueiredo Vilela, P.; Camargo, S.E.; Carvalho, C.A.; Jorge, A.O.; de Oliveira, L.D. Cytotoxicity of Brazilian plant extracts against oral microorganisms of interest to dentistry. *BMC Complement. Altern. Med.* **2013**, *13*, 208. [CrossRef] [PubMed]

54. Waterman, P.G.; Mole, S. *Analysis of Phenolic Plant Metabolites*; Blackwell Scientific: Oxford, UK; Boston, MA, USA, 1994.

55. De Sousa, J.P.; Bueno, P.C.; Gregorio, L.E.; da Silva Filho, A.A.; Furtado, N.A.; de Sousa, M.L.; Bastos, J.K. A reliable quantitative method for the analysis of phenolic compounds in Brazilian propolis by reverse phase high performance liquid chromatography. *J. Sep. Sci.* **2007**, *30*, 2656–2665. [CrossRef] [PubMed]

56. Gorup, L.F.; Longo, E.; Leite, E.R.; Camargo, E.R. Moderating effect of ammonia on particle growth and stability of quasi-monodisperse silver nanoparticles synthesized by the Turkevich method. *J. Colloid Interface Sci.* **2011**, *360*, 355–358. [CrossRef] [PubMed]

57. Das, A.; Kumar, A.; Patil, N.B.; Viswanathan, C.; Ghosh, D. Preparation and characterization of silver nanoparticle loaded amorphous hydrogel of carboxymethylcellulose for infected wounds. *Carbohydr. Polym.* **2015**, *130*, 254–261. [CrossRef] [PubMed]

58. Gillum, A.M.; Tsay, E.Y.; Kirsch, D.R. Isolation of the Candida albicans gene for orotidine-5′-phosphate decarboxylase by complementation of *S. cerevisiae* ura3 and *E. coli* pyrF mutations. *Mol. Gen. Genet. MGG* **1984**, *198*, 179–182. [CrossRef] [PubMed]

59. Kuete, V.; Wiench, B.; Alsaid, M.S.; Alyahya, M.A.; Fankam, A.G.; Shahat, A.A.; Efferth, T. Cytotoxicity, mode of action and antibacterial activities of selected Saudi Arabian medicinal plants. *BMC Complement. Altern. Med.* **2013**, *13*, 354. [CrossRef] [PubMed]

13

Comparative Study on Antistaphylococcal Activity of Lipopeptides in Various Culture Media

Maciej Jaśkiewicz * [ID], Damian Neubauer and Wojciech Kamysz

Department of Inorganic Chemistry, Faculty of Pharmacy, Medical University of Gdańsk, 80-416 Gdańsk, Poland; dneu@gumed.edu.pl (D.N.); kamysz@gumed.edu.pl (W.K.)
* Correspondence: mj@gumed.edu.pl

Academic Editor: Naresh Kumar

Abstract: *Staphylococcus aureus* bacteria are one of the leading microorganisms responsible for nosocomial infections as well as being the primary causative pathogen of skin and wound infections. Currently, the therapy of staphylococcal diseases faces many difficulties, due to a variety of mechanisms of resistance and virulence factors. Moreover, a number of infections caused by *S. aureus* are connected with biofilm formation that impairs effectiveness of the therapy. Short cationic lipopeptides that are designed on the basis of the structure of antimicrobial peptides are likely to provide a promising alternative to conventional antibiotics. Many research groups have proved a high antistaphylococcal potential of lipopeptides, however, the use of different protocols for determination of antimicrobial activity may be the reason for inconsistency of the results. The aim of this study was to learn how the use of various bacteriological media as well as solvents may affect activity of lipopeptides and their cyclic analogs. Obtained results showed a great impact of these variables. For example, cyclic analogs were more effective when dissolved in an aqueous solution of acetic acid and bovine serum albumin (BSA). The greater activity against planktonic cultures was found in brain-heart infusion broth (BHI) and tryptic-soy broth (TSB), while the antibiofilm activity was higher in the Mueller-Hinton medium.

Keywords: antimicrobial peptides; lipopeptides; cyclic lipopeptides; *Staphylococcus aureus*; biofilm; culture media

1. Introduction

Staphylococcus aureus is one of the major pathogens responsible for variety of community- and hospital-acquired infections ranging from topical and harmless skin infections to severe systemic disorders such as endocarditis, necrotizing pneumonia, osteomyelitis or even sepsis [1,2]. Prevalence of staphylococcal diseases is related to the fact that some strains of the genus *Staphylococcus* such as *S. aureus* and *S. epidermidis* are typical skin colonizers. It has been determined that between 10% and 35% of healthy individuals are persistent carriers of *S. aureus*, and anterior nares are indicated as the most consistent sites from which these organisms can be cultured [3]. Moreover, there is a strong link between nasal carriage and increased risk of nosocomial infections [4]. Despite the fact that *S. aureus* and *S. epidermidis* are likely to belong to skin physiological flora, in some cases they can lead to opportunistic diseases. Moreover, those two strains have also been shown to be the most frequent causative factors of nosocomial infections on indwelling devices [5]. Treatment of staphylococcal diseases faces many difficulties, mainly because of a facile transmission (e.g., through exposure of the hands of healthcare workers), a variety of virulence factors, development of resistance to antibiotics, and the ability to adhere and form biofilm [4,6]. Biofilm can be defined as a microbial sessile community embedded within a self-produced matrix of extracellular polymeric substances that can be attached to biotic and abiotic surfaces. It seems likely that bacteria in some conditions prefer to form biofilm, firstly because extracellular matrix is capable of sequestrating and concentrating environmental nutrients, and secondly because it provides protection from exogenous stress factors such as antimicrobial substances or activity of immune system of invaded the organism. Another characteristic feature of the biofilm is a quorum-sensing. This term is referred to as the ability of bacteria to secrete low-molecular-weight signaling molecules that affect transcription patterns throughout local biofilm population. As a result of that activity, a better adaptation to rapid environmental changes is provided [7]. Since approximately 80% of all human bacterial infections are associated with biofilm, it is reasonable to consider antibiofilm activity of new antimicrobials [8]. Recently, various approaches to treat biofilm-related infections have been developed including antibodies, anti-adhesion strategies, the use of bacteriophages or quorum-sensing inhibitors [9]. Antimicrobial peptides (AMPs) are compounds with proven in vitro and in vivo antibiofilm activities [10]. These compounds are evolutionarily conserved molecules of the innate immune system of almost all organisms, playing an important role in warding off invading microbial pathogens [11]. To date, AMPs have been studied for their antimicrobial properties as they are targeting a broad spectrum of pathogens including bacteria, fungi, viruses, and protozoa [12,13]. Naturally occurring AMPs can vary in size and most of them do not have more than 50 amino acids in sequence. The majority are cationic molecules containing about 50% of hydrophobic amino acids [14]. Such properties allow them to electrostatically interact with a negatively charged bacterial surface, which leads to disruption of a cell membrane. Many attempts have been made to improve the activity and bioavailability of AMPs such as synthesis of short synthetic analogs, the use of D- or unnatural amino acids, fatty acid acylation or cyclization. Short cationic lipopeptides are compounds designed on the basis of AMPs amphiphilic character to imitate their antimicrobial properties. Net positive charge of these compounds as well as amphipathicity was obtained by combining the hydrophobic fragment of a fatty acid with a cationic peptide chain. The antimicrobial properties of short cationic lipopeptides have also been proven in several studies as a promising alternative for currently used antimicrobials [15,16]. Broth microdilution method is one of the leading procedures used in the in vitro susceptibility testing for bacteria, whereas the protocol issued by Clinical and Laboratory Standards Institute (CLSI) is being commonly used in scientific studies [17]. CLSI protocol is standardized and is internationally accepted by i.e., the European Committee on Antimicrobial Susceptibility Testing, the British Society for Antimicrobial Chemotherapy, the Deutsches Institut für Normung, and the Comité de l'Antibiogramme de la Société Française de Microbiologie. Owing to this assay the minimum inhibitory concentration (MIC) can be determined. However, since some peptides have a tendency to precipitate or bind to polystyrene, methods for evaluating their antimicrobial activity are being discussed. For instance, the most popular one was described by Hancock (University of British Columbia, Vancouver, BC, Canada) which involves different preparation of the peptide stock solution [18]. Despite the fact that there are reference protocols for MIC determination (which is actually conducted for planktonic forms of bacteria), there are no unified procedures used to determine antibiofilm activity. The aim of this study was to evaluate and to compare the results of antistaphylococcal activity (against both planktonic and biofilm forms) of short cationic lipopeptides and their cyclic analogs in three different microbiological media: Mueller Hinton Broth (which is used in CLSI and Hancock protocol), Brain-Heart Infusion Broth, and Tryptic Soy-Broth. Stock solutions of lipopeptides were prepared in both PBS and aqueous solution of BSA and AcOH.

2. Results

Lipopeptides used in this study are based on previously described compounds with high antistaphylococcal activity (i.e., Pal-KKKK-NH$_2$, Pal-RRR-NH$_2$) [16,19,20]. All of the lipopeptides are palmitoylated at N-terminus and contain three or four basic amino acid residues. Moreover, compounds are amidated at C-termini to maximize positive charge. Arginine residue was introduced at different positions to learn if this simple procedure may provide more active compounds. Arginine, as a basic amino acid, introduce positive charge; however, it has more hydrogen donor atoms and is more basic (pKa~12.5) than lysine (pKa~10.5). Interestingly, plenty of naturally occurring lipopeptides are cyclic. This fact inspired us to design cyclic analogs and evaluate the relevance of disulfide cyclization in case of antimicrobial activity of simple short cationic lipopeptides. In this study, each linear lipopeptide has its cyclic counterpart with a intramolecular disulfide bridge where cationic amino acid residues are placed between two cysteine residues. As a result, all compounds have well defined hydrophobic and hydrophilic regions. The identity of all compounds was confirmed by LC-MS analysis (ESI-MS) and all mass spectra are included in the supplementary materials.

Short cationic lipopeptides and their cyclic analogs were active against all tested strains of *S. aureus*. However, the antistaphylococcal activity depended on the type of medium as well as the solvent used for compound solubilization. MIC values for linear lipopeptides were lower in the BHI and TSB media than in MH (Figure 1). It was only in the case of non-cyclized Pal-CKKKRC-NH$_2$ that this dependence was not observed. In the case of cyclic lipopeptides, the influence of medium type was irrelevant (Pal-CKKRKC-NH$_2$ and Pal-CRKKKC-NH$_2$ were slightly more active in MH). Despite this fact, all cyclic compounds dissolved in acetic acid/BSA were as a rule more active in comparison to those dissolved in PBS. The antibiofilm activity was highest in the MH medium (Figure 2) and cyclic analogs were as active as the linear forms or twofold more active (but only with compounds dissolved in BSA/acetic acid solution). Interestingly, the activity of cyclic lipopeptides was related to the medium and stock solution type. The antibiofilm activity improved in the order MH > TSB > BHI. Moreover, cyclic lipopeptides were even fourfold more active when dissolved in the AcOH/BSA solution. With linear lipopeptides, the type of stock solution seems to be less relevant. Biofilms formed in BHI exhibited resistance to almost all tested compounds, while in the case of TSB medium, cyclic analogs dissolved in PBS did not eradicate the staphylococcal biofilm.

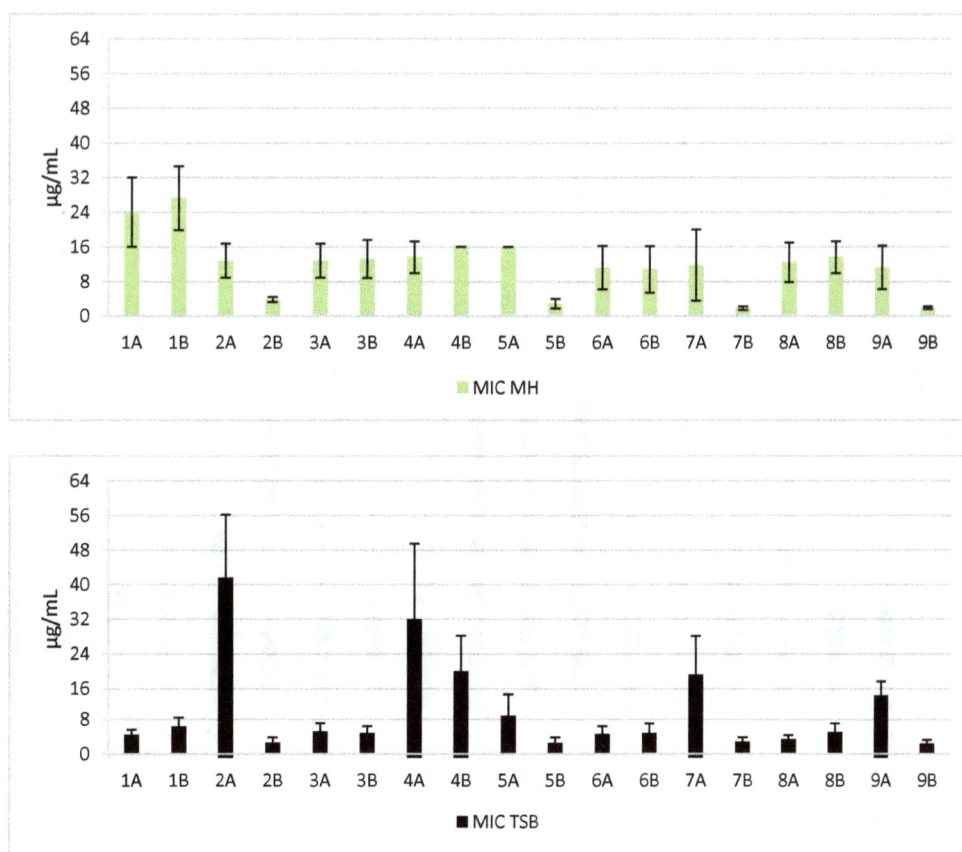

Figure 1. *Cont.*

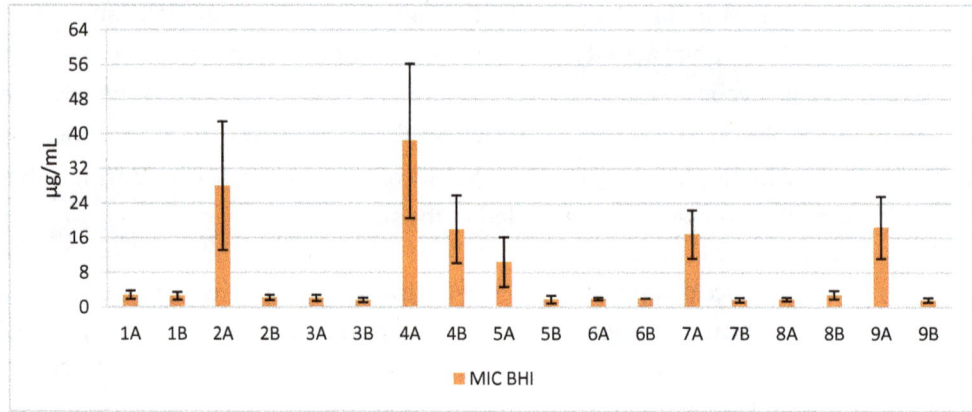

Figure 1. Mean MIC values against clinical and reference strains of *Staphylococcus aureus*. 1—Pal-KKK-NH$_2$; 2—Pal-CKKKC-NH$_2$; 3—Pal-KKKR-NH$_2$; 4—Pal-CKKKRC-NH$_2$ (linear); 5—Pal-CKKKRC-NH$_2$; 6—Pal-KKRK-NH$_2$; 7—Pal-CKKRKC-NH$_2$; 8—Pal-RKKK-NH$_2$; 9—Pal-CRKKKC-NH$_2$ (cyclic); Solvents: A—PBS; B—AcOH/BSA.

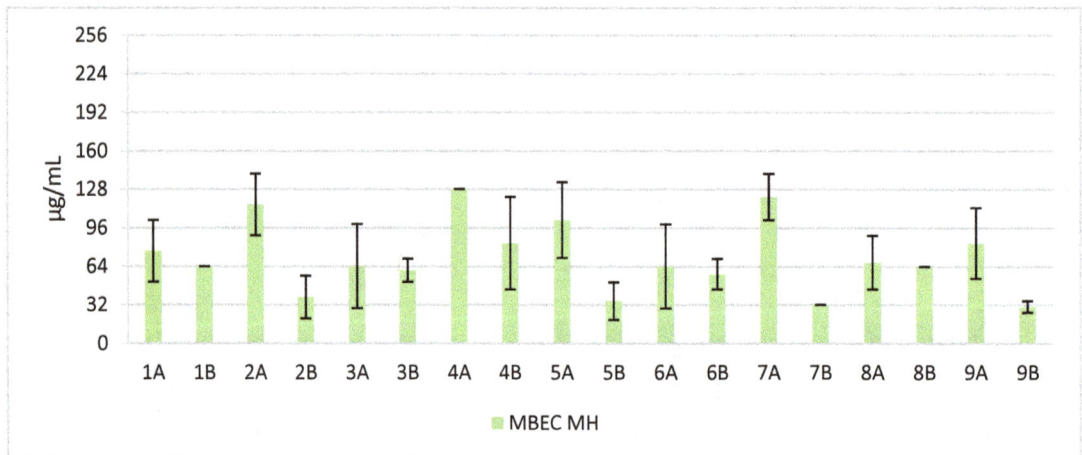

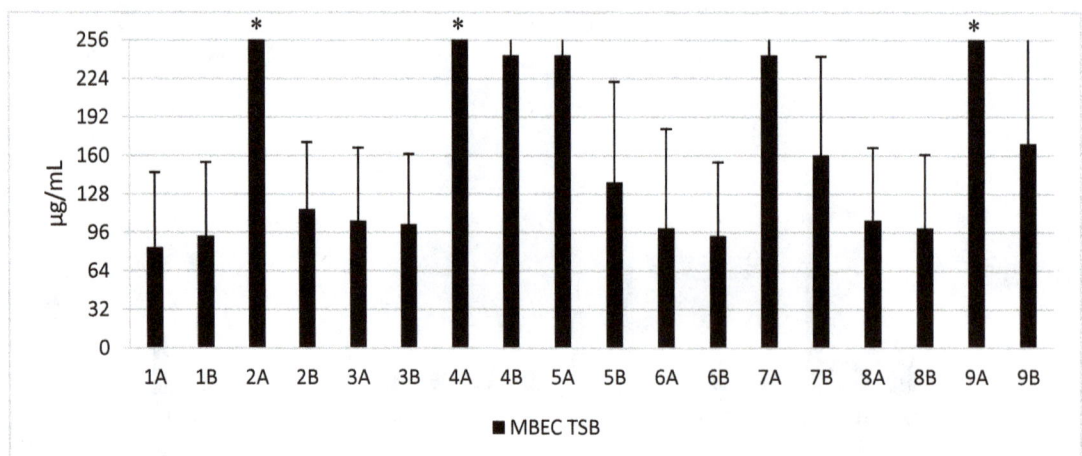

Figure 2. *Cont.*

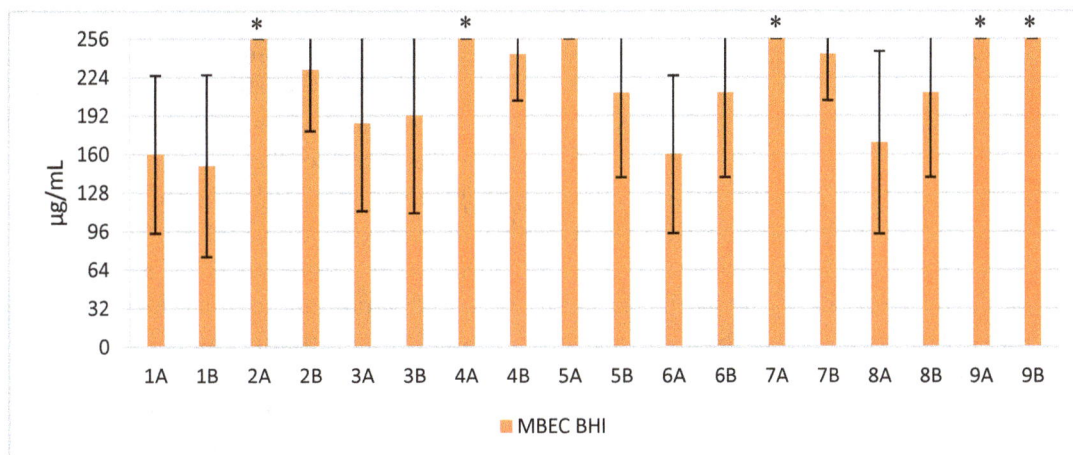

Figure 2. Mean MBEC values against clinical and reference strains of *Staphylococcus aureus*. 1—Pal-KKK-NH$_2$; 2—Pal-CKKKC-NH$_2$; 3—Pal-KKKR-NH$_2$; 4—Pal-CKKKRC-NH$_2$ (linear); 5—Pal-CKKKRC-NH$_2$; 6—Pal-KKRK-NH$_2$; 7—Pal-CKKRKC-NH$_2$ (cyclic); 8—Pal-RKKK-NH$_2$; 9—Pal-CRKKKC-NH$_2$; Solvents: A—PBS; B—AcOH/BSA; *—concentration > 256 µg/mL.

3. Discussion

Such comprehensive research on antimicrobial activity of lipopeptides has not yet been conducted. In this study, many factors were taken into account, including the type of microbiological medium, the use of various peptide stock solution solvents, and the impact of lipopeptide cyclization as well. Moreover, the verification of the activity conducted on 10 strains of *S. aureus* (5 reference and 5 clinical ones) revealed a significant difference in antimicrobial activity of the lipopeptides in miscellaneous microbiological media. The reason of this difference may be associated with environment-dependent plasticity of lipid composition of *S. aureus* membranes. Sen et al. (2016) proved that the membranes of staphylococci grown in MH were less fluid than cells grown in BHI or TSB, which was related to a higher content of branched-chain fatty acids (BCFAs) and carotenoids [21]. These findings may be much more interesting as the staphyloxanthin, a carotenoid pigment, is one of the most potent virulence factors of *S. aureus* [22]. Staphyloxanthin provides integrity of the cell membrane and improves the resistance to reactive oxygen species this enhancing bacterial survival [23–25]. Furthermore, the influence of carotenoid content on susceptibility to host defense peptides was also investigated. In an in vitro study conducted by Mishra et al. (2011), the carotenoid-overproducing strains were less susceptible to daptomycin and cationic antimicrobial peptides such as human neutrophil defensin-1 (hNP-1), platelet microbicidal proteins (PMPs), and polymyxin B [26]. These results are consistent with the findings that higher carotenoid concentrations in *S. aureus* cell membrane cultivated in MH medium might suppress the activity of the tested compounds. In our study, the susceptibility of *S. aureus* biofilms in various growth media was examined. Biofilms formed in the BHI and TSB mediums were insensitive toward lipopeptides. The reason for this situation might be related to the impact of the glucose content on biofilm formation. In contrast to the MH medium (starch 1.50 g/L), BHI and TSB are supplemented with D-glucose (2.00 g/L and 2.50 g/L, respectively). Some studies proved the role of glucose in adhesion induction and modulation of biofilm formation [27,28]. Waldrop et al. (2014) have found that the mass of *S. aureus* biofilms rises with an increasing concentration of glucose with a threshold at 2.00–2.40 g/L [29]. Moreover, the catabolite control protein A (CcpA), which is responsible for regulation of various staphylococcal virulence determinants and resistance to antibiotics, is also regulated by the presence of the glucose [30]. Another factor that may have an impact on the activity of antimicrobials is the salt content of the media. BHI and TSB, in contrast to MH, are supplemented with NaCl (5.0 g/L) and this difference should be taken into account. In fact, the antistaphylococcal activity of some antibiotics such as aminoglycosides or oxacillin decreases in a concentration-dependent manner [31,32]. Nevertheless, our previous studies (2016) on the influence of several salts on antimicrobial activity of lipopeptides showed no difference in the MIC values against *S. aureus* strains for the wide range of NaCl concentration. Moreover, among all tested salts, only sodium acetate and sodium trifluoroacetate were found to increase the activity of tested compounds [33]. Different pH values of the media may also be crucial for the antimicrobial properties. However, the impact of pH differences may not be relevant in the case of BHI, MH and TSB since these culture media have almost the same pH (7.4, 7.4 and 7.3, respectively).

It should be noted that conclusions drawn from the in vitro studies are not always consistent with those determined in vivo. Nevertheless, these "not-ideal" conditions may reveal an unexpected activity of new compounds. For example, the study conducted by Citterio et al. (2016) showed the synergy between human plasma and antimicrobial peptidomimetics, AMPs, and antibiotics against several bacterial pathogens [34]. In this case, the MIC values decreased down to sixteenfold in the presence of plasma. The synergistic effect may be connected with complement proteins or clotting factors, as the activity of all compounds in heat-inactivated plasma were significantly decreased. Another factor included in our study was the use of various solvents for peptide stock solution. Interestingly, lipopeptides dissolved in an aqueous solution of acetic acid and bovine serum albumin (compounds marked with the letter B) were generally more effective than those dissolved in PBS. This approach was supported by a hypothesis that the type of solvent used in stock solution might have an impact on peptide solubility even after serial dilution in culture medium. For example, Steinberg et al. (1997) conducted a study on antimicrobial properties of protegrin-1 using a reference protocol issued by CLSI (formerly NCCLS) and modified a method wherein the peptide was prepared in an aqueous solution of acetic acid and BSA. Interestingly, the MIC values obtained using this modification were significantly lower; 5-times against *S. aureus* and *Enterococcus faecalis* and up to 30-times against *Escherichia coli* and *Pseudomonas aeruginosa* [35]. Similar observations were reported by Giacometti et al. (2000), who compared several methods for the determination of the activity of AMPs such as buforin II, cecropin, indolicidin, magainin II, nisin, and ranalexin [18]. Generally, our observation is inconsistent with the previously determined impact of BSA which is known to reduce lipopeptide antibacterial activity due to strong binding of fatty acids [36,37]. However, in our study, the concentration of BSA was relatively low and thus lipopeptides remained active. BSA may have a negative influence on the antimicrobial activity of lipopeptides and in our study its application gives even better results than PBS stock solution; this shows that phosphate ion should be considered as an activity suppressor, especially in the case of cyclic lipopeptides. Hypothetically, rigid cyclic structure and amino acids side chain orientation promote electrostatic interactions between amine and guanidine moieties with phosphate ion. Cyclization of AMPs is a popular approach to improve the activity and/or selectivity of the parent molecule [38]. For example, in research conducted by Unger et al. (2001), the cyclization of melittin analogs resulted in an increased antibacterial activity. Interestingly, the cyclization also resulted in decreased hemolytic properties; this suggests a lower toxicity towards mammalian cell lines [39]. It has been shown that disulfide cyclization may result in enhanced peptide activity, selectivity, and stability [40]. In our study, cyclic lipopeptides were found to be more effective against all tested staphylococci, but only if they were dissolved in an aqueous solution of acetic acid and BSA. Interestingly, the cyclization did not improve the antibiofilm activity in BHI or TSB. Nevertheless, it remains difficult to indicate which method provides more reliable data. Moreover, different positioning of arginine residue along the peptide chain of both linear and cyclic lipopeptides seems to be irrelevant for antistaphylococcal activity. Despite the fact that protocols utilized for the determination of antimicrobial activity are standardized, the influence of different factors such as solvents for stock solutions or culture media used for in vitro studies may play a pivotal role in selecting promising antimicrobial compounds; this is especially true when taking into account the activity against biofilm. This study indicated the relevance of each variable, despite the overall chemical similarities between lipopeptides.

4. Materials and Methods

4.1. Synthesis of Lipopeptides

The compounds were obtained by manual synthesis on solid support (polystyrene AM-RAM resin) using Fmoc/t-Bu strategy. Coupling reactions were carried out in DCM and DMF mixture using DIC as a coupling reagent and OxymaPure as racemisation suppressant. All reagents were used in fourfold excess based on the resin. Deprotection was performed with 20% piperidine solution in DMF for 15 m. Cleavage from the resin was accomplished in TFA and scavengers mixture—TFA:TIS:water, 96:2:2 (v/v) for 90 m with agitation. Additionally, EDT was applied as a scavenger if the peptide contained cysteine residues. Cyclic analogs were obtained by intramolecular disulphide bridge formation through oxidation with iodine. The lipopeptides were purified using RP-HPLC. The purity and identity of the peptides were confirmed by LC-MS analysis. The structures of selected lipopeptides used in the study are presented in Figures 3–5.

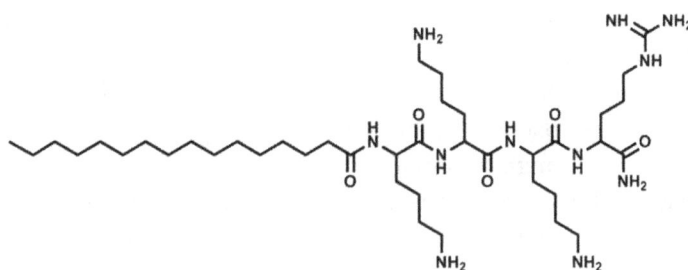

Figure 3. Structure of Pal-KKKR-NH$_2$.

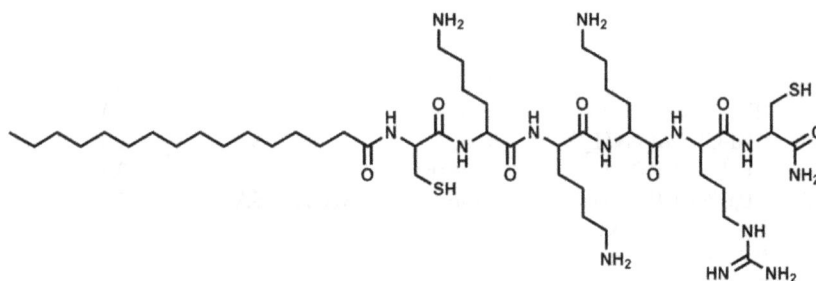

Figure 4. Structure of Pal-CKKKRC-NH$_2$ (linear).

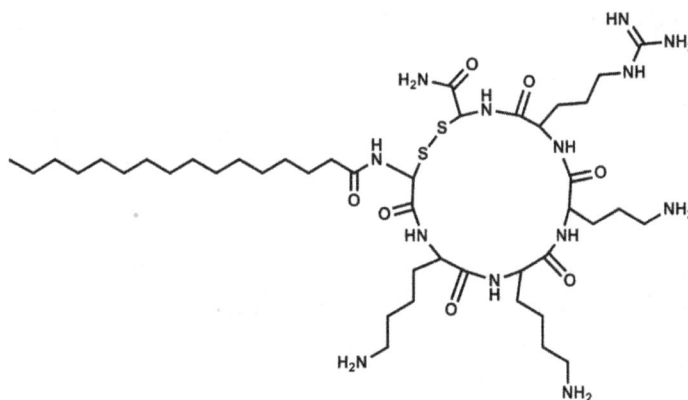

Figure 5. Structure of Pal-CKKKRC-NH$_2$ (cyclic).

4.2. Antimicrobial Assays

4.2.1. MIC Assay

Antimicrobial activity was determined against five reference strains: *S. aureus* ATCC 25923, *S. aureus* ATCC 6538, *S. aureus* ATCC 6538/P, *S. aureus* ATCC 9144, and *S. aureus* ATCC 12598, which were obtained from the Polish Collection of Microorganisms (Polish Academy of Sciences, Wroclaw), and against five clinical strains of *S. aureus*, which were provided by the Department of Oral Microbiology, Medical University of Gdańsk (Poland). These strains were also characterized in terms of methicillin resistance. Preliminary identification and detection was conducted on the ChromID MRSA/ChromID *S. aureus* biplate (bioMérieux) for simultaneous detection of *S. aureus* and methicillin-resistant *S. aureus* (MRSA). All tested strains (both reference and clinical *S. aureus*) were stored in cryo-vials (Roti®-Store, Carl Roth) and recultivated before all microbiological tests. All strains were cultured in three different media: Brain-Heart Infusion Broth (BHI, Biocorp, Warsaw, Poland), Mueller Hinton Broth (MH, Biocorp), and Tryptic-Soy Broth (TSB, Biocorp). Moreover, the stock solutions of lipopeptides were prepared in two different solvents: PBS and an aqueous solution of acetic acid/BSA (0.01% and 0.2% respectively). The complete list of compounds used in this study and their signatures are presented in Table 1. MIC was determined by broth microdilution method on polystyrene 96-well plates. Bacteria at initial inoculums of 5×10^5 CFU/mL were exposed to lipopeptides at concentrations ranging from 0.5 to 256 µg/mL and incubated for 18 h at 37 °C. The MIC value was taken as the lowest concentration of the compound that inhibited the growth of the microorganisms. All assays were performed in triplicate and included the growth and sterility control.

Table 1. List of lipopeptides used in this study.

Sequence	Structure	Solvent	Signature
Pal-KKK-NH$_2$	Linear	PBS	1A
Pal-KKK-NH$_2$	Linear	AcOH/BSA	1B
Pal-CKKKC-NH$_2$	Cyclic	PBS	2A
Pal-CKKKC-NH$_2$	Cyclic	AcOH/BSA	2B
Pal-KKKR-NH$_2$	Linear	PBS	3A
Pal-KKKR-NH$_2$	Linear	AcOH/BSA	3B
Pal-CKKKRC-NH$_2$	Linear	PBS	4A
Pal-CKKKRC-NH$_2$	Linear	AcOH/BSA	4B
Pal-CKKKRC-NH$_2$	Cyclic	PBS	5A
Pal-CKKKRC-NH$_2$	Cyclic	AcOH/BSA	5B
Pal-KKRK-NH$_2$	Linear	PBS	6A
Pal-KKRK-NH$_2$	Linear	AcOH/BSA	6B
Pal-CKKRKC-NH$_2$	Cyclic	PBS	7A
Pal-CKKRKC-NH$_2$	Cyclic	AcOH/BSA	7B
Pal-RKKK-NH$_2$	Linear	PBS	8A
Pal-RKKK-NH$_2$	Linear	AcOH/BSA	8B
Pal-RKKK-NH$_2$	Cyclic	PBS	9A

4.2.2. MBEC Assay

S. aureus biofilms were cultured on polystyrene 96-well flat bottom plates. Bacteria at initial inoculum of 5×10^8 CFU/mL in BHI, MH or TSB were added to the plates and incubated at 37 °C. After 24 h of incubation, all *S. aureus* cultures were rinsed three times with PBS (pH 7.4) and a fresh medium was added. Subsequently, all biofilms were exposed to lipopeptides at concentrations ranging from 0.5 to 256 µg/mL for 24 h at 37 °C. After incubation, resazurin (7-hydroxy-3*H*-phenoxazin-3-one 10-oxide, Sigma Aldrich, Steinheim, Germany) was added as a cell viability reagent and the MBEC was read. All assay were performed in triplicate and included the growth and sterility control.

Supplementary Materials:
Table S1: MIC values [μg/mL] of Staphylococcus aureus strains (SA) in Mueller-Hinton Broth (MH), Table S2: MIC values [μg/mL] of Staphylococcus aureus strains (SA) in Brain-Heart Infusion Broth (BHI), Table S3: MIC values [μg/mL] of Staphylococcus aureus strains (SA) in Tryptic Soy Broth (TSB), Table S4: MBEC values [μg/mL] of Staphylococcus aureus strains (SA) in Mueller-Hinton Broth (MH), Table S5: MBEC values [μg/mL] of Staphylococcus aureus strains (SA) in Brain-Heart Infusion Broth (BHI), Table S6: MBEC values [μg/mL] of Staphylococcus aureus strains (SA) in Tryptic Soy Broth (TSB), Table S7: Measured and calculated m/z of lipopeptides, Figure S1: Mass spectrum of Pal-KKK-NH$_2$, Figure S2: Mass spectrum of Pal-CKKKC-NH$_2$, Figure S3: Mass spectrum of Pal-RKKK-NH$_2$, Figure S4: Mass spectrum of Pal-CRKKKC-NH$_2$, Figure S5: Mass spectrum of Pal-KKRK-NH$_2$, Figure S6: Mass spectrum of Pal-CKKRKC-NH$_2$, Figure S7: Mass spectrum of Pal-KKKR-NH$_2$, Figure S8: Mass spectrum of Pal-CKKKRC-NH$_2$ (cyclic), Figure S9: Mass spectrum of Pal-CKKKRCNH$_2$ (linear).

Acknowledgments: The study was supported by the Polish Ministry of Science and Higher Education Grant for Young Investigators, no. 01-0221/08/508 and by a grant from the Polish National Science Centre (Project No. 2011/03/B/NZ7/00548).We wish to thank Katarzyna Garbacz, M.D., Ph.D., the head of Department of Oral Microbiology for providing the clinical strains of *S. aureus*. Moreover, we wish to thank Ryszard Piękoś for his invaluable help in preparing the manuscript.

Author Contributions: M.J. designed the experiments, performed the microbiological tests and wrote the paper, D.N. performed synthesis and purification of the compounds and wrote the manuscript; W.K. arranged materials and analytical tools and supervised the peptide synthesis and microbiological assays.

Abbreviations

The following abbreviations are used in this manuscript:

AcOH	Acetic acid
AMPs	antimicrobial peptides
BSA	Bovine serum albumin
CFU	Colony forming unit
CLSI	Clinical and Laboratory Standards Institute
DCM	Dichloromethane
DIC	*N,N'*-diisopropylcarbodiimide
DMF	*N,N*-dimethylformamide
EDT	1,2-ethanedithiol
Fmoc	9-fluorenylmethoxycarbonyl
MBEC	Minimum biofilm eradication concentration
MIC	Minimum inhibitory concentration
Pal	Palmitic acid
PBS	Phosphate buffer saline
TIS	Triisopropylsilane
TFA	Trifluoroacetic acid

References

1. Kahl, B.C.; Becker, K. Clinical significance and pathogenesis of staphylococcal small colony variants in persistent infections. *Clin. Microbiol. Rev.* **2016**, *29*, 401–427. [CrossRef] [PubMed]
2. Lin, J.; Lin, D.; Xu, P.; Zhang, T.; Ou, Q.; Bai, C.; Yao, Z. Non-hospital environment contamination with *Staphylococcus aureus* and methicillin-resistant *Staphylococcus aureus*: Proportion meta-analysis and features of antibiotic resistance and molecular genetics. *Environ. Res.* **2016**, *150*, 528–540. [CrossRef] [PubMed]
3. Kluytmans, J.A.J.W.; Wertheim, H.F.L. Nasal carriage of *Staphylococcus aureus* and prevention of nosocomial infections. *Infection* **2005**, *33*, 3–8. [CrossRef] [PubMed]
4. Archer, N.K.; Mazaitis, M.J.; Costerton, J.W.; Leid, J.G.; Powers, M.E.; Shirtliff, M.E. *Staphylococcus aureus* biofilms. *Virulence* **2011**, *2*, 445–459. [CrossRef] [PubMed]
5. Otto, M. Staphylococcus colonization of the skin and antimicrobial peptides. *Expert Rev. Dermatol.* **2010**, *5*, 183–195. [CrossRef] [PubMed]
6. Lowy, F.D. *Staphylococcus aureus* Infections. *N. Engl. J. Med.* **1998**, *339*, 520–532. [CrossRef] [PubMed]
7. Novick, R.P.; Geisinger, E. Quorum sensing in staphylococci. *Annu. Rev. Genet.* **2008**, *42*, 541–564. [CrossRef] [PubMed]

8.   Nusbaum, A.G.; Kirsner, R.S.; Charles, C.A. Biofilms in Dermatology. *Skin Therapy Lett.* **2012**, *17*, 1–5. [PubMed]

9.   Lynch, A.S.; Abbanat, D. New antibiotic agents and approaches to treat biofilm-associated infections. *Expert Opin. Ther. Pat.* **2010**, *20*, 1373–1387. [CrossRef] [PubMed]

10. Dawgul, M.; Maciejewska, M.; Jaśkiewicz, M.; Karafova, A.; Kamysz, W. Antimicrobial peptides as potential tool to fight bacterial biofilm. *Acta Pol. Pharm. Drug Res.* **2014**, *71*, 39–47.

11. Mansour, S.C.; Pena, O.M.; Hancock, R.E. Host defense peptides: Front-line immunomodulators. *Trends Immunol.* **2014**, *35*, 443–450. [CrossRef] [PubMed]

12. Zasloff, M. Antimicrobial peptides of multicellular organisms. *Nature* **2002**, *415*, 389–395. [CrossRef] [PubMed]

13. Phoenix, D.A.; Dennison, S.R.; Harris, F. Antimicrobial peptides: Their history, evolution, and functional promiscuity. *Antimicrob. Pept.* **2013**, 1–37. [CrossRef]

14. Hancock, R.E.; Lehrer, R. Cationic peptides: A new source of antibiotics. *Trends Biotechnol.* **1998**, *16*, 82–88. [CrossRef]

15. Laverty, G.; McLaughlin, M.; Shaw, C.; Gorman, S.P.; Gilmore, B.F. Antimicrobial activity of short, synthetic cationic lipopeptides. *Chem. Biol. Drug Des.* **2010**, *75*, 563–569. [CrossRef] [PubMed]

16. Dawgul, M.; Baranska-Rybak, W.; Kamysz, E.; Karafova, A.; Nowicki, R.; Kamysz, W. Activity of short lipopeptides and conventional antimicrobials against planktonic cells and biofilms formed by clinical strains of *Staphylococcus aureus*. *Future Med. Chem.* **2012**, *4*, 1541–1551. [CrossRef] [PubMed]

17. Clinical and Laboratory Standards Institute (CLSI). *Methods for Dilution Antimicrobial Susceptibility Tests for Bacteria That Grow Aerobically; Approved St andard—Ninth Edition*; Clinical and Laboratory Standards Institute (CLSI): Wayne, PA, USA, 2012; Volume 32, ISBN 1562387839.

18. Giacometti, A.; Cirioni, O.; Barchiesi, F.; Del Prete, M.S.; Fortuna, M.; Caselli, F.; Scalise, G. In Vitro Susceptibility Tests for Cationic Peptides: Comparison of Broth Microdilution Methods for Bacteria That Grow Aerobically. *Antimicrob. Agents Chemother.* **2000**, *44*, 1694–1696. [CrossRef] [PubMed]

19. Greber, K.E.; Dawgul, M.; Kamysz, W.; Sawicki, W. Cationic net charge and counter ion type as antimicrobial activity determinant factors of short lipopeptides. *Front. Microbiol.* **2017**, *8*, 123. [CrossRef] [PubMed]

20. Makovitzki, A.; Avrahami, D.; Shai, Y.; Sela, M. Ultrashort antibacterial and antifungal lipopeptides. *Proc. Natl. Acad. Sci. USA* **2006**, *103*, 15997–16002. [CrossRef] [PubMed]

21. Sen, S.; Sirobhushanam, S.; Johnson, S.R.; Song, Y.; Tefft, R.; Gatto, C.; Wilkinson, B.J. Growth-environment dependent modulation of *Staphylococcus aureus* branched-chain to straight-chain fatty acid ratio and incorporation of unsaturated fatty acids. *PLoS ONE* **2016**, *11*, e0165300. [CrossRef] [PubMed]

22. Leejae, S.; Hasap, L.; Piyawan, S.; Correspondence, V.; Voravuthikunchai, S.P. Inhibition of staphyloxanthin biosynthesis in *Staphylococcus aureus* by rhodomyrtone, a novel antibiotic candidate. *J. Med. Microbiol.* **2013**, *62*, 421–428. [CrossRef] [PubMed]

23. Kahlon, A.K.; Roy, S.; Sharma, A. Molecular docking studies to map the binding site of squalene synthase inhibitors on dehydrosqualene synthase of *Staphylococcus aureus*. *J. Biomol. Struct. Dyn.* **2010**, *28*, 201–210. [CrossRef] [PubMed]

24. Clauditz, A.; Resch, A.; Wieland, K.-P.; Peschel, A.; Götz, F. Staphyloxanthin plays a role in the fitness of *Staphylococcus aureus* and its ability to cope with oxidative stress. *Infect. Immun.* **2006**, *74*, 4950–4953. [CrossRef] [PubMed]

25. Pelz, A.; Wieland, K.-P.; Putzbach, K.; Hentschel, P.; Albert, K.; Gö Tz, F. Structure and biosynthesis of staphyloxanthin from *Staphylococcus aureus* *. *J. Biol. Chem.* **2005**, *280*, 32493–32498. [CrossRef] [PubMed]

26. Mishra, N.N.; Liu, G.Y.; Yeaman, M.R.; Nast, C.C.; Proctor, R.A.; McKinnell, J.; Bayer, A.S. Carotenoid-related alteration of cell membrane fluidity impacts *Staphylococcus aureus* susceptibility to host defense peptides. *Antimicrob. Agents Chemother.* **2011**, *55*, 526–531. [CrossRef] [PubMed]

27. Lim, Y.; Jana, M.; Luong, T.T.; Lee, C.Y. Control of glucose—and NaCl-induced biofilm formation by rbf in *Staphylococcus aureus*. *J. Bacteriol.* **2004**, *186*, 722–729. [CrossRef] [PubMed]

28. Fluckiger, U.; Ulrich, M.; Steinhuber, A.; Döring, G.; Mack, D.; Landmann, R.; Goerke, C.; Wolz, C. Biofilm formation, icaADBC transcription, and polysaccharide intercellular adhesin synthesis by staphylococci in a device-related infection model. *Infect. Immun.* **2005**, *73*, 1811–1819. [CrossRef] [PubMed]

29. Waldrop, R.; McLaren, A.; Calara, F.; McLemore, R. Biofilm growth has a threshold response to glucose in vitro. *Clin. Orthop. Relat. Res.* **2014**, *472*, 3305–3310. [CrossRef] [PubMed]

30. Seidl, K.; Goerke, C.; Wolz, C.; Mack, D.; Berger-Bächi, B.; Bischoff, M. *Staphylococcus aureus* CcpA affects biofilm formation. *Infect. Immun.* **2008**, *76*, 2044–2050. [CrossRef] [PubMed]

31. Campos, J.M.; Gill, C.J.; Hare, R.S.; Miller, G.H. Effect of NaCl supplementation of Mueller-Hinton broth on susceptibility of staphylococci to aminoglycosides. *Antimicrob. Agents Chemother.* **1986**, *29*, 152–154. [CrossRef]

32. Huang, M.B.; Elaine Gay, T.; Baker, C.N.; Banerjee, S.N.; Tenoverl, F.C. Two percent sodium chloride is required for susceptibility testing of staphylococci with oxacillin when using agar-based dilution methods. *J. Clin. Microbiol.* **1993**, *31*, 2683–2688. [PubMed]

33. Migoń, D.; Neubauer, D.; Sikora, K.; Jaśkiewicz, M.; Kamysz, W. Badanie aktywności przeciwdrobnoustrojowej lipopeptydów w środowisku wybranych soli. In *Nauka i Przemysł. Metody Spektroskopowe w praktyce. Nowe wyzwania i możliwości. Tom I*; UMCS: Lublin, Poland, 2016; pp. 336–338. ISBN 978-83-945225-0-6. (In Polish)

34. Citterio, L.; Franzyk, H.; Palarasah, Y.; Andersen, T.E.; Mateiu, R.V.; Gram, L. Improved in vitro evaluation of novel antimicrobials: Potential synergy between human plasma and antibacterial peptidomimetics, AMPs and antibiotics against human pathogenic bacteria. *Res. Microbiol.* **2016**, *167*, 72–82. [CrossRef] [PubMed]

35. Steinberg, D.A.; Hurst, M.A.; Fujii, C.A.; Kung, A.H.C.; Ho, J.F.; Cheng, F.-C.; Loury, D.J.; Fiddes, J.C. Protegrin-1: A broad-spectrum, rapidly microbicidal peptide with in vivo activity. *Antimicrob. Agents Chemother.* **1997**, *41*, 1738–1742. [PubMed]

36. Findlay, B.; Szelemej, P.; Zhanel, G.G.; Schweizer, F.; Beyermann, M. Guanidylation and tail effects in cationic antimicrobial lipopeptoids. *PLoS ONE* **2012**, *7*, e41141. [CrossRef] [PubMed]

37. Svenson, J.; Brandsdal, B.-O.; Stensen, W.; Svendsen, J.S. Albumin binding of short cationic antimicrobial micropeptides and its influence on the in vitro bactericidal effect. *J. Med. Chem.* **2007**, *50*, 3334–3339. [CrossRef] [PubMed]

38. Matsuzaki, K. Control of cell selectivity of antimicrobial peptides. *Biochim. Biophys. Acta—Biomembr.* **2009**, *1788*, 1687–1692. [CrossRef] [PubMed]

39. Unger, T.; Oren, Z.; Shai, Y. The Effect of cyclization of magainin 2 and melittin analogues on structure, function, and model membrane interactions: Implication to their mode of action. *Biochemistry* **2001**. [CrossRef]

40. Góngora-Benítez, M.; Tulla-Puche, J.; Albericio, F. Multifaceted roles of disulfide bonds. Peptides as therapeutics. *Chem. Rev.* **2014**, *114*, 901–926. [CrossRef] [PubMed]

14

Bacteria from Animals as a Pool of Antimicrobial Resistance Genes

Maria Angeles Argudín [1,*], **Ariane Deplano** [1], **Alaeddine Meghraoui** [1], **Magali Dodémont** [1], **Amelie Heinrichs** [1], **Olivier Denis** [1,2], **Claire Nonhoff** [1] and **Sandrine Roisin** [1]

[1] National Reference Centre—*Staphylococcus aureus*, Department of Microbiology, Hôpital Erasme, Université Libre de Bruxelles, Route de Lennik 808, 1070 Brussels, Belgium; Ariane.Deplano@erasme.ulb.ac.be (A.D.); Alaeddine.Meghraoui@erasme.ulb.ac.be(A.M.); Magali.Dodemont@erasme.ulb.ac.be (M.D.); Amelie.Heinrichs@erasme.ulb.ac.be (A.H.); odenis@ulb.ac.be (O.D.); Claire.Nonhoff@erasme.ulb.ac.be(C.N.); Sandrine.Roisin@erasme.ulb.ac.be (S.R.)

[2] Ecole de Santé Publique, Université Libre de Bruxelles, Avenue Franklin Roosevelt 50, 1050 Bruxelles, Belgium

[*] Correspondence: maria.argudin@erasme.ulb.ac.be

Academic Editor: Mary Barton

Abstract: Antimicrobial agents are used in both veterinary and human medicine. The intensive use of antimicrobials in animals may promote the fixation of antimicrobial resistance genes in bacteria, which may be zoonotic or capable to transfer these genes to human-adapted pathogens or to human gut microbiota via direct contact, food or the environment. This review summarizes the current knowledge of the use of antimicrobial agents in animal health and explores the role of bacteria from animals as a pool of antimicrobial resistance genes for human bacteria. This review focused in relevant examples within the ESC(K)APE (*Enterococcus faecium*, *Staphylococcus aureus*, *Clostridium difficile* (*Klebsiella pneumoniae*), *Acinetobacter baumannii*, *Pseudomonas aeruginosa*, and *Enterobacteriaceae*) group of bacterial pathogens that are the leading cause of nosocomial infections throughout the world.

Keywords: *mec*; *cfr*; *mcr*

1. Introduction

The discovery of antimicrobial agents in the mid-twentieth century revolutionized the management and therapy of bacterial infections. Infections that would normally have been fatal became curable. Ever since then, the antimicrobial agents have saved the lives of millions of people. However, these gains are now seriously jeopardized by the rapid emergence and spread of antimicrobial-resistant bacteria [1]. Antimicrobial resistance (AMR) is a major health problem rapidly spreading across the world. The *Review on Antimicrobial Resistance* report [2] estimates that at least 700,000 annual deaths are due to infections by drug-resistant strains of common bacterial infections, human immunodeficiency virus (HIV), tuberculosis and malaria. Numbers suggested that up to 50,000 lives are lost each year due to antibiotic-resistant infections in Europe and the US alone [2]. The inappropriate use of antibiotics in food animals, as well as in the medical practice has potentiated the risk of untreatable infections. Due to the free movement of people and goods between countries, and the intensive international transport of livestock, the problem of AMR is becoming by nature a global problem. Moreover, the AMR emergence is accompanied with a decline in the discovery of new antimicrobial agents. It has been estimated that most of the antibiotics used presently for common human and animal infections will be useless within five to ten years, turning back the clock to the pre-antibiotic era [1].

Antimicrobial agents are principally used for therapy and prevention of human and animal diseases, but they are still used in some countries for growth-promotion in food animal productions [3].

Their indiscriminate use has contributed to the emergence of bacterial resistance, in hospitals, community and livestock settings. AMR may spread from animals to humans and vice versa; directly by the spread of the resistant bacteria or indirectly by the spread of resistance genes from animal bacteria to human bacteria. In this manuscript, we overview the current knowledge about the use of antimicrobial agents of critical importance in veterinary medicine, and investigate the potential of bacteria from animals as an AMR-gene reservoir. We have also underlined some resistance genes that were firstly described in bacteria from animals and later were found in human bacteria. This review focused in relevant examples within the ESKAPE (*Enterococcus faecium, Staphylococcus aureus, Klebsiella pneumoniae, Acinetobacter baumannii, Pseudomonas aeruginosa*, and *Enterobacter* spp.) or ESCAPE (*E. faecium, S. aureus, Clostridium difficile, A. baumannii, P. aeruginosa*, and Enterobacteriaceae) bacterial pathogens that are the leading cause of nosocomial infections throughout the world [4,5].

2. Use of Antimicrobials in Animal Health

Antimicrobial agents play a key role in the treatment of bacterial infections in human and veterinary medicine. In fact, AMR has been considered the quintessential One Health issue [6]. This One Health approach recognizes that the human health is connected to the animal health and the environment [7].

The use of antimicrobials in veterinary medicine creates a selective pressure for the emergence of antimicrobial resistant bacteria, including animal pathogens, human pathogens that have animal reservoirs and commensal bacteria from animals [8] The bacteria selected by this pressure can spread to humans either by direct contact with animals or food products, or indirectly via environmental pathways and/or non-food producing animals [8] (Figure 1).

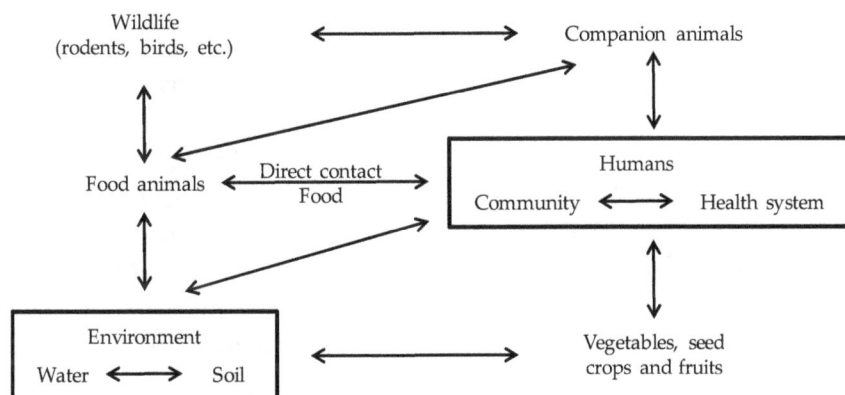

Figure 1. Interactions between groups. Antimicrobial-resistant bacteria can spread to humans either by the food supply, direct contact with food or companion animals or, more indirectly, through environmental pathways, including waterways, soils and vegetables contaminated with human or animals waste, and vectors such as rodents, insects, and birds. Based on da Costa et al. [8] and McEwen et al. [9] with modifications.

The antimicrobial use in animals selects for AMR in commensal and zoonotic bacteria [9]. Soil treated with manure represents a "hot spot" of bacteria carrying AMR-genes [10]. However, soil itself is also a natural reservoir for antimicrobial-resistant bacteria [10]. The fecal wastes from animals contaminate groundwater, streams and other waterways, contributing to the spread of bacteria carrying AMR-genes [9]. Human wastes from homes, hospitals and offices also contribute to contaminate rivers and waterways with antimicrobial-resistant bacteria [9]. In fact, treated wastewater and lake water have been shown to contain AMR-genes and antimicrobial-resistant bacteria [10]. Soils and irrigation water are contamination sources for vegetables and fruits, in which resistant bacteria have been detected [10]. Antimicrobial-resistant bacteria may also spread between farms via infected carrier animals, companion animals or wildlife vectors [9]. Finally, there is a flow of patients and bacteria between community and hospital environments (Figure 1).

These complex transmission routes within farm animals, between farm animals and humans and the transfer of AMR-genes among bacteria, make it challenging to prove whether a reservoir of AMR-genes in livestock poses a risk for animal or human health [10]. However, some antimicrobial-resistant bacteria are zoonotic agents or can colonize and/or infect several hosts. In this sense, the current approach to evaluate the reservoir of AMR-genes in farm animals is to study the AMR-level of commensal bacteria and zoonotic agents in healthy farm animals and slaughter [10]. Reports from the European Food Safety Authority (EFSA) and the European Centre for Disease Prevention and Control (ECDC) monitoring AMR in animals are increasing. Yet, there are some limitations in the current data, and Thanner et al. [10] have recently suggested a voluntary monitoring program by researchers.

In order to underline the importance of the current available antimicrobials classes, the World Health Organization (WHO) started categorizing the most important antimicrobials in human medicine. The last revision of the list was done in 2016 [11]. The importance of each antimicrobial group is based on two criteria: C1, "the antimicrobial class is the sole, or one of limited available therapies, to treat serious bacterial infections in people"; and C2, "the antimicrobial class is used to treat infections in people caused by either: (i) bacteria that may be transmitted to humans from nonhuman sources, or (ii) bacteria that may acquire resistance genes from non-human sources". Antimicrobials that meet both criteria are considered "critically important" in human medicine, antimicrobials that meet one of the criteria are considered "highly important", and antimicrobials that meet none of the two criteria are considered "important" [11].

Similarly to the WHO, the World Organization for Animal Health (also named *Organisation mondiale de la santé animale*, OIE) [12] has developed a list of the antimicrobial agents of veterinary importance [13]. Since in veterinary medicine, many different species have to be treated the criteria to classify the antimicrobials were different than for the human medicine. The OIE criteria were based on a questionnaire prepared by the ad hoc group, which was sent to the OIE delegates of all member countries and international organizations which had signed a co-operation agreement with the OIE. The responses were analyzed by the ad hoc group and discussed in some international committees. The criterion C1 was based on the response rate to the questionnaire: "This criterion was met when a majority of the respondents (more than 50%) identified the importance of the antimicrobial class in their response to the questionnaire". The criterion C2 was based on the treatment of each serious animal disease and the availability of alternative antimicrobial agents: "This criterion was met when compounds within the class were identified as essential against specific infections and there was a lack of sufficient therapeutic alternatives". Similarly to the WHO list, antimicrobials that meet both criteria are considered "critically important" in veterinary medicine, antimicrobials that meet one of the criteria are considered "highly important", and antimicrobials that meet none of the two criteria are considered "important".

After the ban of antimicrobial growth promoters, antimicrobial agents are still allowed with veterinary prescription [10]. Around 37% of the antimicrobials (mainly ionophores) used in food animal production do not have equivalent drugs used for human therapeutic purposes [14]. Similarly, tetracyclines, that are not considered a first-line antimicrobial therapy in human medicine, make up another 44% of total antimicrobial used in animal agriculture [14]. While not all antimicrobial agents used in animal health are used in human medicine, most antimicrobials used in food animals are analogs to those used in human medicine [10]. In both WHO and OIE lists, substances belonging to certain groups (aminoglycosides, cephalosporins of third generation, macrolides, penicillins, and quinolones) were considered critical important antimicrobial groups [11,13]. In fact, some specific antibiotics are critically and/or highly important in both human and veterinary medicine (Table 1). Interestingly, the antibiotic streptomycin is also used in plant agriculture in the prevention of fire blight disease in apple and pear tree caused by the phytopathogenic *Erwinia amylovora* [10].

Table 1. Antimicrobials used in both human and veterinary medicine.

Group	Antimicrobial Agent(s)	Categorization in Human Medicine [1]	Categorization in Veterinary Medicine [2]
Aminoglycosides	Amikacin, dihydrostreptomycin, framycetin, gentamicin, kanamycin, neomycin, tobramycin, streptomycin	CIA	CIA
	Spectinomycin	IA	CIA
Ansamycins	Rifampicin, rifamixin	CIA	HIA [4]
Cephalosporins (1st and 2nd generation)	Cefacetrile, cefalexin, cefalotin, cefapyrin, cefazolin, cefuroxime	HIA [3]	HIA
Cephalosporins (3rd generation)	Cefoperazone, ceftriaxone	CIA	CIA
Macrolides	Erythromycin, oleandomycin, josamycin, spiramycin	CIA	CIA
Penicillins	Benzylpenicillin (penicillin G), amoxicillin, ampicillin, hetacillin, ticarcillin, phenoxymethylpenicillin (penicillin V), phenethicillin	CIA	CIA
	Cloxacillin, dicloxacillin, mecillinam, nafcillin, oxacillin	HIA [3]	CIA
Penicillins + β-lactamase inhibitors	Amoxicillin-Clavulanic acid, Ampicillin-Sulbactam	CIA	CIA
Polymixins	Bacitracin	IA	HIA
	Colistin, polymyxin B	CIA	HIA
Quinolones (1st generation)	Flumequine, nalidixic acid, oxolinic acid	CIA	HIA
Quinolones (2nd generation)	Ciprofloxacin, norfloxacin, ofloxacin	CIA	CIA
Sulfonamides	Sulfadiazine, sulfadimethoxine, sulfadimidine, sulfafurazole (sulfisoxazole), sulfamerazine, sulfamethoxazole, sulfamethoxypyridazine, sulfanilamide, sulfapyridine	HIA [3]	CIA
Tetracyclines	Chlortetracycline, doxycycline, oxytetracycline, tetracycline	HIA [3]	CIA
Others	Fusidic acid	HIA [3]	IA
	Fosfomycin	CIA	HIA [4]
	Lincomycin	HIA	HIA
	Thiamphenicol	HIA [3]	CIA
	Trimethoprim	HIA [3]	CIA

[1] Based on Anonymous [11]. [2] Based on Anonymous [13]. [3] In certain geographic settings this/these antimicrobial(s) can be considered CIA. [4] Only authorized in few countries and with a limited number of indications. CIA, critically important antimicrobial agent(s); HIA, highly important antimicrobial agent(s); IA, important antimicrobial agent(s).

The use of antimicrobial agents in human medicine is restricted to therapy and prophylaxis. However, the antimicrobials in farm animals have therapeutic, prophylactic, metaphylactic and sub-therapeutic uses [9,15]. Therapeutic treatments are planned for individual animals that are diseased, but in food animal productions it is often more efficient to treat entire groups by medicating feed or water [9,15]. This metaphylactic use is particularly common and it implies the use of antimicrobials in the whole herd or flock for disease prophylaxis and/or therapy in case of presence of clinical illness in one individual of the group [3,15]. Moreover, for some animals (poultry and fish) this mass medication is the only feasible means of treatment [9]. This metaphylactic use results in the frequent exposition of entire groups of animals, healthy and diseased, to antimicrobial agents [10]. Prophylactic antimicrobial treatments are typically used during high-risk periods for infectious disease such as after weaning or transport [9]. Antimicrobials may also be administered in relatively low (sub-therapeutic) concentrations to food animals to promote growth and to enhance feed efficiency [9,15]. A ban on the use of growth promoters was implemented in Europe in 2006, but it has not led to any consistent decrease in antimicrobials consumption since this ban has been compensated by metaphylactic and prophylactic uses [3].

In addition to antimicrobials, metals compounds, such as zinc and copper, are also used to supplement animal (mainly in pigs) feed for the prevention of post-weaning diarrhea and the stimulation of growth. Resistance to these compounds is often associated to resistance to antimicrobial drugs such as methicillin in staphylococci, or macrolides and glycopeptides in enterococci [16]. It has been shown that these metal resistance genes are frequent in animal-associated bacteria [16–19]. The use of antimicrobials, biocides and metal compounds in animal productions in sub-therapeutic doses and with long exposure periods, may promote that bacteria fix genes that confer AMR [6,10]. These resistance genes can subsequently be transmitted to human-adapted pathogens or to human gut microbiota via people, contaminated food or the environment [6,10].

The multiple pathways involved in AMR-genes dissemination and exchange within the agriculture, the environment and the food processing industry (Figure 1) make difficult to track the movement of these genes in vivo [10]. In this regard, Thanner et al. [10] underlined some gaps regarding our current knowledge about AMR in plant and animal agriculture, and proposed a worldwide surveillance program of soil, plants, animals, water and wastewater treatment plants using the same methods that for AMR monitoring of human hospitals isolates. As for AMR in human bacteria, a better knowledge of the AMR in animal bacteria will help to achieve an effective and controlled use of antimicrobials in animals, thereby avoiding the dissemination of known and novel AMR-genes [10].

3. Presence of AMR-Genes in Animals: The Metagenomics Evidence

Although some bacterial species (such as *Mycobacterium tuberculosis* and *Streptococcus pneumoniae*) are specialist human pathogens, a larger number of species are opportunistic pathogens (such as *Escherichia coli*) causing disease in humans and other hosts including livestock and wildlife species, and are also present in the wider environment [3]. The interplay of these ecologies is important, since animals and the environment represent a major AMR reservoir. Through evolution, microorganisms have synthetized antibiotics and/or develop resistance methods for microbial competition in the environment [20]. In fact, AMR-genes have been found in soils not exposed to antimicrobials [21,22]. However, the human activity is increasing and changing this environmental resistome [20]. Indeed, animal microbiomes have acquired genes over years of exposure to antimicrobial agents and heavy metals compounds used as therapeutics, metaphylactics, prophylactics and growth promoters [3,23].

Current studies based on metagenomics and/or real-time polymerase chain reaction (PCR) approaches have given diverse results regarding the human, animal and environmental resistome. These novel technologies offer the possibility to elucidate the presence of AMR-genes in human, animal and environmental microbiomes and to identify the factors causing their persistence, selection and spread [10].

Some studies have suggested that human and animal microbiomes are different [21]. Agga et al. [21] compared environments related to animal (cattle and swine) and municipal (human) waste and saw that antimicrobial-resistant bacteria populations associated with animal agriculture were distinct from those associated to human activity. However, regarding the gene content, 25 out of 61 unique AMR-genes identified were common between municipal waste and animal samples. The half of the AMR-genes detected in another study [24], were only found in external environments. These genes from external environment microbiomes were mainly related to biocide and metal resistance [24]. Human microbiota had the highest abundance and diversity of AMR-genes, and the lowest taxonomic diversity [24]. Nevertheless, it was seen that tetracycline resistance genes dominated in both human and animal microbiomes [24]. Moreover, 20.5% of the AMR-genes detected were found in human, animal and environmental samples [24]. A recent study based on the comparison of published data on metagenomics made similar conclusions [25]. This study showed that the environment is a reservoir of the basic forms of resistance genes (such as bla_{TEM}), while both the human and mammalian gut microbiomes contained the widest diversity of clinically relevant resistance genes [25].

Some studies have identified AMR-genes in animal samples regardless of the antibiotic exposure. Sequence-based metagenomics analysis of conventionally raised cattle without therapeutic antibiotics exposure revealed that 3.7% of the sequences encoded resistance to antibiotics and toxic compounds, and nearly half of these genes encoded multidrug resistance efflux pumps [26]. A similar metagenomics study in chicken ceca, revealed that around 2% of the sequences encoded resistance to antibiotics and toxic compounds [27]. At least one quarter of these genes were related to tetracycline and fluoroquinolones resistance [27]. Studies in swine fecal samples revealed the existence of at least 149 AMR-genes in non-medicated animals [28,29].

Although non-exposed animals may already carry bacteria with resistance genes, some studies have underlined that their resistome can change after antibiotic exposure. Diverse studies have shown that antibiotic treatment increased diversity of antibiotic resistance genes [28,29]. Moreover, some enriched genes, such as an aminoglycoside O-phosphotransferase, confer resistance to antibiotics that were not administered, demonstrating the potential for indirect selection of resistance to classes of antibiotics not fed [28]. The effects of administering sub-therapeutic concentrations of antimicrobials to beef cattle were investigated in a recent study, showing that the antimicrobial treatment differentially affected the abundance of certain resistance genes in fecal deposits, but not their persistence [30]. In other study, the administration of the third generation cephalosporin ceftiofur in dairy cows increased the β-lactam and multidrug resistance genes in feces [31]. Nevertheless, another study identified approximately the same number (21–26) of unique AMR-genes in manure samples of four dairy cows despite different prior exposure to antibiotics [32].

Some metagenomics studies have underlined the dominance of tetracycline resistance genes in animal microbiomes [24,33]. These results may be partially explained by the historical and current exposure to tetracyclines in the animal husbandry. Yet, a metagenomics study in pigs reared in an antibiotic-free environment revealed also the presence of diverse tetracycline resistance genes including novel genes, as well as a gene [tet(40)] not previously observed outside the human gut microbiome [34].

Although the metagenomics studies seem promising, they have some limitations. Since, some annotated genes (ex. efflux pumps) that confer AMR, perform other basic functions, more research on gene expression and functional analysis is needed to determine whether these genes can confer phenotypical resistance to antimicrobials [23]. Moreover, the sequence-based metagenomics approach does not provide information about the genetic context [23]. Nevertheless, some promising plasmid metagenomics studies have showed a broad dissemination of plasmid carrying AMR-genes in pig and bovine samples [35,36]. The functional genomics study about the tetracycline resistome of the pig gut has shown that most of the genes resided on putative mobile genetic elements (MGEs), which may contribute to the maintenance and dissemination of antibiotic resistance in antibiotic-free environments [34]. Nevertheless, other studies have probed that the presence of MGEs is also affected by antibiotic exposure [31,37]. It has been seen that the antimicrobial exposure increased the abundance of phage integrase-encoding genes (that may carry virulence or AMR-genes) in the viromes of swine, demonstrating the induction of prophages with antibiotic treatment [37]. In the study based on the administration of ceftiofur in dairy cows, an increase in gene sequences associated with phages, prophages, transposable elements and plasmids was observed [31].

Some metagenomics studies have proven that the animal microbiome is different of the human microbiome, but, interestingly, their shared a part of their resistome. Acquired resistance genes seem disseminated in the absence of selective pressure, but their abundance is affected by antibiotic exposition. These findings confirm that continue antimicrobial selective pressure in both humans and animals may benefit the dissemination of acquired resistance genes [23]. As other authors have concluded, a prudent use of antibiotics in human and veterinary health is needed to slow down the AMR spread and prevent the emergence of novel AMR-genes [23].

4. AMR-Genes in Gram-Positive Bacteria from Animals

Three Gram-positive species are considered members of the ESC(K)APE group: *C. difficile*, *E. faecium*, and *S. aureus*. This section focuses on the current knowledge about these pathogens regarding their AMR in animals, particularly on the genes common within these species (Table 2).

Table 2. Examples of common AMR-genes found in *Clostridium*, Enterococci and Staphylococci.

Antimicrobial Agent(s) Group	Resistance Mechanism	Resistance Gene	Species Group
Chloramphenicol	Active efflux (MFS transporter)	*fexA*	Enterococci, Staphylococci
MLS$_B$	Target site modification (rRNA methylation)	*erm*(A)	*Clostridium*, Enterococci, Staphylococci
		erm(B)	*Clostridium*, Enterococci, Staphylococci
Oxazolidinones	Active efflux (ABC transporter)	*optrA*	Enterococci, Staphylococci
PhLOPSA$_A$	Target site modification (rRNA methylation)	*cfr*	Enterococci, Staphylococci
		cfr(B)	*Clostridium*, Enterococci
Tetracycline	Target site protection (ribosome protective protein)	*tet*(M)	*Clostridium*, Enterococci, Staphylococci
Trimethoprim	Target replacement (trimethoprim resistant dihydrofolate reductase)	*dfrK*	Enterococci, Staphylococci
Glycopeptides	Target replacement (modified peptidoglycan precursor)	*vanA*	Enterococci, Staphylococci

Based on Brenciani et al. [38], Deshpande et al. [39], He et al. [40], Fan et al. [41]; Liu et al. [42], Lopez et al. [43], Roberts et al. [44], Shen et al. [45], Spigaglia et al. [46], Van Hoek et al. [47] and Wendlandt et al. [48]. ABC, ATP-binding cassette; MFS, Major Facilitator Superfamily; MLS$_B$, macrolide-lincosamide-streptogramin B; PhLOPSA$_A$, phenicols, lincosamides, oxazolidinones, pleuromutilins and streptogramin A.

4.1. Clostridium difficile

C. difficile is an ubiquitous environmental organism widespread in rivers, lakes and soils. It is also found in the hospital environment where it is difficult to eradicate, as well as in meat products and animals including diverse species (calves, ostriches, chickens, elephants, dogs, horses and pigs) [49]. Although there are some current genomic updates of the clostridial phylogeny [50,51], in this review we use the classical nomenclature of *Clostridium difficile*.

C. difficile is recognized as the major cause of healthcare antibiotic-associated diarrhea [46]. Over the last decade, an alarming increase in incidence of *C. difficile* infection was observed across the USA, Canada and Europe, and it has been associated with the emergence of the highly virulent (hypervirulent) clone BI/NAP1/027 [named according to its restriction enzyme analysis (REA), pulsed-field gel electrophoresis (PFGE) and PCR Ribotype (RT)] [46,52]. This dramatic increase in *C. difficile* infections was associated to the fluoroquinolone resistance of this clone [52]. Fluoroquinolones are broad-spectrum antimicrobials highly effective for the treatment of bacterial infections in animals and humans. Most RT027 isolates harbored mutations in the quinolone-resistance determining region (QRDR) of the DNA gyrase subunit gene, *gyrA*, that confer resistance to fluoroquinolones [52]. Nevertheless, clinical *C. difficile* strains acquire fluoroquinolone resistance due to alterations in the QRDR of either GyrA or GyrB DNA gyrase subunits [46].

C. difficile infection has also emerged as a cause of diarrhea in the community, especially in populations previously considered at low risk, such as young people, antibiotic-naive patients or people without healthcare exposure [46]. Studies in the community indicated that up to 13% healthy human subjects are asymptomatically colonized with *C. difficile* [52]. In addition to RT027, a number of emergent hypervirulent RTs have recently been identified, notably the hypervirulent RT078 recognized as infection cause in hospitals, the community and animals [46]. The use of fluoroquinolones in the pork industry may have also contributed to the emergence of the multidrug-resistant RT078 [53]. In a study by Keessen et al. [53], most human and porcine isolates were resistant to ciprofloxacin (96%), and some were also resistant to moxifloxacin (16% for both human and porcine isolates). Resistance to moxifloxacin in this study was associated with a *gyrA* mutation [53]. Moreover, the use of fluoroquinolones [ciprofloxacin in humans, and enrofloxacin in pigs] was significantly associated with isolation of moxifloxacin-resistant isolates in both populations [53]. The authors proposed that the increased fluoroquinolone use could have contributed to the spread of *C. difficile* RT078 [53].

RT078 is commonly isolated from swine and other food animals [52]. It is likely that RT078 is an important pathogen of piglet diarrhea worldwide [49,54]. Molecular genotyping has suggested that RT078 isolates of human and swine origin are highly related and may therefore represent a potential zoonotic transmission [52]. Several studies have suggested that transmission from swine to humans may occur in farms or in large integrated swine operations, and moreover, the aerial dissemination of *C. difficile* from pig farms has been shown [52,54]. Due to the increased incidence of *C. difficile* infection outside the hospital environment and the presence of the same genetic lineage in food animals and its products, some authors have suggested that *C. difficile* may be considered as a foodborne pathogen [52]. Although RT078 is predominant in studies on swine, other RTs have been described in animals [52]. For example, RT046 has been found in both piglets and humans in Sweden [55].

AMR in *C. difficile* has been less intensively investigated than in other Gram-positive pathogens (such as *S. aureus*). In fact, few AMR-genes [such as *erm*(A), *erm*(B), *tet*(M), *tet*(44), *tet*(W), *ant(6)-Ib*, *catD* and *cfr*(B)] have been characterized in *C. difficile* isolates [46]. Resistance to cephalosporins is still uncharacterized, although most clinical *C. difficile* strains are resistant to these antibiotics. Similarly, some *C. difficile* human and animal isolates with reduced susceptibility to metronidazole have been found, although the resistance mechanism is not completely understood [46].

The most widespread mechanism of resistance to the antibiotics of the macrolide-lincosamide-streptogramin B (MLS$_B$) group in *C. difficile* is ribosomal methylation due to the erythromycin ribosomal methylases (*erm*) genes of class B [46]. It is to note, that *erm*(B) is the *erm* gene with the widest bacteria host range, and it has been found in both Gram-positive and Gram-negative bacteria, aerobic, and anaerobic genera and in most ecosystems [56]. However, *erm*-negative *C. difficile* strains resistant to both erythromycin and clindamycin or only to erythromycin have been also described [46]. Alterations in the 23S rRNA or ribosomal proteins (L4 or L22) have been found in some of these strains, but the presence of these changes in susceptible isolates had excluded their role in resistance [46]. Interestingly, a multidrug resistant *cfr*-like gene, *cfr*(B), that modifies the 23S rRNA has been recently found in clinical *C. difficile* isolates [57,58] (see Section 4.3.2).

The *tet*(M) gene is the most frequent tetracycline resistance determinant in *C. difficile* isolates [46]. Interestingly, most RT078 isolates carry the transposon Tn916 harboring *tet*(M) [52]. Nevertheless, other *tet* genes [*tet*(W), *tet*(44)] have been identified in *C. difficile* [46,59]. The *tet*(W) gene has been found together with *tet*(M) in *C. difficile* isolates recovered from animals and humans [46]. The *tet*(44) gene has been associated to the transposon Tn6164 in human and environmental isolates [46,59].

4.2. Enterococcus faecium

Enterococci are commensal bacteria of the gastrointestinal tract of mammals and other animals that can also be detected in the environment [60,61]. In adult people, enterococci account for about 1% of the intestinal microbiota, being *E. faecium* and *Enterococcus faecalis* the most prevalent enterococci in the human gastrointestinal tract [61]. These species are opportunistic human pathogens that are implicated in life-threatening hospital acquired infections such as bacteremia and infective endocarditis [60,61].

Enterococci are intrinsically resistant to a number of first-line antimicrobial agents. They have resistance against cephalosporins and cotrimoxazole, as well as low-level resistance to β-lactams and aminoglycosides [60]. Moreover, clinical and animal *Enterococcus* isolates with resistance to other antimicrobials such as macrolides, tetracyclines, streptogramins and glycopeptides have been described [60,62]. Antimicrobials such as linezolid, daptomycin and tigecycline can be used in the treatment of enterococcal infections [63,64]. Nevertheless, resistance against these former antimicrobials has been reported, mainly in the clinical setting [63,64].

Nowadays, the vancomycin-resistant enterococci (VRE) pose a major therapeutic challenge due to their difficult treatment [61]. VRE were found in the hospital setting in the 80s [61,64], while the first description of animal reservoirs of vancomycin-resistant *E. faecium* was published in 1993 [65]. Later on, VRE have been described in diverse animals and environmental sources [60]. As vancomycin has not been used in veterinary medicine, it was hypothesized that the use of another glycopeptide, the avoparcin, as additive in farm animals feed, has influenced the emergence of VRE in animals since the 70s [60]. This correlation has been criticized and several studies have shown that vancomycin-resistant *E. faecium* persisted in animals for an extended time after the banning of avoparcin in the 90s [54,60]. However, this persistence has been related to co-selection with other antimicrobials (such as tetracycline or the macrolide tylosine) and metals (such as copper sulphate) [54,60]. It has been suggested that VRE strains are predominately host-specific, being hospital isolates genetically different from animal strains [60]. However, some research, based on multilocus sequence typing (MLST) showed that certain isolates from diverse clonal complexes (CCs) are present in animals, healthy humans and patients [54,60,61]. Moreover, the same variants of *Tn*1546 carrying the glycopeptide-resistant gene *vanA* have been detected in enterococci from human and animal origin, underlying that *E. faecium* from animals can act as a donor of AMR-genes for other pathogenic enterococci [54,60].

Similar to glycopeptides, the use of other antimicrobials as grown promotors may have influenced the emerging of enterococci resistant strains in food animals. In 1999, the streptogramin combination quinupristin/dalfopristin (RP59500, Synercid) was approved for clinical use. The mixture of type B streptogramin (quinupristin) and type A streptogramin (dalfopristin) in a 30:70 ratio showed good activity against multiresistant *E. faecium* strains [66]. Nevertheless, before its approval for clinical use, in 1997, quinupristin/dalfopristin-resistant *E. faecium* isolates were found in both human patients and chicken samples [66]. The use of virginiamycin, a streptogramin licensed for growth promotion in animals (including chickens and other poultry), was associated to the development of resistance to streptogramin combinations by enterococci [66]. In this sense, diverse streptogramin A resistance genes [such as *vat*(D), *vat*(E), *vga*(D) and *vat*(H)] have been detected in *E. faecium* from animals in Europe, USA and/or Asia [60].

Regarding other antimicrobials, human and animal *E. faecium* isolates frequently harbored genes conferring resistance against aminoglycosides [*aph(3′)IIIa*], tetracycline [*tet*(M)], and macrolides [*erm*(B)] [61]. Recently, a novel gene, *optrA*, which encodes for an ABC transporter that confers resistance to oxazolidinones and phenicols has been found in *E. faecalis* and *E. faecium* of human and animal origin [67]. This gene has been found chromosomally and plasmid located in Enterococci [40], but also in *Staphylococcus sciuri* [41,68]. The *optrA*-carrying plasmids in enterococci have also other AMR-genes against antibiotics such as MLS$_B$ [*erm*(A)-like)] and/or phenicol (*fexA*) [40]. Retrospective analysis of genome sequences has revealed that *optrA* has a wide dissemination in Gram-positive bacteria and it has also been found in diverse *Streptococcus* species (including *S. suis*, *S. agalactiae* and *S. pyogenes*) [69].

Some genes (*cfr* and *dfrK*) first discovered in animal-related staphylococci have recently been found in enterococci (see Sections 4.3.2 and 4.3.3). The trimethoprim resistance gene *dfrK*, encoding a trimethoprim resistant dihydrofolate reductase, was recently detected in *E. faecium* [43] (see Section 4.3.3). The multi-resistance gene *cfr* encodes a RNA methyltransferase that modifies the 23S rRNA gene conferring resistance to ribosome-targeting antimicrobials [44]. It has been detected in *E. faecalis* from animals and humans, *E. thailandicus* from pigs and farm environment, *E. casseliflavus* and *E. gallinarum* from pigs [42,45]. A non-functional *cfr*, due to a deletion in the regulatory region upstream, has been detected together with *optrA* in a clinical *E. faecium* isolate [38]. As for *C. difficile*, a functional *cfr*(B) has recently been found in *E. faecium* clinical isolates [39] (see Section 4.3.2).

4.3. Staphylococcus aureus and Related Species

S. aureus is part of the normal and transit human microbiota, and it is usually present in the nasopharyngeal mucosa, but also in the skin and other corporal areas [70–72]. The general carrier rate in humans is estimated between 20 and 30 percent for persistent colonization [73]. *S. aureus* is an opportunistic pathogen, which produces a wide spectrum of diseases, ranging from minor's skin to deep infections, as well as potentially-fatal diseases such as diverse invasive infections and toxin-mediated diseases [74,75]. As in humans, *S. aureus* is a commensal bacterium for animals but it is also able to cause diverse infections including abscesses, chondronecrosis, dermatitis, mastitis, pyaemia, osteomyelitis, pneumonia, septicemia and skin and wound infections [76].

Staphylococci of animal origin harbor a wide variety of AMR-genes [48,77–83]. Recent reviews by Wendlandt et al. [48,81] have underlined that at least 44 AMR-genes in staphylococci have been detected in both human and animal isolates (Table 3). Interestingly, some shared genes were firstly described in isolates from animal origin [such as *tet*(L), *erm*(T), *dfrK*, *fexA*, *cfr*] or possibly originated from *Staphylococcus* species related to animals (as the methicillin resistance gene *mecA*). Next sub-sections are focused on those genes originated from animal related staphylococci.

4.3.1. *mec* Genes in Staphylococci: Origin and Reservoirs

One of the most important acquired resistance in staphylococci is methicillin resistance. This resistance is mainly due to the acquisition of the *mecA* gene, encoding a β-lactam low affinity penicillin binding protein (PBP) called PBP2a. This gene is carried on a MGE termed staphylococcal cassette chromosome *mec* (SCC*mec*). This MGE has been more extensively studied for *S. aureus*, since this is the most important *Staphylococcus* species for the human health. To date, eleven major SCC*mec* types carrying *mecA* have been described in methicillin resistant *S. aureus* (MRSA), which have been assigned on the characterization of its two essential components the *mec* and *ccr* complexes [84–86]. The *mec*-gene complex corresponded to the *mecA* operon variants, which can include functional and/or truncated regulatory genes. The *ccr* complex includes the recombinase(s) involve in the excision and integration of the element into the chromosome. The remaining regions of the SCC*mec* on which subtypes are based are called junkyard or joining regions, and they can contain MGEs, as well as heavy metal [arsenate (*ars* operon), cadmium (*cadD-cadX*), cadmium and zinc (*ccrC*), copper (*copB*), mercury (*mer* operon)] and other AMR (amynoglicosides (*aadD*, *aad9/spc*, *aacA-aphD*), bleomycin (*ble*), erythromycin [*erm*(A)], tetracycline [*tet*(K)]) resistance genes. Many non-typable SCC*mec* cassettes exist, and non-*S. aureus* staphylococci carry similar SCC*mec* and novel *mec-ccr* combinations as those found in *S. aureus* [17,87–90]. This suggests horizontal transfer and recombination events within Staphylococci species. In fact, the *mecA* is widely distributed among methicillin resistant coagulase negative Staphylococci (MRCoNS) [17,87–91].

Table 3. Examples of AMR-genes identified in Staphylococci from animal and/or human origin.

Antimicrobial Agent(s) Group	Resistance Mechanism	Resistance Gene(s)	Staphylococci Origin
B-lactams	Enzymatic inactivation (hydrolization)	*blaZ*	A, H
	Target site replacement (alternative PBP)	*mecA*, *mecC* (*mecA*$_{LGA251}$)	A, H
Aminoglycosides	Enzymatic inactivation (acetylation and phosphorylation)	*aacA-aphD*	A, H
	Enzymatic inactivation (adenylation)	*aadD*, *aadE*, *str*	A, H
	Enzymatic inactivation (phosphorylation)	*aphA3*	A, H

Table 3. *Cont.*

Antimicrobial Agent(s) Group	Resistance Mechanism	Resistance Gene(s)	Staphylococci Origin
Aminocylitols	Enzymatic inactivation (adenylation)	*spc, spd, spw*	A, H
	Enzymatic inactivation (acetylation)	*apmA*	A
Bleomycin	Bleomycin binding protein	*ble*	A, H
Fosfomycin	Enzymatic inactivation (metallothiol-transferase)	*fosD* (*fosB*)	A, H
Fusidic acid	Target site protection (ribosome protective protein)	*fusB, fusC*	A, H
Macrolides	Active efflux (MFS transporter)	*mef*(A)	H
	Enzymatic inactivation (phosphorylation)	*mph*(C)	A, H
Macrolides, streptogramin B	Active efflux (ABC transporter)	*msr*(A)	A, H
MLS$_B$	Target site modification (rRNA methylation)	*erm*(A), *erm*(B), *erm*(C), *erm*(F), *erm*(T), *erm*(43)	A, H
		erm(33), *erm*(44), *erm*(45)	A
		erm(G), *erm*(Q), *erm*(Y), *erm*(44)v	H
Mupirocin	Target replacement (mupirocin-insensitive isoleucyl-tRNA synthase)	*mupA* (*ileS2*)	A, H
		mupB	H
Lincosamides	Enzymatic inactivation (nucleotidylation)	*lnu*(A), *lnu*(B)	A, H
	Active efflux (ABC transporter)	*lsa*(B)	A
Lincosamides, streptogramin A	Active efflux (ABC transporter)	*sal*(A)	A
LPS$_A$	Active efflux (ABC transporter)	*vga*(A), *vga*(A)v, *lsa*(E)	A, H
		vga(B)	H
		vga(C), *vga*(E), *vga*(E)$_{variant}$	A
Phenicols	Enzymatic inactivation (acetylation)	*cat*$_{pC221}$, *cat*$_{pC223}$, *cat*$_{pC194}$	A, H
	Active efflux (MFS transporter)	*fexA*	A, H
PhLOPSA$_A$	Target site modification (rRNA methylation)	*cfr*	A, H
Streptogramin A	Enzymatic inactivation (acetylation)	*vat*(A)	H
		vat(B)	A, H
		vat(C)	H
Streptogramin B	Enzymatic inactivation (hydrolization)	*vgb*(A)	H
		vgb(B)	A, H
Streptothricins	Enzymatic inactivation (acetylation)	*sat4*	A, H
Tetracyclines	Active efflux (MFS transporter)	*tet*(K), *tet*(L)	A, H
	Target site protection (ribosome protective protein)	*tet*(M)	A, H
		tet(O)	A
Oxazolidinones-phenicols	Active efflux (ABC transporter)	*optrA*	A
Trimethoprim	Target replacement (trimethoprim resistant dihydrofolate reductase)	*dfrA* (*dfrS1*), *dfrD, dfrG, dfrK*	A, H
Vancomycin	Target replacement (modified peptidoglycan precursor)	*vanA*	H

Based on Argudín et al. [82,84,92,93], Fan et al. [41], Li et al. [68], Schwarz et al. [80], Seah et al. [94], Strauss et al. [95], Wendlandt et al. [48,81] and Wipf et al. [96,97]. A, animal origin; ABC, ATP-binding cassette; H, human origin; LPS$_A$, lincosamides-pleuromutilins-streptogramin A; MFS, Major Facilitator Superfamily; MLS$_B$, macrolide-lincosamide-streptogramin B; PBP, penicillin binding protein; PhLOPSA$_A$, phenicols, lincosamides, oxazolidinones, pleuromutilins and streptogramin A.

Closed related *mecA* allotypes have been described in members of the *S. sciuri* group [98–100]. The members of the *S. sciuri* group are mainly considered commensal animal-associated bacteria with a broad range of hosts, although they have also been found in the environment and occasionally causing disease in humans and other hosts [98–100]. The *mecA* variants found in members of the *S. sciuri* species group are chromosomal located without being part of a SCC*mec*, and are usually phenotypically susceptible to β-lactams or show a heterogeneous resistance [91]. In this sense, a member of the *S. sciuri* group, the commensal animal-related *S. fleurettii*, has been suggested as the highly probable origin of the *mecA* gene [101]. The *mecA*-containing regions of *S. fleurettii* strains recovered from animals or its products are similar to the *mec* region of the *S. aureus* SCC*mec* type II. Moreover, the analysis of the corresponding gene loci region (with *mecA* gene homologues) of *S. sciuri* and *S. vitulinus* (which evolved from a common ancestor with that of *S. fleurettii*), probed that the *mecA* gene of *S. fleurettii* descended from its ancestor and was not recently acquired [101]. These findings suggested that the SCC*mec* in *S. aureus* was generated by acquiring this intrinsic *mecA* region of *S. fleurettii*.

Recently, two *mecA* gene homologs (*mecB* and *mecC*) have been discovered [102–104]. The gene *mecB* (formerly named *mecAm*) was found in 2009 in a *Macrococcus caseolyticus* isolated from a chicken [102]. This gene is located in a typical *mec* operon (*blaZb-mecB-mecR1b-mecIb*) with similar regulatory genes but also accompanied of a *blaZ* homologue encoding for a putative β-lactamase [85]. The *mecB* operon has been found on a transposon (*Tn6045*) either plasmid or chromosomal located [102], as well as in SCC*mec* elements [102,105]. Nowadays, *mecB* has not been detected in staphylococci. However, there is a potential risk of transmission since staphylococci and macrococci are closely related members of the same family (*Staphylococcaceae*). Moreover, these bacteria share a common niche, since *M. caseolyticus* is a commensal bacterium colonizing animal skin as staphylococci. Additionally, this *mec* variant is located in different MGEs, including a plasmid, which is a more mobile vehicle within bacteria than the SCC*mec* [85].

The gene *mecC* (formerly named *mecA*$_{LGA251}$) was discovered in 2011 in *S. aureus* by two different working groups [103,104]. It was described from isolates originating from mastitis in cows and from humans in the United Kingdom, Ireland and Denmark [103,104]. Even if this gene was first described in 2011, a retrospective analysis in Denmark has shown that *mecC*-positive MRSA strains have been circulating before [106]. The *mecC* gene has a wide distribution and positive strains have been found in humans from both infection cases and carriage state, as well as in animals including livestock (dairy cattle, beef cattle, sheep, farmed rabbits), companion (cats, dogs, guinea pigs), wildlife (birds, mammals) and zoo (mara) animals [91,107]. Generally, there is a low occurrence of *mecC*-positive human isolates (ex. less than 1% in clinical MRSA from Belgium, [108]). This gene has mainly been associated with *S. aureus* lineages related to infections and colonization in animals [91]. The gene *mecC* in *S. aureus* is located on the SCC*mec* XI, which as few other SCC*mec* types also carried heavy metal resistance genes [104]. *mecC* homologues have been found in other staphylococci (*S. xylosus*, *S. sciuri*, and *S. stepanovicii*), associated to cassettes similar to SCC*mec* XI or to composite SCC*mec* together with *mecA* [109–111]. New *mecC* allotypes have been identified: *mecC1* in *S. xylosus* related to bovine mastitis [109] and *mecC2* in *Staphylococcus saprophyticus* from common shrew [112].

4.3.2. The Multi-Resistance Gene *cfr*

Linezolid, the first member of the oxazolidinone class of antibiotics, is considered to be a last-resort antimicrobial for the treatment of infections caused by VRE, MRSA and penicillin-resistant pneumococci [45]. Several mechanisms conferring linezolid resistance have been described in staphylococci, including point mutations in genes encoding 23S rRNA and mutations in ribosomal proteins L3, L4 and L22 [113,114]. In 2000, the gene *cfr* was identified in a bovine *S. sciuri* recovered in 1997 [115]. This gene encodes an RNA methyltransferase that modifies the 23S rRNA gene conferring combined resistance to phenicols, lincosamides, oxazolidinones, pleuromutilins and streptogramin A antimicrobials (known as PhLOPSA$_A$ phenotype). It also confers decreased susceptibility to the 16-membered macrolides (josamycin and spiramycin) [45]. Afterwards, this gene has been identified in methicillin-susceptible *S. aureus* (MSSA), MRSA, various coagulase negative staphylococci (CoNS) and in the coagulase-variable *S. hyicus* [45].

Although linezolid resistance mediated by *cfr* is not frequent in the clinical environment [116], reports of clinical outbreaks by *cfr*-containing *S. aureus* strains have been reported [117,118]. Recently, a clinical case due to a *cfr*-positive livestock-associated (LA-) MRSA CC398 has been described [119]. This gene has been found in important MRSA pandemic lineages such as the sequence type (ST)22/SCC*mec* IV, the Panton-Valentine leukocidin (PVL) positive ST8/SCC*mec* IV/USA300 or the ST125-MRSA-IVc [114,120,121]. It has also been detected in clinical strains of *S. capitis* [122] and methicillin-resistant *S. epidermidis* (MRSE) [123].

In staphylococci from animals, the *cfr* gene has been identified in isolates from different sources including pigs (in *S. aureus*, *S. arlettae*, *S. cohnii*, *S. equorum*, *S. haemolyticus*, *S. hyicus*, *S. saprophyticus*, *S. sciuri*, *S. simulans* and *S. warneri*), bovine (in *S. aureus*, *S. lentus*, *S. sciuri* and *S. simulans*), poultry (in *S. arlettae*, *S. cohnii*, *S. equorum*, *S. rostri*, *S. sciuri* and *S. simulans*), and companion animals (in *S. pseudintermedius*) [45,81,124,125]. The *cfr* gene has been described as chromosomally and plasmid located, linked to specific insertions sequences (IS) [45]. Moreover, the genetic elements of staphylococci with *cfr* usually carried additional resistance genes, including β-lactam (*blaZ*), aminoglycosides [*aacA-aphD, aadD, ant(4')-Ia*], aminocytitols (*spc*), bleomycin (*ble*), fosfomycin (*fosB*), MLS$_B$ [*erm*(A), *erm*(B), *erm*(C), *erm*(33)], lincosamides-pleuromutilins-streptogramin A [*lsa*(B)], phenicol (*fexA*), tetracycline [*tet*(L)], oxazolidinones-phenicols (*optrA*) and/or trimethoprim (*dfrK*) resistance genes (Table 4). The immediate genetic environment within the diverse *cfr*-carrying elements is similar, therefore it has been suggested that a limited number of acquisition events explain the diversity seen among the plasmidic or chromosomal structures [45].

Recent studies have described the *cfr* gene or a variant in other Gram-positive (including *Bacillus* spp., *C. difficile*, *Enterococcus* spp., *Macrococcus caseolyticus*, *Jeotgalicoccus pinnipedialis* and *S. suis*) and Gram-negative (*Proteus vulgaris* and *E. coli*) species (Table 4). With the exception of *Clostridium* and *Enterococcus* isolates, the *cfr*-positive isolates of the other non-*Staphylococcus* genera were obtained exclusively from livestock and related farm environments [39,45,57,58].

In *Bacillus* spp., the gene *cfr* has been identified in three related plasmids from pig isolates from China, one (PBS-01) of these plasmids being previously reported in *S. cohnii* [45]. The *cfr*-carrying plasmid PSS-03 has been detected in both *M. caseolyticus* and *S. cohnii* [45], while the plasmid pJP1 or variants type pJP1-like have been found in *M. caseolyticus*, *J. pinnipedialis*, and *S. lentus* isolates [45]. Interestingly, some of these *cfr*-plasmids found in Gram-positive bacteria carried additional resistance genes against aminoglycosides (*aadD, aadY*), bleomycin (*ble*), MLS$_B$ [*erm*(B), *erm*(C)] and/or phenicol (*fexB*). In fact, a new multiresistance plasmid pWo28-3 related to pJP1, harbouring *aacA-aphD, aadD, ble, optrA, cfr* and *fexA*, has been identified in *S. sciuri* [68]. The *cfr* has also been found associated to a novel IS (IS*Enfa5*) truncating a novel lincosamide resistance gene *lnu*(E) in the plasmid pStrcfr of *S. suis* [126].

Recently, the *cfr* variant gene, designated *cfr*(B), was identified in *C. difficile* and *E. faecium* clinical isolates [39,57,58]. The nomenclature and functionally of this gene has been extensively discussed [127]. The Cfr proteins detected in other Gram-positive (*Bacillus*, *Macrococcus*, *Jeotgalicoccus*, *Staphylococcus* and *Streptococcus*) and in Gram negative (*Proteus* and *Escherichia*) bacteria were indistinguishable or similar (99% identity) from the original *S. sciuri* Cfr protein [127]. However, the *cfr*(B) shared only 75% amino acid identity with the original Cfr protein [39,58,127]. Schwarz et al. [127] suggested that the protein encoded by *cfr*(B) was structurally distantly related to the original Cfr. However, further research proved that the *cfr*(B) product does function as a Cfr protein [58], and therefore may be considered as a variant.

Table 4. Examples of the genetic environments of *cfr* genes.

Genetic Environment	Strain or Plasmid Name	Accession Number	Species	Additional Resistance Genes
Chromosomal region	Strain CM05	JN849634	*S. aureus*	*erm*(B)
	Strain FSEC-02	KR779900	*E. coli*	-
	Strain Ox3196 (*Tn6218*)	HG002389	*C. difficile*	-
	Strain PV-01	JF969273	*P. vulgaris*	-
Plasmid	P3-38	JQ911740	*E. thailandicus*	-
	p004-737X	EU598691	*S. aureus*	-
	p7LC	JX910899	*S. epidermidis*	*aacA–aphD*
	pBD-01	GU591497	*S. cohnii*	*erm*(B)
	pBS-01	GU591497	*Bacillus* spp.	*erm*(B)
	pBS-02	HQ128580	*Bacillus* spp.	-
	pBS-03	JQ394981	*Bacillus* spp.	*aadY*
	pEC-01	JN982327	*E. coli*	-
	pEF-01 [1]	NC_014508	*E. faecalis*	*fexB*
	pERGB	JN970903	*S. aureus*	*aadD, tet*(L), *dfrK*
	pFSEC-01	KR779901	*E. coli*	-
	pGXEC3	KM580532	*E. coli*	*bla*$_{CTX-M-14b}$
	pGXEC6	KM580533	*E. coli*	-
	pHNEP28	KT845955	*E. coli*	-
	pHOU-*cfr*	JQ660368	*E. faecalis*	-
	pMHZ	JX232067	*S. capitis*	-
	pMSA16	JQ246438	*S. aureus*	*erm*(A)
	pSCEC2	KF152885	*E. coli*	*floR, tet*(A)*-tetR, strA/str, sul*
	pSS-01	JQ041372	*S. cohnii*	*aacA–aphD, fexA*
	pSS-02	JF834910	*S. saprophyticus*	*fexA*
	pSS-03	JQ219851	*S. cohnii,* *M. caseolyticus*	*erm*(C)
	pSCFS1	NC_005076	*S. sciuri*	*erm*(33), *lsa*(B), *spc*
	pSCFS3	AM086211	*S. aureus*	*fexA*
	pSCFS6	AM408573	*S. warneri*	*fexA, lsa*(B)
	pSCFS7	FR675942	*S. aureus*	*fexA*
	pSD11	KM212169	*E. coli*	-
	pSP01	KR230047	*S. epidermidis*	*blaZ, lsa*(B), *msr*(A), *aad*
	pStrcfr	KC844846	*S. suis*	Δ*lnu*(E)
	pJP1	JQ320084	*J. pinnipedialis*	*aadD, ble*
	pJP1-like	KF129408	*S. lentus*	*aacA–aphD, aadD, ble, fexA*
	pJP2	KC989517	*S. rostri*	*aacA–aphD, aadD, ble, fexA, fosD*
	pW3	JQ911739	*E. thailandicus*	*erm*(B)
	pW9-2	JQ911741	*E. faecalis*	-
	pWo28-3	KT601170	*S. sciuri*	*aacA-aphD, aadD, ble, fexA, optrA*
Possible plasmids	Strains UW10882 and UW12712 (*Tn6218*-like)	SRP078305	*E. faecium*	-

Based on Bender et al. [128], Brenciani et al. [129], Gopegui et al. [121], Li et al. [68], Liu et al. [130], Shen et al. [45], Sun et al. [131], Wang et al. [126], Wendlandt et al. [81] and Zhang et al. [132–134]. [1] *cfr*-carriying plasmids related to pEF-01 have been found in *E. casseliflavus* and *E. gallinarum* [42].

Regarding *Enterococcus*, *cfr*-carrying plasmids have been described in *E. faecalis* from animals and humans, as well as in pig-related isolates of *E. thailandicus*, *E. casseliflavus* and *E. gallinarum* [42,45]. The *cfr* gene has also been detected chromosomally located in *E. casseliflavus* from pigs [42]. As mentioned in Section 4.2, a non-functional *cfr* gene has been detected together with *optrA* in clinical *E. faecium* isolates [38]. However, recently a *cfr*(B) gene sharing 99.9% sequence identity with the corresponding gene in *C. difficile* has been identified in *E. faecium* clinical isolates [39,128]. Deshpande et al. [39] described two copies of *cfr*(B) chromosomally located and embedded in a *Tn*6218 similar to the *cfr*-carrying transposon described in *C. difficile*. While the *cfr*(B) described by Bender et al. [128] was found in *Tn*6218-like elements possible linked to plasmids.

It has been shown that the gene *cfr* is functionally active in Gram-negative hosts [45]. Furthermore, it has been identified chromosomally located (inserted into the chromosomal *fimD* gene) in *P. vulgaris* from pigs, and in diverse plasmids in *E. coli* from pigs [45,130–134] or food of animal origin [135]. The IS26 appears to play an important role in the transfer of this multiresistance gene in Gram-negative bacteria, since it appears in the *cfr*-carrying plasmids detected in *E. coli* [45,130–135]. One of these *cfr*-carrying plasmids from *E. coli* of swine origin carried also the extended-spectrum-β-lactamase (ESBL) gene *bla*$_{CTX-M-14b}$ [133].

4.3.3. Other Genes in Animal-Associated *S. aureus*

S. aureus from animals can be related to various CCs [90,136,137]. However, animals are considered the main reservoir of the specific *S. aureus* lineage CC398, which has been the subject of numerous studies during recent years [18,19,82,138–143]. Studies based on the phylogenetic analysis of genome-wide single nucleotide polymorphisms (SNPs) supported the existence of two subpopulations in CC398: an ancestral human-adapted clade and an animal-associated clade [144,145]. Nevertheless, LA-MRSA CC398 isolates of the animal-associated clade are able to infect humans [119,145]. Analysis of genes present in CC398 has revealed numerous genes in common with clinical *S. aureus* and/or other staphylococci, but also some novel or rare resistance genes have been found in animal-related isolates from this lineage [79,81]. Some of these rare or novel genes are often on plasmids encoding for other AMR-genes such as the multi-resistance gene *cfr* (Table 5).

One interesting gene, found in animal-associated *S. aureus*, is the phenicol exporter gene *fexA*. It was first described in a bovine *S. lentus* isolate, but later it has been found in diverse plasmids of LA-MRSA CC398 from pigs, cattle and horses, as well as on plasmids from the also animal-related *S. aureus* CC9 [79,81]. This gene has been related to the non-conjugative transposon *Tn*558 that has been detected (partially or complete) in plasmids or in the chromosome of various CoNS of animal origin [79]. The *fexA* is co-located in plasmids with additional resistance genes (Table 5). Interestingly, the *fexA* gene has been described in *cfr*-carrying plasmids of clinical important MRSA pandemic lineages [114,120].

The tetracycline gene *tet*(L) was found initially in the 80s in diverse plasmids from *Bacillus*. In staphylococci, it was first described in the early 90s on a plasmid from a porcine *S. hyicus*. In addition, subsequently, it was detected on structurally diverse plasmids of staphylococci of animal origin [77,79]. This gene has been found co-located on plasmids from staphylococci with other additional antimicrobial and heavy metals resistance genes (Table 5). Regarding LA-MRSA CC398, the gene *tet*(M) is the most frequent tetracycline-resistant gene found in these isolates, although it is accompanied frequently by *tet*(K) and *tet*(L) [139]. The gene *tet*(L) has also been described in clinical *S. aureus* in the 90s [146], and recently in a *cfr*-carrying plasmid with additional antimicrobial genes [*dfrK* and *aadD*] in a clinical *S. aureus* ST125 strain [121].

The trimethoprim resistance gene *dfrK* was discovered co-located on a plasmid with *tet*(L) in LA-MRSA CC398 [79,81]. Similar to other genes in staphylococci, the *dfrK* has been found on diverse plasmids co-located with other antimicrobial and heavy metals resistance genes (Table 5). The *dfrK* gene is widely disseminated in LA-MRSA CC398 and it has been found in isolates from pigs, cattle and poultry [79]; but it has also been found chromosomally located on the transposon *Tn*559 of MSSA CC398 [147]. Additionally, the *Tn*559 carrying *dfrK* has been found in *E. faecium* [43].

Table 5. Examples of resistance genes co-located on plasmids from Staphylococci.

AAG	Gene(s)	apmA	spc	aacA-aphD	aadD	blaZ	ble	fosD	cadXD	copA	mco	erm(A)	erm(B)	erm(C)	erm(T)	erm(33)	lnu(B)	lsa(B)	lsa(E)	vga(A)	vga(C)	fexA	cfr	tet(K)	tet(L)	tet(M)	optrA	dfrK
AC	apmA	/			■				■	■	■		■												■			■
	spc		/												■	■						■						
AG	aacA-aphD			/	■	■	■	■					■				■	■		■	■	■	■		■	■	■	
	aadD	■			/		■	■					■							■	■	■	■	■	■	■		
BL	blaZ			■		/		■					■					■							■			
BM	ble			■		■	/	■												■						■		
FM	fosD			■	■	■	■	/															■					
HM	cadXD	■		■	■				/	■	■			■											■			■
	copA	■			■				■	/	■																	
	mco	■			■				■	■	/																	
	erm(A)											/											■					
MLSB	erm(B)	■		■					■	■	■		/				■	■		■					■			■
	erm(C)								■	■				/	■										■			
	erm(T)				■				■	■				■	/										■			■
	erm(33)			■												/	■											
LN	lnu(B)			■					■				■				/	■							■			
	lsa(B)	■			■								■		■			/	■									
LPSA	lsa(E)			■											■				/	■					■			
	vga(A)				■															/					■	■	■	
	vga(C)				■																/	■						
Ph	fexA			■	■								■		■							/	■		■			
PhLOPSAA	cfr			■	■	■	■	■	■		■	■										■	/		■			
TC	tet(K)			■					■															/				
	tet(L)	■			■								■									■			/	■		■
	tet(M)																			■					■	/	■	
OP	optrA			■	■															■						■	/	■
TM	dfrK	■			■				■	■			■		■										■		■	/

A black square indicates that the corresponding resistance gene(s) can be found co-located together in plasmids. This table is based on the plasmids described by Fan et al. [41], Gómez-Sanz et al. [148], Gopegui et al. [121], Kadlec et al. [79], Li et al. [68], Shen et al. [45], Schwarz et al. [78,80] and Wendlandt et al. [81]. AAG, antimicrobial agent(s) group; AC, aminocylitols; AG, aminoglycosides; BL, B-lactams; BM, bleomycin; FM, fosfomycin; HM, heavy metals; LN, lincosamides; LPSA, lincosamides-pleuromutilins-streptogramin A; MLSB, macrolide-lincosamide-streptogramin B; OP, oxazolidinones-phenicols; Ph, phenicol; PhLOPSAA, phenicols, lincosamides, oxazolidinones, pleuromutilins and streptogramin A; TC, tetracycline; TM, trimethoprim.

The *erm*(T) gene has been previously identified in other Gram-positive bacteria (such as *Streptococcus* and *Lactobacillus*) [79]. In staphylococci, this gene has been originally found in animal-associated CC398, but further research suggested that it is particularly associated to the MRSA and MSSA CC398 from the ancestral human clade [79,149,150]. Nevertheless, a recent study comparing *erm*(T)-carrying plasmids from *S. aureus* ST398 from pig and humans, showed that these plasmids are quite similar and all carried additional tetracycline [*tet*(L)] and heavy metal (*cadD-cadX*, *copA*, *mco*) resistance genes [148]. The plasmid (pUR1902) recovered from a pig isolate carried also *aadD* as a plasmid (pUR2941) from a human isolate, while the remaining plasmid (pUR2940) from a human isolate additionally carried *erm*(C) and *dfrK* [148].

A recent review by Wendlandt et al. [81] underlined the presence of diverse multidrug resistance (MDR) genes co-located together or with other resistance genes on plasmids in staphylococci from animal origin. These genes included MLS$_B$ [*erm*(A), *erm*(B), *erm*(C), *erm*(T), *erm*(33)], lincosamides-pleuromutilins-streptogramin A [*lsa*(E), *vga*(A), *vga*(C)] and PhLOPSA$_A$ (*cfr*) resistance genes [81]. The main resistance mechanisms conferred by these MDR genes included target modification by methylation (*erm* and *cfr* genes) and active efflux via ABC transporters [*vga* and *lsa*(E) genes] [81]. Their location on plasmids, co-located with other AMR-genes, may potentiate their co-selection and persistence in animal staphylococci, and furthermore represent an important pool of resistance against critically and highly important antimicrobial agents [81].

5. AMR-Genes in Gram-Negative Bacteria from Animals

The Gram-negative members of the ESC(K)APE group are *A. baumannii*, *P. aeruginosa*, and the members of Enterobacteriaceae. A large number of antimicrobial resistance genes have been described in Gram-negative bacteria [44,47]. Since this area is extremely large and complex, in this section, we summarize part of the current knowledge about AMR in *A. baumannii*, *P. aeruginosa* and Enterobacteriaceae from animals, with special attention to the emergence of carbapenemase-producing Gram-negative bacteria in animals (Table 6) and the emergence of the colistin resistance.

Table 6. Examples of carbapenemase genes found in Gram-negative bacteria from animals.

Gene	Species	Origin
bla$_{IMP-4}$	*P. aeruginosa*	Dog
bla$_{NDM-1}$	*A. baumannii*	Pig
	E. coli, S. enterica	Various livestock and wildlife animals
bla$_{NDM-5}$	*E. coli*	Fowl
bla$_{NDM-9}$	*E. coli*	Chicken
bla$_{OXA-23}$	*A. baumannii*	Various livestock and companion animals
	A. lwoffi	Poultry
bla$_{OXA-48}$	*E. coli, K. pneumoniae*	Companion animals
bla$_{OXA-58}$	*A. baumannii*	Fowl
bla$_{OXA-497}$	*A. baumannii*	Dairy cattle
bla$_{VIM-1}$	*E. coli, S. enterica*	Various livestock, companion and wildlife animals
bla$_{VIM-2}$	*P. aeruginosa*	Cattle, fowl

Based on Al Bayssari et al. [151], Fisher et al. [152], Guerra et al. [153], Michael et al. [154], Schwarz et al. [155], Wang et al. [156], Webb et al. [157] and Zhang et al. [158].

5.1. Acinetobacter baumannii

A. baumannii is an important nosocomial pathogen that usually affects immunocompromised patients suffering from various underlying diseases [159]. Nosocomial infection with this bacterium has been associated with increased morbidity, mortality and health care costs [160]. It is responsible of hospital outbreaks, and it has a remarkable ability to survive for prolonged periods throughout hospital environments [160]. It is well established that the members of the genus *Acinetobacter* are ubiquitous microorganisms. However, *A. baumannii* as a highly prevalent microorganism in nature, is a misconception because the difficulties encountered in its identification [159,160]. In fact, *A. baumannii* is phenotypically and genotypically closely related to other *Acinetobacter* species (*A. pittii*, *A. nosocomialis* and *A. calcoaceticus*), making the species identification challenging [159].

A. baumannii has been related with community-acquired infections (single events or case series) [160], and has been isolated from various environmental locations: soils contaminated with petroleum hydrocarbons, vegetables, inanimate surfaces in contact with humans, manured agricultural soil, pig slurry and aquaculture environments [160]. Multi-susceptible *Acinetobacter* isolates were commonly found in the 70s–80s in soil and in the hospital setting, clinical *A. baumannii* being easily treated with common antibiotics during this period [20,159]. However, this bacterium has an extraordinary ability to upregulate or acquire resistance determinants, and nowadays infections with multidrug or even pandrug resistant isolates are increasing [159].

During the last decade, *A. baumannii* strains have also been isolated from animals, mainly causing outbreaks in veterinary clinics or hospitals [160]. *A. baumannii* strains have been isolated from diverse animals including ducks, pigeons, chickens, donkeys, rabbits, pets (cats and dogs), mules, livestock (cattle, caws, goats, pigs), horses, lice and arthropods [161]. In a study based on PFGE, it was seen that isolates from livestock were different than *A. baumannii* human strains [162]. Yet, isolates recovered from pig fecal samples harbored bla_{OXA-51}, which has already been reported in human clinical isolates [162]. In the same study new bla_{OXA-51}-like genes ($bla_{OXA-148}$, $bla_{OXA-149}$ and $bla_{OXA-150}$), not previously detected in human isolates, were described in bacteria from cattle [162]. However, it is important to underline that the bla_{OXA-23} and bla_{OXA-51}-like genes may be naturally occurring in *A. baumannii* [163]. On the other hand, the studies in companion animals have reported *A. baumannii* isolates genetically similar to the nosocomial European (also called International) clones I, II and III, suggesting its spread from humans to animals directly or via the environment [159,160,164,165].

Regarding the distribution of AMR-genes in *A. baumannii* in animals, some studies have reported the emergence of carbapenemase producing *A. baumannii* in livestock and companion animals [153,159] (Table 6). The bla_{OXA-23} is a wide distributed carbapenemase gene in *A. baumannii* isolates, which has been described recently in livestock and/or pets [151,153,154,159,165]. The bla_{OXA-23} gene has also been found in *A. lwoffi* from poultry [154]. In *A. baumannii* this gene has been found in STs not previously reported in humans, as well as in *A. baumannii* strains belonging to ST2, which has been previously related to hospitals outbreaks [151]. The bla_{OXA-58} has been found together with bla_{OXA-23} in *A. baumannii* from fowl [151]. Similarly, a bla_{NDM-1} positive *A. baumannii* isolate has been recovered from a pig suffering from pneumonia and sepsis [158]. This bla_{NDM-1} was harbored by a plasmid also carrying other AMR-genes [*aphA6*, *ble* and *msr*(E)-*mph*(E)] [158]. The bla_{NDM-1} has been found in other *Acinetobacter* species [*A. junii* (from a pig farm) and *A. calcoaceticus* (from around a cow farm)] recovered from environmental samples and farm animals [155,166]. A new carbapenemase ($bla_{OXA-497}$) has been found in *A. baumannii* from dairy cattle [157]. A class 1 integron similar to an integron of a human isolate has been also identified in an equine *A. baumannii* isolate [167].

Currently, there are some reports underlying the emergence of *A. baumannii* strains resistant to both carbapenems and polymyxins (colistin and polymyxin B) in the clinical setting [168]. Resistance rates against polymyxins varied from 0.7% to 6.5% depending on the country [168]. Most polymyxin resistant strains from Europe have been recovered in Greece and Italy [168]. Interestingly, recent reports have also underlined the presence of colistin and polymyxin B resistant *A. baumannii* and other *Acinetobacter* spp. isolates in meat (chicken, turkey, beef and pork) [169,170]. Resistance to polymyxins in *A. baumannii* is mediated by mutations in the genes *pmrA* and/or *pmrB* [168]. Nevertheless, a new colistin resistance mechanism mediated by plasmids (the *mcr*-genes, see Section 5.3.4) has emerged in Enterobacteriaceae [168]. Although no clinical or environmental *A. baumannii* isolates carrying *mcr*-genes have yet been described, a recent study has proved that *A. baumannii* transformed with *mcr-1* carrying plasmids had increased colistin resistance [171]. This finding highlights the threat of a possible dissemination of these *mcr*-genes to multidrug resistant *A. baumannii* [171].

5.2. Pseudomonas aeruginosa

P. aeruginosa is an opportunistic pathogen often found in water and soil that is pathogenic to plants, humans, farm animals and companion animals. In humans, it is a cause of community and nosocomial infections, especially in patients immunocompromised and/or with cystic fibrosis. In animals, it caused pyoderma, otitis and urinary tract infections in companion animals, mastitis in dairy cows, endometritis in horses and hemorrhagic pneumoniae in fur-bearing animals [172–176]. Due to the presence of several drug efflux systems and porins, as well as its cell wall with low permeability, *P. aeruginosa* is intrinsically resistant to a wide range of antimicrobials including benzylpenicillins, aminobenzylpenicillins, carboxypenicillins, first and second generation cephalosporins, chloramphenicol and tetracycline [172,173]. Moreover, this bacterium is able to form biofilms and to acquire diverse resistance mechanisms.

The studies about AMR in animals are scarce, and mainly have focused in companion animals. A study has shown that *P. aeruginosa* isolates recovered from diverse veterinary samples during 1994–2003 have high resistance rates against β-lactams (70–100%) and sulphonamides (80–90%), while resistance against quinolones an aminoglycosides are more variable, with resistances ranging from 5 to 98% depending of the antibiotic [173]. Similar results were found in a study with canine isolates recovered between 2003 and 2006, although an increase in quinolone resistance was seen [174]. Resistance rates to the former antimicrobials are also similar in current studies among companion animals, although higher resistance rates against the aminoglycoside gentamicin [177] and the quinolone enrofloxacin [176] have been found. In *P. aeruginosa* from companion animals, the resistance to quinolones has been related to point mutations in *gyrA*, *gyrB*, *parC* and/or *parE* genes [172,176], and the resistance to aminoglycoside has been associated to diverse resistance genes (such as *aacA4* and *aadA6*) [172,176]. Resistance rates are generally lower in *P. aeruginosa* from livestock comparing to strains from companion animals [174,175].

Regarding its potential as zoonotic pathogen, a recent study by Haenni et al. [174] confirmed that the *P. aeruginosa* population in veterinary samples from France has a non-clonal epidemic structure. There was a poor association between an animal species and a specific clone, even though certain clones, possibly correlating with higher pathogenicity, seem to be more prevalent than others [174]. Clones associated to human outbreaks were detected, but not the most frequent epidemic clones associated to MDR in humans (also called "high risk clones") [174].

The presence of ESBLs (via phenotypic methods) has been confirmed in *P. aeruginosa* isolates from animals [176,178]. Moreover, some reports have underlined the emergence of *P. aeruginosa* isolates with carbapenemases in animals (Table 6). The gene bla_{IMP-4} has been found in *P. aeruginosa* from dog [156], and the gene bla_{VIM-2} has been found in *P. aeruginosa* from cattle and fowl [151].

Similar to *A. baumannii*, recent reports have underlined the emergence of polymyxin-resistant *P. aeruginosa* [168]. Resistance rates are low (0.5% to 1.1%) in most countries, although, the situation is worrying in China where 22.2% of extensively drug-resistant bacteraemic *P. aeruginosa* isolates are resistant to polymyxin B [168]. Diverse mechanisms of polymyxin resistance have been described in *P. aeruginosa*, even though no clinical or environmental strains carrying *mcr*-genes have been reported [168]. Nevertheless, the recent study by Liu et al. [171] showed that *P. aeruginosa* isolates transformed with plasmids carrying *mcr-1* only had moderate changes in colistin susceptibility.

5.3. Enterobacteriaceae

As some Enterobacteriaceae (Ex. *Salmonella enterica*, *Yersinia enterocolitica*) are typically food-borne pathogens, this section will mainly focus on some transmissible AMRs-genes that have emerged in Enterobacteriaceae from animals (Table 7). The recent discover of the *cfr* gene in Enterobacteriaceae has been discussed at Section 4.3.2.

Table 7. Examples of important plasmid-associated resistance mechanisms in Enterobacteriaceae from animals.

Antimicrobial Group	Resistance Mechanism	Example Gene(s)
Aminoglycosides	Enzymatic inactivation (acetylation)	*acc(3)-IV*
Aminoglycosides/Quinolones	Enzymatic inactivation (acetylation)	*aac(6′)-Ib-cr*
β-lactams	Enzymatic inactivation (hydrolization)	*bla*$_{CTX-M}$
Quinolones	Target replacement (pentapeptide repeat protein)	*qnr*
	Active efflux (MFS transporter)	*qepA*
	Active efflux (RND transporter)	*oqxAB*
PhLOPSA$_A$	Target site modification (rRNA methylation)	*cfr*
Polymyxins	Target site modification (PEtN transferase)	*mcr*

Based on Baron et al. [179], Rodríguez-Martínez et al. [180] and Shen et al. [45]. MFS, Major Facilitator Superfamily; PEtN, phosphoethanolamine; PhLOPSA$_A$, phenicols, lincosamides, oxazolidinones, pleuromutilins and streptogramin A; RND, resistance-nodulation-cell division family.

5.3.1. Emergence of Streptothricin-Resistant *E. coli* in the 1980s

Similarly to Gram-positive bacteria, the use of antibiotics as grown promotors in the animal husbandry may potentiate the emergence of resistant Enterobacteriaceae isolates in food animals. A good example is the emergence of streptothricin-resistant *E. coli* in the 1980s. The aminoglycosidic growth promoter nourseothricin (streptothricin) was used in farm animals in Germany during the 1980s, while no equivalent antimicrobials were used in humans over this period [49]. Resistance emerged in *E. coli* from pigs the second year after the introduction of this antibiotic. It was mediated by a plasmid containing a transposon coding for a streptothricin acetyltransferase [181]. Subsequently, this resistance was found in *E. coli* isolated from pig farmers, in the community and in other Enterobacteriaceae from humans (*Salmonella* and *Shigella*) [49]. Nowadays, streptothricin-resistance is extensively extended and it is also characteristic of Gram-positive bacteria such as enterococci and staphylococci [182].

5.3.2. ESBL/AmpC-Carrying Enterobacteriaceae in Animals

Bacteria carrying ESBLs are a worldwide clinical problem. ESBLs are mainly plasmid-encoded enzymes providing an extended resistance to β-lactam antibiotics, due to their ability to inactivate cephalosporins [49,183]. They can be produced by a variety of different bacteria including Enterobacteriaceae or no-fermenting bacteria (such as *P. aeruginosa*), *E. coli* and *K. pneumoniae* being the most frequently found ESBL-producing bacteria. ESBL-producing bacteria are known as nosocomial pathogens and since the late 1990s they have been increasingly found as a causal agent of infections in the community [183]. Until the 90s, the vast majority of ESBLs identified in human clinical isolates were SHV (sulfhydryl-variable) or TEM (named Temoneira for the first patient from whom the pathogen was isolated) types [184]. However, later, CTX-M (cefotaximase) β-lactamases have emerged and currently they are the most prevalent ESBLs in human Enterobacteriaceae [184].

The occurrence of ESBL-producing bacteria has been broadly recognized in veterinary medicine since the 2000s [183,184]. ESBL-producing bacteria have been found as disease agents and/or colonizers in livestock, companion animals, zoo animals and wild animals [54,183–186]. *E. coli* and *Klebsiella* spp. are cause of mastitis in dairy cattle, but most often livestock animals are asymptomatic carriers of ESBLs producers [54,187]. The first ESBL-producing *E. coli* was isolated from a dog with urinary tract infection and it carried SHV-12 [188]. Later on diverse CTX-M, TEM and SHV types have been observed in *E. coli*, *Salmonella* spp. and *K. pneumoniae* from livestock and companion animals [54,155,183,185,186]. The β-lactamases CTX-M-1, CTX-M-14, CTX-M-15, SHV-12 and TEM-52 are the most frequent types in Enterobacteriaceae from animals [54,155,183,185–187]. This distribution is similar in humans, where CTX-M types are the major β-lactamases in *E. coli* and *Klebsiella* spp. [54,183]. Host-range plasmids of different incompatibility groups (such as IncN, IncI, incF and IncK) have been related to these bla_{CTX-M} genes [154].

Identical phylogenic lineages (such as ST131) have been found in *E. coli* isolates from humans and animals [184]. The risk of zoonotic transfer from livestock to people with close contact to these animals is still largely unknown, but some studies have implicated a transfer of ESBL-producing *E. coli* or ESBLs genes from poultry or pigs to farm workers [183] Besides this direct zoonotic transfer, other routes as foods of animal origin may be a risk factor for human colonization or infection. In a recent study 70.6% of tested farms were ESBL-positive [183]. In one case the same isolate was detected in human and cattle samples, indicating a zoonotic transfer. In few other cases, pig and human isolates shared the same ESBLs genes, although the isolates belonged to different lineages suggesting horizontal gene transfer.

In contrast to the situation in Europe, ESBL genes have not been commonly reported in animal isolates in North America [154]. In North America, the plasmid-encoded AmpC B-lactamases genes are more frequently found [154], but these genes have also been described in Europe [54]. The broad-spectrum cephalosporinases (AmpC) were the first β-lactamases described in *E. coli* [47], and nowadays they have emerged worldwide [184]. As for ESBLs, *E. coli* carrying AmpC (bla_{CMY-2}) has been identified in animals during the 2000s [184]. These β-lactamases have been detected in *E. coli* and *Salmonella* spp. from livestock and companion animals, being CMY-2 the most frequent one [184,185]. Other AmpC β-lactamases encoding by bla_{ACC} type genes have also been detected in *Salmonella* spp. from livestock [153,184].

5.3.3. Carbapenemase-Producing Enterobacteriaceae in Animals

The carbapenemases are β-lactamases able of degrading carbapenems [153]. The epidemiologically most important carbapenemases are class B metallo-β-lactamases (MBLs) such as VIM (Verona integron-encoded MBL), IMP (imipenemase) and NDM (New Delhi MBL), class A, such as, KPC (*K. pneumoniae* carbapenemase), and class D including OXA (Carbapenem-hydrolysing oxacillinase) carbapenemases [153]. Resistance due to carbapenemases is mainly linked to the nosocomial setting, since carbapenems are not approved for use in veterinary medicine. However, they may be use for companion animals under certain conditions [154]. Although they are not used in livestock, carbapenem-resistant bacteria have been isolated from farm animals in recent years [154]. In animals, the first carbapenemase gene, bla_{VIM-1}, was found in a porcine *E. coli* and it was linked to a multiresistance class 1 integron [152]. Later on, this and other carbapenemases have been found in livestock, wildlife and companion animals (Table 6), notably bla_{VIM-1} in *S. enterica* serovar Infantis and *E. coli* from livestock; bla_{NDM-1} in *S. enterica* sevorar Corvallis and *E. coli* from wild animals and/or livestock; bla_{OXA-48} in *E. coli* and *K. pneumoniae* from companion animals [153,155]. Carbapenemases have been detected in other Gram-negative bacteria including *A. baumannii* (see Section 5.1) and *P. aeruginosa* (see Section 5.2). However, the limited reports suggested that carbapenem-resistant bacteria are still at a very low prevalence in livestock [154].

5.3.4. *mcr*-Genes Mediating Colistin Resistance

Colistin, also named polymyxin E, is currently used as a last-line drug against MDR Gram-negative bacteria [168,179]. However, resistance against colistin has even emerged in humans without contact to this antibiotic [189]. Moreover, since the 60s colistin has been used in pig production for therapeutic (in monotherapy), prophylactic and grown promotions purposes [190]. In addition, to its use in pigs, polymyxins (especially polymyxin B), are used in some countries for the treatment of coliform and *Pseudomonas* mastitis in cows [190]. Polymyxins are used in companion animals (dogs and cats) for topical indications such as otitis and ophthalmic diseases [190].

Colistin resistance is frequently due to chromosomal mutations and it has been detected in *P. aeruginosa*, *A. baumannii* and Enterobacteriaceae [168,179]. Most mechanisms conferring resistance against colistin are related to modifications of its primary target, the lipid A moiety of lipopolysaccharide (LPS) [168,179]. Colistin resistance mechanisms are different across bacterial genera, but most implied lipid A modifications with 4-amino-4-deoxy-L-arabinose (L-ara4N) and/or phosphoethanolamine (PEtN) [168,179].

The chromosomal-related colistin resistance mechanisms have no possibly of horizontal transfer, but plasmid-related genes (*mcr-1*, *mcr-2*) coding for PEtN transferases have recently emerged. The first *mcr*-gene, corresponded to *mcr-1*. It was initially described in an IncI2 plasmid from an *E. coli* from a pig, but in the same study it was soon after found in *E. coli* and *K. pneumoniae* from patients [191]. This gene was discovered in November 2015, but recent research has identified this gene in *E. coli* collections from the 80s [179]. The amino-acid sequence of MCR-1 showed that it was closely related (63%) to the PEtN transferase EptA found in *Paenibacillus sophorae* and *Enhydrobacter aerosaccus* [191]. Interestingly, the polymyxin is biosynthesized in *Paenibacillus* spp. [191]. Structural analysis of the MCR-1 complete protein showed that it was closely related to the PEtN transferases LptA of *Neisseria meningitidis* and EptC of *Campylobacter jejuni*, which are also known to be intrinsically resistant to polymyxin [179,191]. Further research showed that the prevalence of the *mcr-1* gene was 20% in animal strains and 1% in human strains in China, and nowadays it has been also detected in animal and human isolates recovered from other countries covering Europe, Africa and America [168,179,187].

The *mcr-1* gene has been identified in Enterobacteriaceae from humans, food, farm animals, wildlife, and environment samples [190]. Although it has been mainly detected (80%) in *E. coli*, it has also been described in *Klebsiella*, *Salmonella*, *Shigella* and *Enterobacter* [168,179]. In addition, it has recently been detected in *Cronobacter sakazakii* [192]. Interestingly, the *mcr-1* gene has been related to diverse plasmid incompatibility groups including IncFIA, IncFIB, IncFIC, IncFI, IncFII, IncHI2, IncI1, IncI2, IncN, IncP, IncQ1, IncX1, IncX4, IncY and pVT553 [168,179,190]. This gene has also been related to a class 1 integron within an IncFII plasmid [193]. Moreover, *mcr-1* has been identified in ESBL and carbapenamase producing Enterobacteriaceae from animals and humans (Table 8).

Table 8. Associated β-lactam resitances in colistin-resistant *mcr-1* carrying isolates.

Species	Origin	Associated β-Lactam Resitances		
		ESBLs	AmpC	Carbapenemases
C. sakazakii	A	-	-	NDM-9
E. coli	A	CTX-M-1, CTX-M-2, CTX-M-8, CTX-M-15, CTX-M-27, CTX-M-55, TEM-1	CMY-2, LAT-1	NDM-1, NDM-5, NDM-9
	F	CTX-M-1, CTX-M-14, CTX-M-15, CTX-M-55, CTX-M-65, SHV-12, TEM-1, TEM-52	CMY-2	NDM-9, OXA-1
	H	CTX-M-1, CTX-M-2, CTX-M-8, CTX-M-14, CTX-M-15, CTX-M-27, CTX-M-55, CTX-M-65, SHV-12, TEM-1, TEM-52	ACT-15, CMY-2, DHA-1	KPC-2, NDM-1, NDM-5, OXA-1, OXA-48, VIM-1
	E	SHV-12, TEM-1	-	-
	W	CTX-M-2, CTX-M-14	-	-
Enterobacter spp.	H	CTX-M-15, TEM-1	-	KPC-2, OXA-1
K. pneumoniae	H	CTX-M-1, SHV-11, TEM-1	-	KPC-3, NDM-5
S. enterica	A	TEM-1	-	-
	F	CTX-M-1, TEM-1	-	-
	H	TEM-1	CMY-2	-

Based on Delgado-Blas et al. [194], Di Pilato et al. [195], Jeannot et al. [168], Kong et al. [196], Liu et al. [192] and Mediavilla et al. [197]. A, animal origin; E, environmental origin; F, food origin; H, human origin; W, wildlife origin.

A variant (with only a SNP of difference) of *mcr-1*, *mcr-1.2* has been detected on a transferable IncX4 plasmid in a *K. pneumoniae* recovered from a patient [195]. This *mcr-1.2* strain also carried β-lactamases genes (*bla*TEM-1, *bla*SHV-11, and *bla*KPC-3) [195]. Very recently, a novel plasmid mediated colistin resistance gene, *mcr-2* has been discovered [198]. This *mcr-2* has been found in an IncX4 plasmid of *E. coli* from porcine and bovine origin in Belgium [198]. This gene corresponded to a new *mcr*-gene, since MCR-1 and MCR-2 shared 80.7% of similarity [198]. It has been seen that the *mcr-2* gene had higher prevalence than *mcr-1* in *E. coli* isolates from porcine origin [198].

Food animals seem the main source of human contamination by the *mcr*-genes [190]. However, the *mcr-1* gene has also been detected in *E. coli* carried or infecting humans without animal contact [190]. These findings underlined that this gene, which probably has emerged in the animal sector, is already widespread in the environment and it is transmissible via various routes to humans [190,199].

5.3.5. Other AMR-Genes in Enterobacteriaceae from Animals

Increasing levels of quinolone resistance among Enterobacteriaceae and other bacteria (*Campylobacter* spp.) have been a particular case of concern since the 90s [155]. The extended use of quinolones to treat poultry infections has increased the quinolone resistance among *E. coli* strains in poultry industry [200]. Although quinolone resistance is generally not highly frequent in animal farming, high and/or moderate levels of quinolone resistance have been reported in poultry [200].

The mechanisms of quinolone resistance in Enterobacteriaceae from animals are similar to those described in isolates from humans [201]. Mutations at *gyrA* (DNA gyrase) and/or *parC* (topoisomerase IV) genes were responsible of quinolone resistance in *E. coli* and *Salmonella* spp. isolates from animals [155,201]. Moreover, reports about plasmid-mediated quinolone resistance (PMQR) genes [*qnr*, *acc(6)-Ib-cr*, *qepA*, *oqxAB*] in bacteria from animal origin have been published since 2000s [155,180].

The Qnr proteins are encoded by several variants of *qnr* genes (*qnrA*, *qnrB*, *qnrC*, *qnrD*, *qnrS*), being the *qnrS1* gene variant the most frequently reported and worldwide diffused in animal and human samples [200] (Table 9). Some *qnr* genes have been described in Enterobacteriaceae (mainly *Salmonella* spp. and *E. coli*) of animal origin [155,180,202]. Their wide distribution suggests an origin prior to the inclusion of quinolones in medicine [180]. It has been suggested that these genes have originated in bacteria from the natural environment [20]. In fact, *qnr* genes have been found in aquatic and waterborne organisms such as *Shewanella*, *Aeromonas* and *Citrobacter* species, and in the Vibrionaceae family [20,180].

As the *qnr* genes, PMQR efflux pump genes (*qepA* and *oqxAB*) have also a wide distribution, and they have been found in diverse Enterobacteriaceae from animals and humans [155,180] (Table 9). These genes are related to transmissible plasmids, although *oqxAB* is also commonly found in the chromosome of *K. pneumoniae* [180]. Other plasmid-mediated efflux pumps affecting quinolones have been described sporadically [180].

The *cr* variant of the aminoglycoside *aac(6′)-Ib* resistance gene was discover in 2006 [203]. The *aac(6′)-Ib* gene encodes a aminoglycoside acetyltransferase able to confer resistance against kanamycin, tobramycin and amikacin. The two mutations present at *aac(6′)-Ib-cr* confer low level ciprofloxacine resistance, with a slightly cost to the levels of aminoglycoside resistance [203]. Hence, it acts additively together with Qnr proteins to generate quinolone resistance [201]. This gene is widely distributed in Gram-negative bacteria (Table 9).

Regarding other aminoglycoside resistance genes, the gene *aac(3)-IV*, which confers cross-resistance between gentamicin and apramycin, need to be underlined [204]. It was originally isolated in 1981 from an *E. coli* recovered from farm animals in France. Although apramycin has only veterinary use, this gene has been detected in Enterobacteriaceae from human patients and wastewater from a residential area [204]. It has been suggested that apramycin consumption at farm level has increased the occurrence of *aac(3)-IV* positive *E. coli* in pigs [204].

Table 9. Examples of distribution of certain PMQR-genes.

Gene	Species	Origin
	Aeromonas spp.	E, W
	C. freundii, C. koseri, Enterobacter spp., *P. aeruginosa, P. mirabilis, Stenothrophomonas maltophilia, Shigella* spp.	H
acc(6)-Ib-cr	*E. coli*	C, E, F, H, L, W, Z
	Haemophilus parasuis	L
	K. pneumoniae	C, H, Z
	Laribacter hongkongensis	E, W
	Salmonella spp.	E, F, H, L, W
	E. coli	E, F, H, L, W, Z
oqxAB	*K. pneumoniae*	H
	Salmonella spp.	F, H, L
	E. coli	C, E, H, L
qepA	*K. pneumoniae*	H
	Salmonella spp.	F, H
	Shigella spp.	H, E
	C. freundii, E. cloacae, K. pneumoniae, P. aeruginosa, P. mirabilis	H
qnrA1	*E. coli*	C, L
	H. parasuis	L
	Salmonella spp.	H, L
qnrA3	*Shewanella algae*	E
qnrA6	*E. coli, K. pneumoniae, Morganella morganii, P. mirabilis*	H
qnrB1	*C. freundii, K. pneumoniae*	H
	E. coli	H, W
	C. freundii, K. pneumoniae	H
qnrB2	*E. coli*	C, H, L
	Salmonella spp.	E, H, L
	C. freundii	H
qnrB4	*E. coli*	L
	Salmonella spp.	H, L
qnrB5	*Salmonella* spp.	F
	E. coli	E, L
qnrB6	*H. parasuis*	L
	K. pneumoniae	H
	Salmonella spp.	W
qnrB7	*Salmonella* spp.	H
qnrB8-variant	*C. freundii*	H
qnrB9	*C. freundii*	E
qnrB10	*C. freundii, K. pneumoniae*	H
	E. coli	L

Table 9. *Cont.*

Gene	Species	Origin
qnrB12	*Salmonella* spp.	H, L
qnrB17	*Aeromonas* spp.	E, W
	E. coli	L
qnrB19	*E. coli*	C, E, H, L
	K. pneumoniae	H
	Salmonella spp.	F, H, L, W
qnrB24	*C. freundii*	H
qnrD	*E. coli*	E, L
	P. mirabilis	C, H, E
	Salmonella spp.	F, H, L
qnrS1	*E. coli*	C, E, F, H, L, W, Z
	Enterobacter spp.	E
	K. pneumoniae, Shigella spp.	H
	Salmonella spp.	E, F, H, L, W
qnrS2	*Aeromonas* spp.	E, W
	E. coli	F
	Pseudomonas spp., *Pseudoalteromonas* spp.	E
qnrS5	*Aeromonas* spp.	E, W

Based on Rodriguez–Martinez et al. [180], Schwarz et al [155] and Veldman et al. [202]. C, companion animals origin; E, environmental origin; F, food origin; H, human origin; L, livestock origin; W, wildlife origin; Z, zoo animals.

Several other aminoglycoside resistance genes [such as *aac(3)-II, aac(3)-III, aadA1, aadA2, aadA5* and *ant(2″)-I*] have been described in *E. coli* from animal origin [200]. Other aminoglycoside resistance genes [*aac(3)-I, ant(2″)-Ia* and *aac(6)-Ib*] are more related to human *E. coli* isolates [200].

Enterobacteriaceae from animals carry other resistance genes. For example, a moderate incidence of chloramphenicol resistance is registered in *E. coli* from food animals in Europe, mainly mediated by genes such as *catA1, floR* and *cmlA1* [200]. Other chloramphenicol resistance genes (such as *catB*) are more frequent in human *E. coli* isolates [200].

E. coli isolates from animals carry also diverse sulfonamide (*sul1, sul2, sul3*), tetracycline [*tet*(A), *tet*(B)], and trimethoprim (*dfrA1, dfrA12, dfrA17*) resistance genes [200,204]. Interestingly, the gene *sul3* was first detected in an *E. coli* isolate from a pig, and later it was found in both healthy and diseased humans [204].

6. Conclusions

The continuous antibiotic selective pressure in human and animal health may contribute to the mobilization of acquired resistance genes. This is illustrated by several facts: (i) some studies have suggested that the *mecA* gene may have originated in animal related staphylococci; (ii) it has recently been observed that two mutiresistance genes (*cfr* and *optrA*) associated to MGEs such as plasmids along with other AMR-genes, have a wide dissemination in Gram-positive bacteria from animals and humans; (iii) typical nosocomial resistances linked to ESBLs and carbapenemases are emerging in Gram-negative bacteria from animals; and (iv) the *mcr*-genes, which may probably have emerged in the animal sector are currently spreading among human and animal *E. coli* isolates. These examples underline the fact that bacteria from animals represent an important pool of resistance genes for human pathogens.

Resistance to antibiotics is escalating, and at the same time the current pipeline of new antimicrobials is running dry, creating an ever increasing gap. Since a complete ban on the use of antimicrobials in farm animals would have serious repercussions for animal health, welfare and productivity, we need to use these agents more prudently in both human and animal medicine [3]. Rapid diagnosis tools are needed to determine therapy strategies more quickly and accurately, as well as the further examination of alternatives to antimicrobials for farm animals (such as phage therapy or vaccines) [3]. We are facing the possibility of a future without effective antibiotics for some infections and a scenario where infections that hitherto were considered harmless, are now a serious health problem and a major cause of morbidity, mortality, together with major financial and social repercussions.

Acknowledgments: We thank members of our laboratories and our microbiologist colleagues for their support to the Belgian National Reference Centre—*Staphylococcus aureus*.

Author Contributions: Maria Angeles Argudín conceived, designed and wrote the manuscript, Ariane Deplano, Alaeddine Meghraou, Magali Dodémont, Amelie Heinrichs, Olivier Denis, Claire Nonhoff and Sandrine Roisin revised the manuscript.

Abbreviations

l-ara4N	4-amino-4-deoxy-l-arabinose
ABC	ATP-binding cassette
AMR	antimicrobial resistance
CC	clonal complex
CoNS	coagulase negative staphylococci
CTX-M	cefotaximase
ECDC	European Centre for Disease Prevention and Control
EFSA	European Food Safety Authority
erm	erythromycin ribosomal methylase
ESBLs	extended spectrum beta-lactamases
ESC(K)APE	*E. faecium, S. aureus, Clostridium difficile, A. baumannii, P. aeruginosa,* and Enterobacteriaceae
ESKAPE	*Enterococcus faecium, S. aureus, Klebsiella pneumoniae, Acinetobacter baumannii, Pseudomonas aeruginosa,* and *Enterobacter* spp.
HIV	human immunodeficiency virus
IMP	imipenemase
IS	insertion sequence
KPC	*K. pneumoniae* carbapenemase
QRDR	quinolone-resistance determining region
LA-MRSA	livestock-associated methicillin resistant *Staphylococcus aureus*
LPS	lipopolysaccharide
MBL	metallo-β-lactamase
MFS	Major Facilitator Superfamily
MGE	mobile genetic element
MLS$_B$	macrolide-lincosamide-streptogramin B
MLST	multilocus sequence typing
MRCoNS	methicillin resistant coagulase negative staphylococci
MDR	multidrug resistance
MRSA	methicillin resistant *Staphylococcus aureus*
MRSE	methicillin-resistant *Staphylococcus epidermidis*
MSSA	methicillin susceptible *S. aureus*
NDM	New Delhi metallo-β-lactamases
OIE	World Organization for Animal Health

OXA   carbapenem-hydrolysing oxacillinase
PBP   penicillin binding protein
PCR   polymerase chain reaction
PEtN   phosphoethanolamine
PFGE   pulsed-field gel electrophoresis
PMQR   plasmid-mediated quinolone resistance
PVL   Panton-Valentine leucocidin
REA   restriction enzyme analysis
RND   resistance-nodulation-cell division family
RT   ribotype
SCC*mec*   staphylococcal cassette chromosome *mec*
SHV   sulfhydryl-variable β-Lactamase
SNP   single nucleotide polymorphism
ST   sequence type
TEM   Temoneira β-Lactamase
VIM   Verona integron-encoded metallo-β-lactamase
VRE   vancomycin-resistant enterococci
WHO   World Health Organization

References

1. Butaye, P.; Argudín, M.A.; Threlfall, J. Introduction to antimicrobial-resistant foodborne pathogens. In *Antimicrobial Resistance and Food Safety: Methods and Techniques*, 1st ed.; Chen, C.Y., Yan, X., Jackson, C.R., Eds.; Academic Press: Cambridge, MA, USA, 2015; pp. 1–18; ISBN 978-0-12-801214-7.

2. O'Neill, J. *Tackling Drug-Resistant Infections Globally: Final Report and Recommendations. The Review on Antimicrobial Resistance*; HM Government and the Wellcome Trust: London, UK, 2016. Available online: https://amr-review.org/sites/default/files/160518_Final%20paper_with%20cover.pdf (accessed on 27 March 2017).

3. Woolhouse, M.; Ward, M.; van Bunnik, B.; Farrar, J. Antimicrobial resistance in humans, livestock and the wider environment. *Philos Trans. R. Soc. Lond. Ser. B Biol. Sci.* **2015**, *370*, 20140083. [CrossRef] [PubMed]

4. Rice, L.B. Federal funding for the study of antimicrobial resistance in nosocomial pathogens: No ESKAPE. *J. Infect. Dis.* **2008**, *197*, 1079–1081. [CrossRef] [PubMed]

5. De Rosa, F.G.; Corcione, S.; Pagani, N.; Di Perri, G. From ESKAPE to ESCAPE, from KPC to CCC. *Clin. Infect. Dis.* **2015**, *60*, 1289–1290. [CrossRef] [PubMed]

6. Robinson, T.P.; Bu, D.P.; Carrique-Mas, J.; Fèvre, E.M.; Gilbert, M.; Grace, D.; Hay, S.I.; Jiwakanon, J.; Kakkar, M.; Kariuki, S.; et al. Antibiotic resistance is the quintessential One Health issue. *Trans. R. Soc. Trop. Med. Hyg.* **2016**, *110*, 377–380. [CrossRef] [PubMed]

7. One Health Initiative Will Unite Human and Veterinary Medicine. Available online: http://www.onehealthinitiative.com/index.php (accessed on 5 January 2017).

8. Da Costa, P.M.; Loureiro, L.; Matos, A.J. Transfer of multidrug-resistant bacteria between intermingled ecological niches: The interface between humans, animals and the environment. *Int. J. Environ. Res. Public Health* **2013**, *10*, 278–294. [CrossRef] [PubMed]

9. McEwen, S.A.; Fedorka-Cray, P.J. Antimicrobial use and resistance in animals. *Clin. Infect. Dis.* **2002**, *34*, S93–S106. [CrossRef] [PubMed]

10. Thanner, S.; Drissner, D.; Walsh, F. Antimicrobial resistance in agriculture. *mBio* **2016**, *7*, e02227. [CrossRef] [PubMed]

11. World Health Organization. *Critically Important Antimicrobials for Human Medicine*, 5th ed.; World Health Organization: Geneva, Switzerland, 2017; ISBN 978-92-4-151222-0.

12. World Organisation for Animal Health. Available online: http://www.oie.int/en/ (accessed on 27 March 2017).

13. Anonymous. OIE List of Antimicrobial Agents of Veterinary Importance. World Organisation for Animal Health (OIE), 2015. Available online: http://www.oie.int/en/our-scientific-expertise/veterinary-products/antimicrobials/ (accessed on 27 March 2017).

14. FDA. Summary Report on Antimicrobials Sold or Distributed for Use in Food Producing Animals. 2015. Available online: http://www.fda.gov/downloads/ForIndustry/UserFees/ AnimalDrugUserFeeActADUFA/UCM534243.pdf (accessed on 27 March 2017).

15. FAO. Drivers, Dynamics and Epidemiology of Antimicrobial Resistance in Animal Production. 2016. Available online: http://www.fao.org/3/a-i6209e.pdf (accessed on 27 March 2017).

16. Yazdankhah, S.; Rudi, K.; Bernhoft, A. Zinc and copper in animal feed—Development of resistance and co-resistance to antimicrobial agents in bacteria of animal origin. *Microb. Ecol. Health Dis.* **2014**, *25*. [CrossRef] [PubMed]

17. Argudín, M.A.; Butaye, P. Dissemination of metal resistance genes among animal methicillin-resistant coagulase-negative staphylococci. *Res. Vet. Sci.* **2016**, *105*, 192–194. [CrossRef] [PubMed]

18. Argudín, M.A.; Lauzat, B.; Kraushaar, B.; Alba, P.; Agerso, Y.; Cavaco, L.; Butaye, P.; Porrero, M.C.; Battisti, A.; Tenhagen, B.A.; et al. Heavy metal and disinfectant resistance genes among livestock-associated methicillin-resistant *Staphylococcus aureus* isolates. *Vet. Microbiol.* **2016**, *191*, 88–95. [CrossRef] [PubMed]

19. Sharma, M.; Nunez-Garcia, J.; Kearns, A.M.; Doumith, M.; Butaye, P.R.; Argudín, M.A.; Lahuerta-Marin, A.; Pichon, B.; AbuOun, M.; Rogers, J.; et al. Livestock-associated methicillin resistant *Staphylococcus aureus* (LA-MRSA) clonal complex (CC) 398 isolated from UK animals belong to European lineages. *Front. Microbiol.* **2016**, *7*, 1741. [CrossRef] [PubMed]

20. Finley, R.L.; Collignon, P.; Larsson, D.G.; McEwen, S.A.; Li, X.Z.; Gaze, W.H.; Reid-Smith, R.; Timinouni, M.; Graham, D.W.; Topp, E. The scourge of antibiotic resistance: The important role of the environment. *Clin. Infect. Dis.* **2013**, *57*, 704–710. [CrossRef] [PubMed]

21. Agga, G.E.; Arthur, T.M.; Durso, L.M.; Harhay, D.M.; Schmidt, J.W. Antimicrobial-resistant bacterial populations and antimicrobial resistance genes obtained from environments impacted by livestock and municipal waste. *PLoS ONE* **2015**, *10*, e0132586. [CrossRef] [PubMed]

22. Chen, B.; Yuan, K.; Chen, X.; Yang, Y.; Zhang, T.; Wang, Y.; Luan, T.; Zou, S.; Li, X. Metagenomic analysis revealing antibiotic resistance genes (ARGs) and their genetic compartments in the Tibetan environment. *Environ. Sci. Technol.* **2016**, *50*, 6670–6679. [CrossRef] [PubMed]

23. Allen, H.K. Antibiotic resistance gene discovery in food-producing animals. *Curr. Opin. Microbiol.* **2014**, *19*, 25–29. [CrossRef] [PubMed]

24. Pal, C.; Bengtsson-Palme, J.; Kristiansson, E.; Larsson, D.G. The structure and diversity of human, animal and environmental resistomes. *Microbiome* **2016**, *4*, 54. [CrossRef] [PubMed]

25. Fitzpatrick, D.; Walsh, F. Antibiotic resistance genes across a wide variety of metagenomes. *FEMS Microbiol. Ecol.* **2016**, *92*, 168. [CrossRef] [PubMed]

26. Durso, L.M.; Harhay, G.P.; Bono, J.L.; Smith, T.P. Virulence-associated and antibiotic resistance genes of microbial populations in cattle feces analyzed using a metagenomic approach. *J. Microbiol. Method* **2011**, *84*, 278–282. [CrossRef] [PubMed]

27. Qu, A.; Brulc, J.M.; Wilson, M.K.; Law, B.F.; Theoret, J.R.; Joens, L.A.; Konkel, M.E.; Angly, F.; Dinsdale, E.A.; Edwards, R.A. Comparative metagenomics reveals host specific metavirulomes and horizontal gene transfer elements in the chicken cecum microbiome. *PLoS ONE* **2008**, *3*, e2945. [CrossRef] [PubMed]

28. Looft, T.; Johnson, T.A.; Allen, H.K.; Bayles, D.O.; Alt, D.P.; Stedtfeld, R.D.; Sul, W.J.; Stedtfeld, T.M.; Chai, B.; Cole, J.R.; et al. In-feed antibiotic effects on the swine intestinal microbiome. *Proc. Natl. Acad. Sci. USA* **2012**, *109*, 1691–1696. [CrossRef] [PubMed]

29. Zhu, Y.-G.; Johnson, T.A.; Su, J.-Q.; Qiao, M.; Guo, G.-X.; Stedtfeld, R.D.; Hashsham, S.A.; Tiedje, J.M. Diverse and abundant antibiotic resistance genes in Chinese swine farms. *Proc. Natl. Acad. Sci. USA* **2013**, *110*, 3435–3440. [CrossRef] [PubMed]

30. Alexander, T.W.; Yanke, J.L.; Reuter, T.; Topp, E.; Read, R.R.; Selinger, B.L.; McAllister, T.A. Longitudinal characterization of antimicrobial resistance genes in feces shed from cattle fed different subtherapeutic antibiotics. *BMC Microbiol.* **2011**, *11*, 19. [CrossRef] [PubMed]

31. Chambers, L.; Yang, Y.; Littier, H.; Ray, P.; Zhang, T.; Pruden, A.; Strickland, M.; Knowlton, K. Metagenomic analysis of antibiotic resistance genes in dairy cow feces following therapeutic administration of third generation cephalosporin. *PLoS ONE* **2015**, *10*, e0133764. [CrossRef] [PubMed]

32. Wichmann, F.; Udikovic-Kolic, N.; Andrew, S.; Handelsman, J. Diverse antibiotic resistance genes in dairy cow manure. *mBio* **2014**, *5*, e01017. [CrossRef] [PubMed]

33. Durso, L.M.; Miller, D.N.; Wienhold, B.J. Distribution and quantification of antibiotic resistant genes and bacteria across agricultural and nonagricultural metagenomes. *PLoS ONE* **2012**, *7*, e48325. [CrossRef] [PubMed]

34. Kazimierczak, K.A.; Scott, K.P.; Kelly, D.; Aminov, R.I. Tetracycline resistome of the organic pig gut. *Appl. Environ. Microbiol.* **2009**, *75*, 1717–1722. [CrossRef] [PubMed]

35. Brown Kav, A.; Sasson, G.; Jami, E.; Doron-Faigenboim, A.; Benhar, I.; Mizrahi, I. Insights into the bovine rumen plasmidome. *Proc. Natl. Acad. Sci. USA* **2012**, *109*, 5452–5457. [CrossRef] [PubMed]

36. Heuer, H.; Binh, C.T.; Jechalke, S.; Kopmann, C.; Zimmerling, U.; Krögerrecklenfort, E.; Ledger, T.; González, B.; Top, E.; Smalla, K. IncP-1ε plasmids are important vectors of antibiotic resistance genes in agricultural systems: Diversification driven by class 1 integron gene cassettes. *Front. Microbiol.* **2012**, *3*, 2. [CrossRef] [PubMed]

37. Allen, H.K.; Looft, T.; Bayles, D.O.; Humphrey, S.; Levine, U.Y.; Alt, D.; Stanton, T.B. Antibiotics in feed induce prophages in swine fecal microbiomes. *mBio* **2011**, *2*, e00260. [CrossRef] [PubMed]

38. Brenciani, A.; Morroni, G.; Vincenzi, C.; Manso, E.; Mingoia, M.; Giovanetti, E.; Varaldo, P.E. Detection in Italy of two clinical *Enterococcus faecium* isolates carrying both the oxazolidinone and phenicol resistance gene *optrA* and a silent multiresistance gene *cfr*. *J. Antimicrob. Chemother.* **2016**, *71*, 1118–1119. [CrossRef] [PubMed]

39. Deshpande, L.M.; Ashcraft, D.S.; Kahn, H.P.; Pankey, G.; Jones, R.N.; Farrell, D.J.; Mendes, R.E. Detection of a new *cfr*-like gene, *cfr*(B), in *Enterococcus faecium* isolates recovered from human specimens in the United States as part of the SENTRY Antimicrobial Surveillance Program. *Antimicrob. Agents Chemother.* **2015**, *59*, 6256–6261. [CrossRef] [PubMed]

40. He, T.; Shen, Y.; Schwarz, S.; Cai, J.; Lv, Y.; Li, J.; Feßler, A.T.; Zhang, R.; Wu, C.; Shen, J.; et al. Genetic environment of the transferable oxazolidinone/phenicol resistance gene *optrA* in *Enterococcus faecalis* isolates of human and animal origin. *J. Antimicrob. Chemother.* **2016**, *71*, 1466–1473. [CrossRef] [PubMed]

41. Fan, R.; Li, D.; Wang, Y.; He, T.; Feßler, A.T.; Schwarz, S.; Wu, C. Presence of the *optrA* gene in methicillin-resistant *Staphylococcus sciuri* of porcine origin. *Antimicrob. Agents Chemother.* **2016**, *60*, 7200–7205. [CrossRef] [PubMed]

42. Liu, Y.; Wang, Y.; Dai, L.; Wu, C.; Shen, J. First report of multiresistance gene *cfr* in *Enterococcus* species *casseliflavus* and *gallinarum* of swine origin. *Vet. Microbiol.* **2014**, *170*, 352–357. [CrossRef] [PubMed]

43. López, M.; Kadlec, K.; Schwarz, S.; Torres, C. First detection of the staphylococcal trimethoprim resistance gene *dfrK* and the *dfrK*-carrying transposon *Tn559* in enterococci. *Microb. Drug Resist.* **2012**, *18*, 13–18. [CrossRef] [PubMed]

44. Roberts, M.C.; Schwarz, S.; Aarts, H.J. Erratum: Acquired antibiotic resistance genes: An overview. *Front. Microbiol.* **2012**, *3*, 384. [CrossRef] [PubMed]

45. Shen, J.; Wang, Y.; Schwarz, S. Presence and dissemination of the multiresistance gene *cfr* in Gram-positive and Gram-negative bacteria. *J. Antimicrob. Chemother.* **2013**, *68*, 1697–1706. [CrossRef] [PubMed]

46. Spigaglia, P. Recent advances in the understanding of antibiotic resistance in *Clostridium difficile* infection. *Ther. Adv. Infect. Dis.* **2016**, *3*, 23–42. [CrossRef] [PubMed]

47. Van Hoek, A.H.; Mevius, D.; Guerra, B.; Mullany, P.; Roberts, A.P.; Aarts, H.J. Acquired antibiotic resistance genes: An overview. *Front. Microbiol.* **2011**, *2*, 203. [CrossRef] [PubMed]

48. Wendlandt, S.; Feßler, A.T.; Monecke, S.; Ehricht, R.; Schwarz, S.; Kadlec, K. The diversity of antimicrobial resistance genes among staphylococci of animal origin. *Int. J. Med. Microbiol.* **2013**, *303*, 338–349. [CrossRef] [PubMed]

49. Hunter, P.A.; Dawson, S.; French, G.L.; Goossens, H.; Hawkey, P.M.; Kuijper, E.J.; Nathwani, D.; Taylor, D.J.; Teale, C.J.; Warren, R.E.; et al. Antimicrobial-resistant pathogens in animals and man: Prescribing, practices and policies. *J. Antimicrob. Chemother.* **2010**, *65*, i3–i17. [CrossRef] [PubMed]

50. Yutin, N.; Galperin, M.Y. A genomic update on clostridial phylogeny: Gram-negative spore formers and other misplaced clostridia. *Environ. Microbiol.* **2013**, *15*, 2631–2641. [CrossRef] [PubMed]

51. Lawson, P.A.; Citron, D.M.; Tyrrell, K.L.; Finegold, S.M. Reclassification of *Clostridium difficile* as *Clostridioides difficile* (Hall and O'Toole 1935) Prévot 1938. *Anaerobe* **2016**, *40*, 95–99. [CrossRef] [PubMed]

52. March, J.W.; Harrison, L.H. *Clostridium difficile*: A food safety concern? In *Antimicrobial Resistance and Food Safety: Methods and Techniques*, 1st ed.; Chen, C.Y., Yan, X., Jackson, C.R., Eds.; Academic Press: Cambridge, MA, USA, 2015; pp. 181–206.

53. Keessen, E.C.; Hensgens, M.P.; Spigaglia, P.; Barbanti, F.; Sanders, I.M.; Kuijper, E.J.; Lipman, L.J. Antimicrobial susceptibility profiles of human and piglet *Clostridium difficile* PCR-ribotype 078. *Antimicrob. Resist. Infect. Control* **2013**, *2*, 14. [CrossRef] [PubMed]

54. Dahms, C.; Hübner, N.O.; Wilke, F.; Kramer, A. Mini-review: Epidemiology and zoonotic potential of multiresistant bacteria and *Clostridium difficile* in livestock and food. *GMS Hyg. Infect. Control* **2014**, *9*. [CrossRef]

55. Norén, T.; Johansson, K.; Unemo, M. *Clostridium difficile* PCR ribotype 046 is common among neonatal pigs and humans in Sweden. *Clin. Microbiol. Infect.* **2014**, *20*, O2–O6. [CrossRef] [PubMed]

56. Roberts, M.C. Update on macrolide-lincosamide-streptogramin, ketolide, and oxazolidinone resistance genes. *FEMS Microbiol. Lett.* **2008**, *282*, 147–159. [CrossRef] [PubMed]

57. Marín, M.; Martín, A.; Alcalá, L.; Cercenado, E.; Iglesias, C.; Reigadas, E.; Bouza, E. *Clostridium difficile* isolates with high linezolid MICs harbor the multiresistance gene *cfr*. *Antimicrob. Agents Chemother.* **2015**, *59*, 586–589. [CrossRef] [PubMed]

58. Hansen, L.H.; Vester, B. A *cfr*-like gene from *Clostridium difficile* confers multiple antibiotic resistance by the same mechanism as the *cfr* gene. *Antimicrob. Agents Chemother.* **2015**, *59*, 5841–5843. [CrossRef] [PubMed]

59. Hargreaves, K.R.; Thanki, A.M.; Jose, B.R.; Oggioni, M.R.; Clokie, M.R. Use of single molecule sequencing for comparative genomics of an environmental and a clinical isolate of *Clostridium difficile* ribotype 078. *BMC Genom.* **2016**, *17*, 1020. [CrossRef] [PubMed]

60. Hammerum, A.M. Enterococci of animal origin and their significance for public health. *Clin. Microbiol. Infect.* **2012**, *18*, 619–625. [CrossRef] [PubMed]

61. Ghosh, A.; Zurek, L. Antibiotic resistance in Enterococci: A food safety perspective. In *Antimicrobial Resistance and Food Safety: Methods and Techniques*, 1st ed.; Chen, C.Y., Yan, X., Jackson, C.R., Eds.; Academic Press: Cambridge, MA, USA, 2015; pp. 155–180.

62. Garrido, A.M.; Gálvez, A.; Pulido, R.P. Antimicrobial Resistance in *Enterococci*. *J. Infect. Dis. Ther.* **2014**, *2*, 150. [CrossRef]

63. Arias, C.A.; Murray, B.E. Emergence and management of drug-resistant enterococcal infections. *Expert Rev. Anti Infect. Ther.* **2008**, *6*, 637–655. [CrossRef] [PubMed]

64. Arias, C.A.; Murray, B.E. The rise of the Enterococcus: Beyond vancomycin resistance. *Nat. Rev. Microbiol.* **2012**, *10*, 266–278. [CrossRef] [PubMed]

65. Bates, J.; Jordens, Z.; Selkon, J.B. Evidence for an animal origin of vancomycin-resistant enterococci. *Lancet* **1993**, *342*, 490–491. [CrossRef]

66. Woodford, N.; Palepou, M.F.; Johnson, A.P.; Chadwick, P.R.; Bates, J. Methicillin-resistant *Staphylococcus aureus* and vancomycin-resistant enterococci. *Lancet* **1997**, *350*, 738. [CrossRef]

67. Wang, Y.; Lv, Y.; Cai, J.; Schwarz, S.; Cui, L.; Hu, Z.; Zhang, R.; Li, J.; Zhao, Q.; He, T.; et al. A novel gene, *optrA*, that confers transferable resistance to oxazolidinones and phenicols and its presence in *Enterococcus faecalis* and *Enterococcus faecium* of human and animal origin. *J. Antimicrob. Chemother.* **2015**, *70*, 2182–2190. [CrossRef] [PubMed]

68. Li, D.; Wang, Y.; Schwarz, S.; Cai, J.; Fan, R.; Li, J.; Feßler, A.T.; Zhang, R.; Wu, C.; Shen, J. Co-location of the oxazolidinone resistance genes *optrA* and *cfr* on a multiresistance plasmid from *Staphylococcus sciuri*. *J. Antimicrob. Chemother.* **2016**, *71*, 1474–1478. [CrossRef] [PubMed]

69. Huang, J.; Chen, L.; Wu, Z.; Wang, L. Retrospective analysis of genome sequences revealed the wide dissemination of *optrA* in Gram-positive bacteria. *J. Antimicrob. Chemother.* **2016**, *72*, 614–616. [CrossRef] [PubMed]

70. Kluytmans, J.; van Belkum, A.; Verbrugh, H. Nasal carriage of *Staphylococcus aureus*: Epidemiology, underlying mechanisms, and associated risks. *Clin. Microbiol. Rev.* **1997**, *10*, 505–520. [PubMed]

71. Kluytmans, J.A.; Wertheim, H.F. Nasal carriage of *Staphylococcus aureus* and prevention of nosocomial infections. *Infection* **2005**, *33*, 3–8. [CrossRef] [PubMed]

72. Wertheim, H.F.L.; Melles, D.C.; Vos, M.C.; van Leeuven, W.; van Belkum, A.; Verbrugh, H.A.; Nouwen, J.L. The role of nasal carriage in *Staphylococcus aureus* infections. *Lancet Infect. Dis.* **2005**, *5*, 751–762. [CrossRef]

73. Van Belkum, A.; Verkaik, N.J.; de Vogel, C.P.; Boelens, H.A.; Verveer, J.; Nouwen, J.L.; Wertheim, H.F. Reclassification of *Staphylococcus aureus* nasal carriage types. *J. Infect. Dis.* **2009**, *199*, 1820–1826. [CrossRef] [PubMed]

74. Mandell, G.L.; Bennett, J.E.; Dolin, R. *Staphylococcus aureus* (including Staphylococcal Toxic Shock). In *Bennett's-Principles and Practice of Infectious Diseases*; Waldvogel, F.A., Ed.; Churchill Livingstone: Philadelphia, PA, USA, 2000.

75. Argudín, M.Á.; Mendoza, M.C.; Rodicio, M.R. Food poisoning and *Staphylococcus aureus* enterotoxins. *Toxins* **2010**, *2*, 1751–1773. [CrossRef] [PubMed]

76. Fitzgerald, J.R.; Penades, J.R. Staphylococci of Animals. In *Staphylococcus Molecular Genetics*, 1st ed.; Lindsay, J., Ed.; Caister Academic Press: Haverhill, UK, 2008; pp. 255–269; ISBN 978-1-904455-29-5.

77. Werckenthin, C.; Cardoso, M.; Martel, J.L.; Schwarz, S. Antimicrobial resistance in staphylococci from animals with particular reference to bovine *Staphylococcus aureus*, porcine *Staphylococcus hyicus*, and canine *Staphylococcus intermedius*. *Vet. Res.* **2001**, *32*, 341–362. [CrossRef] [PubMed]

78. Schwarz, S.; Fessler, A.T.; Hauschild, T.; Kehrenberg, C.; Kadlec, K. Plasmid-mediated resistance to protein biosynthesis inhibitors in staphylococci. *Ann. N. Y. Acad. Sci.* **2011**, *1241*, 82–103. [CrossRef] [PubMed]

79. Kadlec, K.; Fessler, A.T.; Hauschild, T.; Schwarz, S. Novel and uncommon antimicrobial resistance genes in livestock-associated methicillin-resistant *Staphylococcus aureus*. *Clin. Microbiol. Infect.* **2012**, *18*, 745–755. [CrossRef] [PubMed]

80. Schwarz, S.; Shen, J.; Wendlandt, S.; Fessler, A.T.; Wang, Y.; Kadlec, K.; Wu, C.M. Plasmid-mediated antimicrobial resistance in Staphylococci and other firmicutes. *Microbiol. Spectr.* **2014**, *2*. [CrossRef] [PubMed]

81. Wendlandt, S.; Shen, J.; Kadlec, K.; Wang, Y.; Li, B.; Zhang, W.J.; Feßler, A.T.; Wu, C.; Schwarz, S. Multidrug resistance genes in staphylococci from animals that confer resistance to critically and highly important antimicrobial agents in human medicine. *Trends Microbiol.* **2015**, *23*, 44–54. [CrossRef] [PubMed]

82. Argudín, M.A.; Tenhagen, B.A.; Fetsch, A.; Sachsenröder, J.; Käsbohrer, A.; Schroeter, A.; Hammerl, J.A.; Hertwig, S.; Helmuth, R.; Bräunig, J.; et al. Virulence and resistance determinants of German *Staphylococcus aureus* ST398 isolates from nonhuman sources. *Appl. Environ. Microbiol.* **2011**, *277*, 3052–3060. [CrossRef] [PubMed]

83. Argudín, M.A.; Vanderhaeghen, W.; Butaye, P. Diversity of antimicrobial resistance and virulence genes in methicillin-resistant non-*Staphylococcus aureus* staphylococci from veal calves. *Res. Vet. Sci.* **2015**, *99*, 10–16. [CrossRef] [PubMed]

84. International Working Group on the Classification of Staphylococcal Cassette Chromosome Elements (IWG-SCC). Classification of staphylococcal cassette chromosome *mec* (SCC*mec*): Guidelines for reporting novel SCC*mec* elements. *Antimicrob. Agents Chemother.* **2009**, *53*, 4961–4967. [CrossRef]

85. Hiramatsu, K.; Ito, T.; Tsubakishita, S.; Sasaki, T.; Takeuchi, F.; Morimoto, Y.; Katayama, Y.; Matsuo, M.; Kuwahara-Arai, K.; Hishinuma, T.; et al. Genomic Basis for methicillin resistance in *Staphylococcus aureus*. *Infect. Chemother.* **2013**, *45*, 117–136. [CrossRef] [PubMed]

86. Wu, Z.; Li, F.; Liu, D.; Xue, H.; Zhao, X. Novel Type XII Staphylococcal Cassette Chromosome *mec* harboring a new cassette chromosome recombinase, CcrC2. *Antimicrob. Agents Chemother.* 2015 *59*, 7597–7601. [CrossRef] [PubMed]

87. Vanderhaeghen, W.; Vandendriessche, S.; Crombé, F.; Dispas, M.; Denis, O.; Hermans, K.; Haesebrouck, F.; Butaye, P. Species and staphylococcal cassette chromosome *mec* (SCC*mec*) diversity among methicillin-resistant non-*Staphylococcus aureus* staphylococci isolated from pigs. *Vet. Microbiol.* **2012**, *158*, 123–128. [CrossRef] [PubMed]

88. Argudín, M.A.; Vanderhaeghen, W.; Butaye, P. Antimicrobial resistance and population structure of *Staphylococcus epidermidis* recovered from pig farms in Belgium. *Vet. J.* **2015**, *203*, 302–308. [CrossRef] [PubMed]

89. Argudín, M.A.; Vanderhaeghen, W.; Vandendriessche, S.; Vandecandelaere, I.; André, F.X.; Denis, O.; Coenye, T.; Butaye, P. Antimicrobial resistance and population structure of *Staphylococcus epidermidis* recovered from animals and humans. *Vet. Microbiol.* **2015**, *178*, 105–113. [CrossRef] [PubMed]

90. Butaye, P.; Argudín, M.A.; Smith, T.C. Livestock-associated MRSA and its current evolution. *Curr. Clin. Microbiol. Rep.* **2016**, *3*, 19–31. [CrossRef]

91. Becker, K.; Ballhausen, B.; Köck, R.; Kriegeskorte, A. Methicillin resistance in *Staphylococcus* isolates: The "*mec* alphabet" with specific consideration of *mecC*, a *mec* homolog associated with zoonotic *S. aureus* lineages. *Int. J. Med. Microbiol.* **2014**, *304*, 794–804. [CrossRef] [PubMed]

92. Argudín, M.A.; Mendoza, M.C.; González-Hevia, M.A.; Bances, M.; Guerra, B.; Rodicio, M.R. Genotypes, exotoxin gene content, and antimicrobial resistance of *Staphylococcus aureus* strains recovered from foods and food handlers. *Appl. Environ. Microbiol.* **2012**, *78*, 2930–2935. [CrossRef] [PubMed]

93. Argudín, M.A.; Mendoza, M.C.; Martín, M.C.; Rodicio, M.R. Molecular basis of antimicrobial drug resistance in *Staphylococcus aureus* isolates recovered from young healthy carriers in Spain. *Microb. Pathog.* **2014**, *74*, 8–14. [CrossRef] [PubMed]

94. Seah, C.; Alexander, D.C.; Louie, L.; Simor, A.; Low, D.E.; Longtin, J.; Melano, R.G. MupB, a new high-level mupirocin resistance mechanism in *Staphylococcus aureus*. *Antimicrob. Agents Chemother.* **2012**, *56*, 1916–1920. [CrossRef] [PubMed]

95. Strauss, C.; Hu, Y.; Coates, A.; Perreten, V. A Novel *erm*(44) gene variant from a human *Staphylococcus saprophyticus* isolate confers resistance to macrolides and lincosamides but not streptogramins. *Antimicrob. Agents Chemother.* **2016**, *61*, e01655. [CrossRef] [PubMed]

96. Wipf, J.R.; Schwendener, S.; Perreten, V. The novel macrolide-lincosamide-streptogramin B resistance gene *erm*(44) is associated with a prophage in *Staphylococcus xylosus*. *Antimicrob. Agents Chemother.* **2014**, *58*, 6133–6138. [CrossRef] [PubMed]

97. Wipf, J.R.; Schwendener, S.; Nielsen, J.B.; Westh, H.; Perreten, V. The new macrolide-lincosamide-streptogramin B resistance gene *erm*(45) is located within a genomic island in *Staphylococcus fleurettii*. *Antimicrob. Agents Chemother.* **2015**, *59*, 3578–3581. [CrossRef] [PubMed]

98. Nemeghaire, S.; Vanderhaeghen, W.; Argudín, M.A.; Haesebrouck, F.; Butaye, P. Characterization of methicillin-resistant *Staphylococcus sciuri* isolates from industrially raised pigs, cattle and broiler chickens. *J. Antimicrob. Chemother.* **2014**, *69*, 2928–2934. [CrossRef] [PubMed]

99. Nemeghaire, S.; Argudín, M.A.; Haesebrouck, F.; Butaye, P. Molecular epidemiology of methicillin-resistant *Staphylococcus sciuri* in healthy chickens. *Vet. Microbiol.* **2014**, *171*, 357–363. [CrossRef] [PubMed]

100. Nemeghaire, S.; Argudín, M.A.; Feßler, A.T.; Hauschild, T.; Schwarz, S.; Butaye, P. The ecological importance of the *Staphylococcus sciuri* species group as a reservoir for resistance and virulence genes. *Vet. Microbiol.* **2014**, *171*, 342–356. [CrossRef] [PubMed]

101. Tsubakishita, S.; Kuwahara-Arai, K.; Sasaki, T.; Hiramatsu, K. Origin and molecular evolution of the determinant of methicillin resistance in staphylococci. *Antimicrob. Agents Chemother.* **2010**, *54*, 4352–4359. [CrossRef] [PubMed]

102. Tsubakishita, S.; Kuwahara-Arai, K.; Baba, T.; Hiramatsu, K. Staphylococcal cassette chromosome *mec*-like element in *Macrococcus caseolyticus*. *Antimicrob. Agents Chemother.* **2010**, *54*, 1469–1475. [CrossRef] [PubMed]

103. García-Álvarez, L.; Holden, M.T.; Lindsay, H.; Webb, C.R.; Brown, D.F.; Curran, M.D.; Walpole, E.; Brooks, K.; Pickard, D.J.; Teale, C.; et al. Meticillin-resistant *Staphylococcus aureus* with a novel *mecA* homologue in human and bovine populations in the UK and Denmark: A descriptive study. *Lancet Infect. Dis.* **2011**, *11*, 595–603. [CrossRef]

104. Shore, A.C.; Deasy, E.C.; Slickers, P.; Brennan, G.; O'Connell, B.; Monecke, S.; Ehricht, R.; Coleman, D.C. Detection of staphylococcal cassette chromosome *mec* type XI carrying highly divergent *mecA*, *mecI*, *mecR1*, *blaZ*, and *ccr* genes in human clinical isolates of clonal complex 130 methicillin-resistant *Staphylococcus aureus*. *Antimicrob. Agents Chemother.* **2011**, *55*, 3765–3773. [CrossRef] [PubMed]

105. Gómez-Sanz, E.; Schwendener, S.; Thomann, A.; Gobeli Brawand, S.; Perreten, V. First Staphylococcal cassette chromosome *mec* containing a *mecB*-carrying gene complex independent of transposon Tn6045 in a *Macrococcus caseolyticus* isolate from a canine infection. *Antimicrob. Agents Chemother.* **2015**, *59*, 4577–4583. [CrossRef] [PubMed]

106. Petersen, A.; Stegger, M.; Heltberg, O.; Christensen, J.; Zeuthen, A.; Knudsen, L.K.; Urth, T.; Sorum, M.; Schouls, L.; Larsen, J.; et al. Epidemiology of methicillin-resistant *Staphylococcus aureus* carrying the novel *mecC* gene in Denmark corroborates a zoonotic reservoir with transmission to humans. *Clin. Microbiol Infect.* **2013**, *19*, E16–E22. [CrossRef] [PubMed]

107. Espinosa-Gongora, C.; Harrison, E.M.; Moodley, A.; Guardabassi, L.; Holmes, M.A. MRSA carrying *mecC* in captive mara. *J. Antimicrob. Chemother.* **2015**, *70*, 1622–1624. [CrossRef] [PubMed]

108. Deplano, A.; Vandendriessche, S.; Nonhoff, C.; Denis, O. Genetic diversity among methicillin-resistant *Staphylococcus aureus* isolates carrying the *mecC* gene in Belgium. *J. Antimicrob. Chemother.* **2010**, *69*, 1457–1460. [CrossRef] [PubMed]

109. Harrison, E.M.; Paterson, G.K.; Holden, M.T.; Morgan, F.J.; Larsen, A.R.; Petersen, A.; Leroy, S.; De Vliegher, S.; Perreten, V.; Fox, L.K.; et al. A *Staphylococcus xylosus* isolate with a new *mecC* allotype. *Antimicrob. Agents Chemother.* **2013**, *57*, 1524–1528. [CrossRef] [PubMed]

110. Harrison, E.M.; Paterson, G.K.; Holden, M.T.; Ba, X.; Rolo, J.; Morgan, F.J.; Pichon, B.; Kearns, A.; Zadoks, R.N.; Peacock, S.J.; et al. A novel hybrid SCC*mec-mecC* region in *Staphylococcus sciuri*. *J. Antimicrob. Chemother.* **2014**, *69*, 911–918. [CrossRef] [PubMed]

111. Loncaric, I.; Kübber-Heiss, A.; Posautz, A.; Stalder, G.L.; Hoffmann, D.; Rosengarten, R.; Walzer, C. Characterization of methicillin-resistant *Staphylococcus* spp. carrying the *mecC* gene, isolated from wildlife. *Antimicrob. Chemother.* **2013**, *68*, 2222–2225. [CrossRef] [PubMed]

112. Małyszko, I.; Schwarz, S.; Hauschild, T. Detection of a new *mecC* allotype, *mecC2*, in methicillin-resistant *Staphylococcus saprophyticus*. *J. Antimicrob. Chemother.* **2014**, *69*, 2003–2005. [CrossRef] [PubMed]

113. Mendes, R.E.; Deshpande, L.M.; Jones, R.N. Linezolid update: Stable in vitro activity following more than a decade of clinical use and summary of associated resistance mechanisms. *Drug Resist. Updat.* **2014**, *17*, 1–12. [CrossRef] [PubMed]

114. Shore, A.C.; Lazaris, A.; Kinnevey, P.M.; Brennan, O.M.; Brennan, G.I.; O'Connell, B.; Feßler, A.T.; Schwarz, S.; Coleman, D.C. First report of *cfr*-carrying plasmids in the pandemic Sequence Type 22 methicillin-resistant *Staphylococcus aureus* Staphylococcal Cassette Chromosome *mec* Type IV Clone. *Antimicrob. Agents Chemother.* **2016**, *60*, 3007–3015. [CrossRef] [PubMed]

115. Schwarz, S.; Werckenthin, C.; Kehrenberg, C. Identification of a plasmid-borne chloramphenicol-florfenicol resistance gene in *Staphylococcus sciuri*. *Antimicrob. Agents Chemother.* **2000**, *44*, 2530–2533. [CrossRef] [PubMed]

116. Mendes, R.E.; Hogan, P.A.; Jones, R.N.; Sader, H.S.; Flamm, R.K. Surveillance for linezolid resistance via the Zyvox(R) Annual Appraisal of Potency and Spectrum (ZAAPS) programme (2014): Evolving resistance mechanisms with stable susceptibility rates. *J. Antimicrob. Chemother.* **2016**, *71*, 1860–1865. [CrossRef] [PubMed]

117. Morales, G.; Picazo, J.J.; Baos, E.; Candel, F.J.; Arribi, A.; Peláez, B.; Andrade, R.; de la Torre, M.A.; Fereres, J.; Sánchez-García, M. Resistance to linezolid is mediated by the *cfr* gene in the first report of an outbreak of linezolid-resistant *Staphylococcus aureus*. *Clin. Infect. Dis.* **2010**, *50*, 821–825. [CrossRef] [PubMed]

118. Sánchez García, M.; De la Torre, M.A.; Morales, G.; Peláez, B.; Tolón, M.J.; Domingo, S.; Candel, F.J.; Andrade, R.; Arribi, A.; García, N.; et al. Clinical outbreak of linezolid-resistant *Staphylococcus aureus* in an intensive care unit. *JAMA* **2010**, *303*, 2260–2264. [CrossRef] [PubMed]

119. Paridaens, H.; Coussement, J.; Argudín, M.A.; Delaere, B.; Huang, T.D.; Glupczynski, Y.; Denis, O. Clinical case of *cfr*-positive MRSA CC398 in Belgium. *Eur. J. Clin. Microbiol. Infect. Dis.* **2017**. [CrossRef] [PubMed]

120. Shore, A.C.; Brennan, O.M.; Ehricht, R.; Monecke, S.; Schwarz, S.; Slickers, P.; Coleman, D.C. Identification and characterization of the multidrug resistance gene *cfr* in a Panton-Valentine leukocidin-positive sequence type 8 methicillin-resistant *Staphylococcus aureus* IVa (USA300) isolate. *Antimicrob. Agents Chemother.* **2010**, *54*, 4978–4984. [CrossRef] [PubMed]

121. Gopegui, E.R.; Juan, C.; Zamorano, L.; Pérez, J.L.; Oliver, A. Transferable multidrug resistance plasmid carrying *cfr* associated with *tet*(L), *ant(4′)-Ia*, and *dfrK* genes from a clinical methicillin-resistant *Staphylococcus aureus* ST125 strain. *Antimicrob. Agents Chemother.* **2012**, *56*, 2139–2142. [CrossRef] [PubMed]

122. Zhou, W.; Niu, D.; Cao, X.; Ning, M.; Zhang, Z.; Shen, H.; Zhang, K. Clonal dissemination of linezolid-resistant *Staphylococcus capitis* with G2603T mutation in domain V of the 23S rRNA and the *cfr* gene at a tertiary care hospital in China. *BMC Infect. Dis.* **2015**, *15*, 97. [CrossRef] [PubMed]

123. O'Connor, C.; Powell, J.; Finnegan, C.; O'Gorman, A.; Barrett, S.; Hopkins, K.L.; Pichon, B.; Hill, R.; Power, L.; Woodford, N.; et al. 2015. Incidence, management and outcomes of the first *cfr*-mediated linezolid-resistant *Staphylococcus epidermidis* outbreak in a tertiary referral centre in the Republic of Ireland. *J. Hosp. Infect.* **2015**, *90*, 316–321. [CrossRef] [PubMed]

124. Zeng, Z.L.; Wei, H.K.; Wang, J.; Lin, D.C.; Liu, X.Q.; Liu, J.H. High prevalence of Cfr-producing Staphylococcus species in retail meat in Guangzhou, China. *BMC Microbiol.* **2014**, *14*, 151. [CrossRef] [PubMed]

125. Couto, N.; Monchique, C.; Belas, A.; Marques, C.; Gama, L.T.; Pomba, C. Trends and molecular mechanisms of antimicrobial resistance in clinical staphylococci isolated from companion animals over a 16 year period. *J. Antimicrob. Chemother.* **2016**, *71*, 1479–1487. [CrossRef] [PubMed]

126. Wang, Y.; Li, D.; Song, L.; Liu, Y.; He, T.; Liu, H.; Wu, C.; Schwarz, S.; Shen, J. First report of the multiresistance gene *cfr* in *Streptococcus suis*. *Antimicrob. Agents Chemother.* **2013**, *57*, 4061–4063. [CrossRef] [PubMed]

127. Schwarz, S.; Wang, Y. Nomenclature and functionality of the so-called *cfr* gene from *Clostridium difficile*. *Antimicrob. Agents Chemother.* **2015**, *59*, 2476–2477. [CrossRef] [PubMed]

128. Bender, J.K.; Fleige, C.; Klare, I.; Fiedler, S.; Mischnik, A.; Mutters, N.T.; Dingle, K.E.; Werner, G. Detection of a *cfr*(B) variant in german *Enterococcus faecium* clinical isolates and the impact on linezolid resistance in *Enterococcus* spp. *PLoS ONE* **2016**, *11*, e0167042. [CrossRef] [PubMed]

129. Brenciani, A.; Morroni, G.; Pollini, S.; Tiberi, E.; Mingoia, M.; Varaldo, P.E.; Rossolini, G.M.; Giovanetti, E. Characterization of novel conjugative multiresistance plasmids carrying cfr from linezolid-resistant *Staphylococcus epidermidis* clinical isolates from Italy. *J. Antimicrob. Chemother.* **2016**, *71*, 307–313. [CrossRef] [PubMed]

130. Liu, X.Q.; Wang, J.; Li, W.; Zhao, L.Q.; Lu, Y.; Liu, J.H.; Zeng, Z.L. Distribution of *cfr* in *Staphylococcus* spp. and *Escherichia coli* strains from pig farms in China and characterization of a novel *cfr*-carrying F43:A-:B-Plasmid. *Front. Microbiol.* **2017**, *8*, 329. [CrossRef] [PubMed]

131. Sun, J.; Deng, H.; Li, L.; Chen, M.Y.; Fang, L.X.; Yang, Q.E.; Liu, Y.H.; Liao, X.P. Complete nucleotide sequence of *cfr*-carrying IncX4 plasmid pSD11 from *Escherichia coli*. *Antimicrob. Agents Chemother.* **2015**, *59*, 738–741. [CrossRef] [PubMed]

132. Zhang, W.J.; Xu, X.R.; Schwarz, S.; Wang, X.M.; Dai, L.; Zheng, H.J.; Liu, S. Characterization of the IncA/C plasmid pSCEC2 from *Escherichia coli* of swine origin that harbours the multiresistance gene *cfr*. *J. Antimicrob. Chemother.* **2014**, *69*, 385–389. [CrossRef] [PubMed]

133. Zhang, W.J.; Wang, X.M.; Dai, L.; Hua, X.; Dong, Z.; Schwarz, S.; Liu, S. Novel conjugative plasmid from *Escherichia coli* of swine origin that coharbors the multiresistance gene *cfr* and the extended-spectrum-β-lactamase gene *bla*CTX-M-14b. *Antimicrob. Agents Chemother.* **2015**, *59*, 1337–1340. [CrossRef] [PubMed]

134. Zhang, R.; Sun, B.; Wang, Y.; Lei, L.; Schwarz, S.; Wu, C. Characterization of a *cfr*-Carrying Plasmid from Porcine *Escherichia coli* That Closely Resembles Plasmid pEA3 from the Plant Pathogen *Erwinia amylovora*. *Antimicrob. Agents Chemother.* **2016**, *60*, 658–661. [CrossRef] [PubMed]

135. Deng, H.; Sun, J.; Ma, J.; Li, L.; Fang, L.X.; Zhang, Q.; Liu, Y.H.; Liao, X.P. Identification of the multi-resistance gene *cfr* in *Escherichia coli* isolates of animal origin. *PLoS ONE* **2014**, *9*, e102378. [CrossRef] [PubMed]

136. Alba, P.; Feltrin, F.; Cordaro, G.; Porrero, M.C.; Kraushaar, B.; Argudín, M.A.; Nykäsenoja, S.; Monaco, M.; Stegger, M.; Aarestrup, F.M.; et al. Livestock-associated methicillin resistant and methicillin susceptible *Staphylococcus aureus* Sequence Type (CC)1 in European farmed animals: High genetic relatedness of isolates from Italian cattle herds and humans. *PLoS ONE* **2015**, *10*, e0137143. [CrossRef] [PubMed]

137. Feltrin, F.; Alba, P.; Kraushaar, B.; Ianzano, A.; Argudín, M.A.; Di Matteo, P.; Porrero, M.C.; Aarestrup, F.M.; Butaye, P.; Franco, A.; et al. A Livestock-associated, multidrug-resistant, methicillin-resistant *Staphylococcus aureus* Clonal Complex 97 lineage spreading in dairy cattle and pigs in Italy. *Appl. Environ. Microbiol.* **2015**, *82*, 816–821. [CrossRef] [PubMed]

138. Argudín, M.A.; Rodicio, M.R.; Guerra, B. The emerging methicillin-resistant *Staphylococcus aureus* ST398 clone can easily be typed using the Cfr9I SmaI-neoschizomer. *Lett. Appl. Microbiol.* **2010**, *50*, 127–130. [CrossRef] [PubMed]

139. Argudín, M.A.; Fetsch, A.; Tenhagen, B.A.; Hammerl, J.A.; Hertwig, S.; Kowall, J.; Rodicio, M.R.; Käsbohrer, A.; Helmuth, R.; Schroeter, A.; et al. High heterogeneity within methicillin-resistant *Staphylococcus aureus* ST398 isolates, defined by Cfr9I macrorestriction-pulsed-field gel electrophoresis profiles and *spa* and SCC*mec* types. *Appl. Environ. Microbiol.* **2010**, *76*, 652–658. [CrossRef] [PubMed]

140. Crombé, F.; Argudín, M.A.; Vanderhaeghen, W.; Hermans, K.; Haesebrouck, F.; Butaye, P. Transmission Dynamics of Methicillin-Resistant *Staphylococcus aureus* in Pigs. *Front. Microbiol.* **2013**, *4*, 57. [CrossRef] [PubMed]

141. Nemeghaire, S.; Roelandt, S.; Argudín, M.A.; Haesebrouck, F.; Butaye, P. Characterization of methicillin-resistant *Staphylococcus aureus* from healthy carrier chickens. *Avian Pathol.* **2013**, *42*, 342–346. [CrossRef] [PubMed]

142. Nemeghaire, S.; Argudín, M.A.; Haesebrouck, F.; Butaye, P. Epidemiology and molecular characterization of methicillin-resistant *Staphylococcus aureus* nasal carriage isolates from bovines. *BMC Vet. Res.* **2014**, *10*, 153. [CrossRef] [PubMed]

143. Peeters, L.E.; Argudín, M.A.; Azadikhah, S.; Butaye, P. Antimicrobial resistance and population structure of *Staphylococcus aureus* recovered from pigs farms. *Vet. Microbiol.* **2015**, *180*, 151–156. [CrossRef] [PubMed]

144. Price, L.B.; Stegger, M.; Hasman, H.; Aziz, M.; Larsen, J.; Andersen, P.S.; Pearson, T.; Waters, A.E.; Foster, J.T.; Schupp, J.; et al. *Staphylococcus aureus* CC398: Host adaptation and emergence of methicillin resistance in livestock. *mBio* **2012**, *3*, e00305. [CrossRef] [PubMed]

145. Cuny, C.; Abdelbary, M.; Layer, F.; Werner, G.; Witte, W. Prevalence of the immune evasion gene cluster in *Staphylococcus aureus* CC398. *Vet. Microbiol.* **2015**, *177*, 219–223. [CrossRef] [PubMed]

146. Bismuth, R.; Zilhao, R.; Sakamoto, H.; Guesdon, J.L.; Courvalin, P. Gene heterogeneity for tetracycline resistance in *Staphylococcus* spp. *Antimicrob. Agents Chemother.* **1990**, *34*, 1611–1614. [CrossRef] [PubMed]

147. Kadlec, K.; Schwarz, S. dentification of the novel *dfrK*-carrying transposon Tn559 in a porcine methicillin-susceptible *Staphylococcus aureus* ST398 strain. *Antimicrob. Agents Chemother.* **2010**, *54*, 3475–3477. [CrossRef] [PubMed]

148. Gómez-Sanz, E.; Kadlec, K.; Feßler, A.T.; Zarazaga, M.; Torres, C.; Schwarz, S. Novel *erm*(T)-carrying multiresistance plasmids from porcine and human isolates of methicillin-resistant *Staphylococcus aureus* ST398 that also harbor cadmium and copper resistance determinants. *Antimicrob. Agents Chemother.* **2013**, *57*, 3275–3282. [CrossRef] [PubMed]

149. Cuny, C.; Layer, F.; Köck, R.; Werner, G.; Witte, W. Methicillin susceptible *Staphylococcus aureus* (MSSA) of clonal complex CC398, t571 from infections in humans are still rare in Germany. *PLoS ONE* **2013**, *8*, e83165. [CrossRef] [PubMed]

150. Lekkerkerk, W.S.; van Wamel, W.J.; Snijders, S.V.; Willems, R.J.; van Duijkeren, E.; Broens, E.M.; Wagenaar, J.A.; Lindsay, J.A.; Vos, M.C. What is the origin of Livestock-Associated Methicillin-Resistant *Staphylococcus aureus* Clonal Complex 398 isolates from humans without livestock contact? An epidemiological and genetic analysis. *J. Clin. Microbiol.* **2015**, *53*, 1836–1841. [CrossRef] [PubMed]

151. Al Bayssari, C.; Dabboussi, F.; Hamze, M.; Rolain, J.M. Emergence of carbapenemase-producing *Pseudomonas aeruginosa* and *Acinetobacter baumannii* in livestock animals in Lebanon. *J. Antimicrob. Chemother.* **2015**, *70*, 950–951. [CrossRef] [PubMed]

152. Fischer, J.; Rodríguez, I.; Schmoger, S.; Friese, A.; Roesler, U.; Helmuth, R.; Guerra, B. *Escherichia coli* producing VIM-1 carbapenemase isolated on a pig farm. *J. Antimicrob. Chemother.* **2012**, *67*, 1793–1795. [CrossRef] [PubMed]

153. Guerra, B.; Fischer, J.; Helmuth, R. An emerging public health problem: Acquired carbapenemase-producing microorganisms are present in food-producing animals, their environment, companion animals and wild birds. *Vet. Microbiol.* **2014**, *171*, 290–297. [CrossRef] [PubMed]

154. Michael, G.B.; Freitag, C.; Wendlandt, S.; Eidam, C.; Feßler, A.T.; Lopes, G.V.; Kadlec, K.; Schwarz, S. Emerging issues in antimicrobial resistance of bacteria from food-producing animals. *Future Microbiol.* **2015**, *10*, 427–443. [CrossRef] [PubMed]

155. Schwarz, S.; Enne, V.I.; van Duijkeren, E. 40 years of veterinary papers in JAC—What have we learnt? *J. Antimicrob. Chemother.* **2016**, *71*, 2681–2690. [CrossRef] [PubMed]

156. Wang, Y.; Wang, X.; Schwarz, S.; Zhang, R.; Lei, L.; Liu, X.; Lin, D.; Shen, J. IMP-45-producing multidrug-resistant *Pseudomonas aeruginosa* of canine origin. *J. Antimicrob. Chemother.* **2014**, *69*, 2579–2581. [CrossRef] [PubMed]

157. Webb, H.E.; Bugarel, M.; den Bakker, H.C.; Nightingale, K.K.; Granier, S.A.; Scott, H.M.; Loneragan, G.H. Carbapenem-Resistant Bacteria Recovered from Faeces of Dairy Cattle in the High Plains Region of the USA. *PLoS ONE* **2016**, *11*, e0147363. [CrossRef] [PubMed]

158. Zhang, W.J.; Lu, Z.; Schwarz, S.; Zhang, R.M.; Wang, X.M.; Si, W.; Yu, S.; Chen, L.; Liu, S. Complete sequence of the *bla*(NDM-1)-carrying plasmid pNDM-AB from *Acinetobacter baumannii* of food animal origin. *J. Antimicrob. Chemother.* **2013**, *68*, 1681–1682. [CrossRef] [PubMed]

159. Müller, S.; Janssen, T.; Wieler, L.H. Multidrug resistant Acinetobacter baumannii in veterinary medicine—Emergence of an underestimated pathogen? *Berl. Munch. Tierarztl. Wochenschr.* **2014**, *127*, 435–446. [PubMed]

160. Eveillard, M.; Kempf, M.; Belmonte, O.; Pailhoriès, H.; Joly-Guillou, M.L. Reservoirs of *Acinetobacter baumannii* outside the hospital and potential involvement in emerging human community-acquired infections. *Int. J. Infect. Dis.* **2013**, *17*, e802–e805. [CrossRef] [PubMed]

161. Al Atrouni, A.; Joly-Guillou, M.L.; Hamze, M.; Kempf, M. Reservoirs of Non-baumannii Acinetobacter Species. *Front. Microbiol.* **2016**, *7*, 49. [CrossRef] [PubMed]

162. Hamouda, A.; Findlay, J.; Al Hassan, L.; Amyes, S.G. Epidemiology of *Acinetobacter baumannii* of animal origin. *Int. J. Antimicrob. Agents* **2011**, *38*, 314–318. [CrossRef] [PubMed]

163. Cag, Y.; Caskurlu, H.; Fan, Y.; Cao, B.; Vahaboglu, H. Resistance mechanisms. *Ann. Transl. Med.* **2016**, *4*, 326. [CrossRef] [PubMed]

164. Zordan, S.; Prenger-Berninghoff, E.; Weiss, R.; van der Reijden, T.; van den Broeck, P.; Baljer, G.; Dijkshoorn, L. Multidrug-resistant *Acinetobacter baumannii* in veterinary clinics, Germany. *Emerg. Infect. Dis.* **2011**, *17*, 1751–1754. [CrossRef] [PubMed]

165. Ewers, C.; Klotz, P.; Leidner, U.; Stamm, I.; Prenger-Berninghoff, E.; Göttig, S.; Semmler, T.; Scheufen, S. OXA-23 and ISAba1-OXA-66 class D β-lactamases in *Acinetobacter baumannii* isolates from companion animals. *Int. J. Antimicrob. Agents* **2017**, *49*, 7–44. [CrossRef] [PubMed]

166. Wang, B.; Sun, D. Detection of NDM-1 carbapenemase-producing *Acinetobacter calcoaceticus* and *Acinetobacter junii* in environmental samples from livestock farms. *J. Antimicrob. Chemother.* **2015**, *70*, 611–613. [CrossRef] [PubMed]

167. Abbott, Y.; O'Mahony, R.; Leonard, N.; Quinn, P.J.; van der Reijden, T.; Dijkshoorn, L.; Fanning, S. Characterization of a 2.6kbp variable region within a class 1 integron found in an *Acinetobacter baumannii* strain isolated from a horse. *J. Antimicrob. Chemother.* **2005**, *55*, 367–370. [CrossRef] [PubMed]

168. Jeannot, K.; Bolard, A.; Plésiat, P. Resistance to polymyxins in Gram-negative organisms. *Int. J. Antimicrob. Agents* **2017**, *49*, 526–535. [CrossRef] [PubMed]

169. Lupo, A.; Vogt, D.; Seiffert, S.N.; Endimiani, A.; Perreten, V. Antibiotic resistance and phylogenetic characterization of *Acinetobacter baumannii* strains isolated from commercial raw meat in Switzerland. *J. Food Prot.* **2014**, *77*, 1976–1981. [CrossRef] [PubMed]

170. Carvalheira, A.; Casquete, R.; Silva, J.; Teixeira, P. Prevalence and antimicrobial susceptibility of *Acinetobacter* spp. isolated from meat. *Int. J. Food Microbiol.* **2017**, *243*, 58–63. [CrossRef] [PubMed]

171. Liu, Y.Y.; Chandler, C.E.; Leung, L.M.; McElheny, C.L.; Mettus, R.T.; Shanks, R.M.; Liu, J.H.; Goodlett, D.R.; Ernst, R.K.; Doi, Y. Structural Modification of Lipopolysaccharide Conferred by *mcr-1* in Gram-Negative ESKAPE Pathogens. *Antimicrob. Agents Chemother.* **2017**, *61*. [CrossRef] [PubMed]

172. Rubin, J.; Walker, R.D.; Blickenstaff, K.; Bodeis-Jones, S.; Zhao, S. Antimicrobial resistance and genetic characterization of fluoroquinolone resistance of *Pseudomonas aeruginosa* isolated from canine infections. *Vet. Microbiol.* **2008**, *131*, 164–172. [CrossRef] [PubMed]

173. Beier, R.C.; Foley, S.L.; Davidson, M.K.; White, D.G.; McDermott, P.F.; Bodeis-Jones, S.; Zhao, S.; Andrews, K.; Crippen, T.L.; Sheffield, C.L.; et al. Characterization of antibiotic and disinfectant susceptibility profiles among *Pseudomonas aeruginosa* veterinary isolates recovered during 1994–2003. *J. Appl. Microbiol.* **2015**, *118*, 326–342. [CrossRef] [PubMed]

174. Haenni, M.; Hocquet, D.; Ponsin, C.; Cholley, P.; Guyeux, C.; Madec, J.Y.; Bertrand, X. Population structure and antimicrobial susceptibility of *Pseudomonas aeruginosa* from animal infections in France. *BMC Vet. Res.* **2015**, *11*, 9. [CrossRef] [PubMed]

175. Scaccabarozzi, L.; Leoni, L.; Ballarini, A.; Barberio, A.; Locatelli, C.; Casula, A.; Bronzo, V.; Pisoni, G.; Jousson, O.; Morandi, S.; et al. Pseudomonas aeruginosa in Dairy Goats: Genotypic and Phenotypic Comparison of Intramammary and Environmental Isolate. *PLoS ONE* **2015**, *10*, e0142973. [CrossRef] [PubMed]

176. Arais, L.R.; Barbosa, A.V.; Carvalho, C.A.; Cerqueira, A.M. Antimicrobial resistance, integron carriage, and *gyrA* and *gyrB* mutations in *Pseudomonas aeruginosa* isolated from dogs with otitis externa and pyoderma in Brazil. *Vet. Dermatol.* **2016**, *27*, 113–e31. [CrossRef] [PubMed]

177. Ludwig, C.; de Jong, A.; Moyaert, H.; El Garch, F.; Janes, R.; Klein, U.; Morrissey, I.; Thiry, J.; Youala, M. Antimicrobial susceptibility monitoring of dermatological bacterial pathogens isolated from diseased dogs and cats across Europe (ComPath results). *J. Appl. Microbiol.* **2016**, *121*, 1254–1267. [CrossRef] [PubMed]

178. Odumosu, B.T.; Ajetunmobi, O.; Dada-Adegbola, H.; Odutayo, I. Antibiotic susceptibility pattern and analysis of plasmid profiles of *Pseudomonas aeruginosa* from human, animal and plant sources. *Springerplus* **2016**, *5*, 1381. [CrossRef] [PubMed]

179. Baron, S.; Hadjadj, L.; Rolain, J.M.; Olaitan, A.O. Molecular mechanisms of polymyxin resistance: Knowns and unknowns. *Int. J. Antimicrob. Agents,* **2016**, *48*, 583–591. [CrossRef] [PubMed]

180. Rodríguez-Martínez, J.M.; Machuca, J.; Cano, M.E.; Calvo, J.; Martínez-Martínez, L.; Pascual, A. Plasmid-mediated quinolone resistance: Two decades on. *Drug Resist. Updat.* **2016**, *29*, 13–29. [CrossRef] [PubMed]

181. Hummel, R.; Tschäpe, H.; Witte, W. Spread of plasmid-mediated nourseothricin resistance due to antibiotic use in animal husbandry. *J. Basic Microbiol.* **1986**, *26*, 461–466. [CrossRef] [PubMed]

182. Werner, G.; Hildebrandt, B.; Witte, W. Aminoglycoside-streptothricin resistance gene cluster *aadE-sat4-aphA-3* disseminated among multiresistant isolates of *Enterococcus faecium*. *Antimicrob. Agents Chemother.* **2001**, *45*, 3267–3269. [CrossRef] [PubMed]

183. Dahms, C.; Hübner, N.O.; Kossow, A.; Mellmann, A.; Dittmann, K.; Kramer, A. Occurrence of ESBL-producing *Escherichia coli* in livestock and farm workers in Mecklenburg-Western Pomerania, Germany. *PLoS ONE* **2015**, *10*, e0143326. [CrossRef] [PubMed]

184. Ewers, C.; Bethe, A.; Semmler, T.; Guenther, S.; Wieler, L.H. Extended-spectrum β-lactamase-producing and AmpC-producing *Escherichia coli* from livestock and companion animals, and their putative impact on public health: A global perspective. *Clin. Microbiol. Infect.* **2012**, *18*, 646–655. [CrossRef] [PubMed]

185. Doublet, B.; Praud, K.; Nguyen-Ho-Bao, T.; Argudín, M.A.; Bertrand, S.; Butaye, P.; Cloeckaert, A. Extended-spectrum β-lactamase- and AmpC β-lactamase-producing D-tartrate-positive *Salmonella enterica* serovar Paratyphi B from broilers and human patients in Belgium, 2008–10. *J. Antimicrob. Chemother.* **2014**, *69*, 1257–1264. [CrossRef] [PubMed]

186. Pardon, B.; Smet, A.; Butaye, P.; Argudín, M.A.; Valgaeren, B.; Catry, B.; Haesebrouck, F.; Deprez, P. Nosocomial intravascular catheter infections with extended-spectrum Beta-lactamase-producing *Escherichia coli* in calves after strain introduction from a commercial herd. *Transbound. Emerg. Dis.* **2017**, *64*, 130–136. [CrossRef] [PubMed]

187. Alonso, C.A.; Zarazaga, M.; Ben Sallem, R.; Jouini, A.; Ben Slama, K.; Torres, C. Antibiotic resistance in *Escherichia coli* in husbandry animals: The African perspective. *Lett. Appl. Microbiol.* **2017**, *64*, 318–334. [CrossRef] [PubMed]

188. Teshager, T.; Domínguez, L.; Moreno, M.A.; Saénz, Y.; Torres, C.; Cardeñosa, S. Isolation of an SHV-12 beta-lactamase-producing *Escherichia coli* strain from a dog with recurrent urinary tract infections. *Antimicrob. Agents Chemother.* **2000**, *44*, 3483–3484. [CrossRef] [PubMed]

189. Olaitan, A.O.; Morand, S.; Rolain, J.M. Emergence of colistin-resistant bacteria in humans without colistin usage: A new worry and cause for vigilance. *Int. J. Antimicrob. Agents* **2016**, *47*, 1–3. [CrossRef] [PubMed]

190. Rhouma, M.; Beaudry, F.; Thériault, W.; Letellier, A. Colistin in Pig Production: Chemistry, Mechanism of Antibacterial Action, Microbial Resistance Emergence, and One Health Perspectives. *Front. Microbiol.* **2016**, *7*, 1789. [CrossRef] [PubMed]

191. Liu, Y.Y.; Wang, Y.; Walsh, T.R.; Yi, L.X.; Zhang, R.; Spencer, J.; Doi, Y.; Tian, G.; Dong, B.; Huang, X.; et al. Emergence of plasmid-mediated colistin resistance mechanism MCR-1 in animals and human beings in China: A microbiological and molecular biological study. *Lancet Infect. Dis.* **2016**, *16*, 161–168. [CrossRef]

192. Liu, B.T.; Song, F.J.; Zou, M.; Hao, Z.H.; Shan, H. Emergence of colistin resistance gene *mcr-1* in *Cronobacter sakazakii* producing NDM-9 and *Escherichia coli* from the same animal. *Antimicrob. Agents Chemother.* **2016**. [CrossRef]

193. Xavier, B.B.; Lammens, C.; Butaye, P.; Goossens, H.; Malhotra-Kumar, S. Complete sequence of an IncFII plasmid harbouring the colistin resistance gene *mcr-1* isolated from Belgian pig farms. *J. Antimicrob. Chemother.* **2016**, *71*, 2342–2344. [CrossRef] [PubMed]

194. Delgado-Blas, J.F.; Ovejero, C.M.; Abadia-Patiño, L.; Gonzalez-Zorn, B. Coexistence of *mcr-1* and *bla*$_{NDM-1}$ in *Escherichia coli* from Venezuela. *Antimicrob. Agents Chemother.* **2016**, *60*, 6356–6358. [CrossRef] [PubMed]

195. Di Pilato, V.; Arena, F.; Tascini, C.; Cannatelli, A.; Henrici De Angelis, L.; Fortunato, S.; Giani, T.; Menichetti, F.; Rossolini, G.M. *mcr-1.2*, a New *mcr* Variant Carried on a Transferable Plasmid from a Colistin-Resistant KPC Carbapenemase-Producing *Klebsiella pneumoniae* Strain of Sequence Type 512. *Antimicrob. Agents Chemother.* **2016**, *60*, 5612–5615. [CrossRef] [PubMed]

196. Kong, L.H.; Lei, C.W.; Ma, S.Z.; Jiang, W.; Liu, B.H.; Wang, Y.X.; Guan, R.; Men, S.; Yuan, Q.W.; Cheng, G.Y.; et al. Various sequence types of *Escherichia coli* co-harboring *bla*$_{NDM-5}$ and *mcr-1* genes from a commercial swine farm in China. *Antimicrob. Agents Chemother.* **2016**. [CrossRef]

197. Mediavilla, J.R.; Patrawalla, A.; Chen, L.; Chavda, K.D.; Mathema, B.; Vinnard, C.; Dever, L.L.; Kreiswirth, B.N. Colistin- and Carbapenem-Resistant *Escherichia coli* Harboring *mcr-1* and *bla*$_{NDM-5}$, Causing a Complicated Urinary Tract Infection in a Patient from the United States. *mBio* **2016**, *7*. [CrossRef] [PubMed]

198. Xavier, B.B.; Lammens, C.; Ruhal, R.; Kumar-Singh, S.; Butaye, P.; Goossens, H.; Malhotra-Kumar, S. Identification of a novel plasmid-mediated colistin-resistance gene, *mcr-2*, in *Escherichia coli*, Belgium, June 2016. *Euro Surveill.* **2016**, *21*. [CrossRef]

199. Schwarz, S.; Johnson, A.P. Transferable resistance to colistin: A new but old threat. *J. Antimicrob. Chemother.* **2016**, *71*, 2066–2070. [CrossRef] [PubMed]

200. Szmolka, A.; Nagy, B. Multidrug resistant commensal *Escherichia coli* in animals and its impact for public health. *Front. Microbiol.* **2013**, *4*, 258. [CrossRef] [PubMed]

201. Fàbrega, A.; Sánchez-Céspedes, J.; Soto, S.; Vila, J. Quinolone resistance in the food chain. *Int. J. Antimicrob. Agents* **2008**, *31*, 307–315. [CrossRef] [PubMed]

202. Veldman, K.; Cavaco, L.M.; Mevius, D.; Battisti, A.; Franco, A.; Botteldoorn, N.; Bruneau, M.; Perrin-Guyomard, A.; Cerny, T.; De Frutos Escobar, C.; et al. International collaborative study on the occurrence of plasmid-mediated quinolone resistance in *Salmonella enterica* and *Escherichia coli* isolated from animals, humans, food and the environment in 13 European countries. *J. Antimicrob. Chemother.* **2011**, *66*, 1278–1286. [CrossRef] [PubMed]

203. Robicsek, A.; Strahilevitz, J.; Jacoby, G.A.; Macielag, M.; Abbanat, D.; Park, C.H.; Bush, K.; Hooper, D.C. Fluoroquinolone-modifying enzyme: A new adaptation of a common aminoglycoside acetyltransferase. *Nat. Med.* **2006**, *12*, 83–88. [CrossRef] [PubMed]

204. Hammerum, A.M.; Heuer, O.E. Human health hazards from antimicrobial-resistant *Escherichia coli* of animal origin. *Clin. Infect. Dis.* **2009**, *48*, 916–921. [CrossRef] [PubMed]

Permissions

List of Contributors

Tamar Auerbach-Nevo, David Baram, Anat Bashan, Matthew Belousoff, Elinor Breiner, Chen Davidovich, Giuseppe Cimicata, Zohar Eyal, Yehuda Halfon, Miri Krupkin, Donna Matzov, Markus Metz, Mruwat Rufayda, Moshe Peretz, Ophir Pick, Erez Pyetan, Haim Rozenberg, Moran Shalev-Benami, Itai Wekselman, Raz Zarivach, Ella Zimmerman, Nofar Assis, Joel Bloch, Hadar Israeli, Rinat Kalaora, Lisha Lim, Ofir Sade-Falk, Tal Shapira, Leena Taha-Salaime, Hua Tang and Ada Yonath
Department of Structural Biology, Weizmann Institute, Rehovot 76100, Israel

William R. Schwan, Rebecca Polanowski, Sara Medina-Bielski, Michelle Lane, Marc Rott, Lauren Lipker, Amy Wescott and Cassandra Mikel
Department of Microbiology, University ofWisconsin-La Crosse, La Crosse, WI 54601, USA
Emerging Technology Center for Pharmaceutical Development, University ofWisconsin-La Crosse, La Crosse, WI 54601, USA

Paul M. Dunman
School of Medicine and Dentistry, University of Rochester, Rochester, NY 14642, USA
Aaron Monte
Emerging Technology Center for Pharmaceutical Development, University ofWisconsin-La Crosse, La Crosse, WI 54601, USA
Department of Chemistry and Biochemistry, University ofWisconsin-La Crosse, La Crosse, WI 54601, USA

James M. Cook, V.V.N. Phani Babu Tiruveedhula, Christopher M. Witzigmann and Md Tou iqur Rahman
Department of Chemistry and Biochemistry, University of Wisconsin-Milwaukee, Milwaukee, WI 53211, USA

Douglas D. Baumann
Department of Mathematics and Statistics, University of Wisconsin-La Crosse, La Crosse, WI 54601, USA

Márió Gajdács and Gabriella Spengler
Department of Medical Microbiology and Immunobiology, Faculty of Medicine, University of Szeged, 6720 Szeged, Hungary

Edit Urbán
Institute of Clinical Microbiology, Faculty of Medicine, University of Szeged, 6725 Szeged, Hungary

Samudrala Gourinath
School of Life Sciences, Jawaharlal Nehru University, New Delhi 110067, India

Preeti Pandey
School of Life Sciences, Jawaharlal Nehru University, New Delhi 110067, India
Department of Bioscience and Biotechnology, Banasthali University, Rajasthan 304022, India

Suman Kumar Dhar
Special Centre for Molecular Medicine, Jawaharlal Nehru University, New Delhi 110067, India

Vijay Verma
Special Centre for Molecular Medicine, Jawaharlal Nehru University, New Delhi 110067, India
Department of Microbiology, Central University of Rajasthan, Kishangarh 305801, India

James J. Bull
Department of Integrative Biology, University of Texas, Austin, TX 78712, USA
The Institute for Cellular and Molecular Biology, University of Texas, Austin, TX 78712, USA
Center for Computational Biology and Bioinformatics, University of Texas, Austin, TX 78712, USA

Kelly A. Christensen
Department of Mathematics, University of Idaho, Moscow, 83844, USA
Center for Modeling Complex Interactions, University of Idaho, Moscow, 83844, USA

Stephen M. Krone
Department of Mathematics, University of Idaho, Moscow, 83844, USA
Center for Modeling Complex Interactions, University of Idaho, Moscow, 83844, USA
Institute for Bioinformatics and Evolutionary Studies, University of Idaho, Moscow, 83844, USA

Carly Scott
Department of Mathematics, University of Idaho, Moscow, 83844, USA
Department of Biological Sciences, University of Idaho, Moscow, 83844, USA

Cameron J. Crandall
Department of Biological Sciences, University of Idaho, Moscow, 83844, USA

Benjamin R. Jack
The Institute for Cellular and Molecular Biology, University of Texas, Austin, TX 78712, USA

Mallory J. Choudoir, Charles Pepe-Ranney and Daniel H. Buckley
School of Integrative Plant Science, Bradfield Hall 705, Cornell University, Ithaca, NY 14853, USA

Zorik Chilingaryan, Allen T. Y. Lo, Zhi-Qiang Xu, Nicholas E. Dixon and Aaron J. Oakley
Molecular Horizons and School of Chemistry, University of Wollongong, and Illawarra Health and Medical Research Institute, Wollongong, NSW 2522, Australia

Stephen J. Headey and Martin J. Scanlon
Monash Institute of Pharmaceutical Sciences, Monash University, Parkville, VIC 3052, Australia

Gottfried Otting
Research School of Chemistry, Australian National University, Canberra, ACT 2601, Australia

D. İpek Kurtböke
GeneCology Research Centre, Faculty of Science, Health, Education and Engineering, University of the Sunshine Coast, 90 Sippy Downs Drive, Sippy Downs, QLD 4556, Australia

Tuan Son Le
GeneCology Research Centre, Faculty of Science, Health, Education and Engineering, University of the Sunshine Coast, 90 Sippy Downs Drive, Sippy Downs, QLD 4556, Australia
Research Institute for Marine Fisheries, 224 Le Lai, Ngo Quyen, Hai Phong 180000, Vietnam

Thi Hien Nguyen, Hong Phuong Vo, Van Cuong Doan, Hong Loc Nguyen, Minh Trung Tran and Trong Tuan Tran
Research Institute for Aquaculture No. 2, 116 Nguyen Dinh Chieu, District 1, Ho Chi Minh 700000, Vietnam

Paul C. Southgate
Australian Centre for Pacific Islands Research and Faculty of Science, Health, Education and Engineering, University of the Sunshine Coast, Maroochydore, QLD 4556, Australia

George H. Jones
Department of Biology, Emory University, Atlanta, GA 30322, USA

Elisa Binda, Pamela Cappelletti, Flavia Marinelli and Giorgia Letizia Marcone
Department of Biotechnology and Life Sciences, University of Insubria, via J.H. Dunant 3, 21100 Varese, Italy

The Protein Factory Research Center, Politecnico di Milano and University of Insubria, via J.H. Dunant 3, 21100 Varese, Italy

Cassandra E. Nix and Bryan J. Harper
Department of Environmental and Molecular Toxicology, Oregon State University, Corvallis, OR 97331, USA

Stacey L. Harper
Department of Environmental and Molecular Toxicology, Oregon State University, Corvallis, OR 97331, USA
Oregon Nanoscience and Microtechnologies Institute, Corvallis, OR 97330, USA
School of Chemical, Biological and Environmental Engineering, Oregon State University, Corvallis, OR 97331, USA

Cathryn G. Conner, Alexander P. Richter and Orlin D. Velev
Department of Chemical and Biomolecular Engineering, North Carolina State University, Raleigh, NC 27606, USA

Renan Aparecido Fernandes
Department of Dentistry, University Center of Adamantina (UNIFAI), Adamantina 17800-000, São Paulo, Brazil
Department of Dental Materials and Prosthodontics, São Paulo State University (UNESP), School of Dentistry, Araçatuba 16015-050, São Paulo, Brazil

Gabriela Lopes Fernandes, Carla Corrêa Mendes-Gouvêa and Debora Barros Barbosa
Department of Dental Materials and Prosthodontics, São Paulo State University (UNESP), School of Dentistry, Araçatuba 16015-050, São Paulo, Brazil

Andresa Aparecida Berretta, Elina Cassia Torres and Andrei Felipe Moreira Buszinski
Laboratory of Research, Development and Innovation, Apis Flora Industrial e Comercial Ltda., Ribeirão Preto 14020-670, São Paulo, Brazil

Francisco Nunes de Souza-Neto and Emerson Rodrigues de Camargo
Department of Chemistry, Federal University of São Carlos, São Carlos 13565-905, São Paulo, Brazil

Luiz Fernando Gorup
Department of Chemistry, Federal University of São Carlos, São Carlos 13565-905, São Paulo, Brazil
FACET-Department of Chemistry, Federal University of Grande Dourados, Dourados 79804-970, Mato Grosso do Sul, Brazil

Diane Ashiru-Oredope, Anne Doble, Sejal Hansraj and Susan Hopkins
HCAI and AMR Division, Public Health England, London NW9 5EQ, UK

Mary Richard Akpan and Nada Atef Shebl
Department of Clinical and Pharmaceutical Sciences, University of Hertfordshire, Hatfield AL10 9AB, UK

Raheelah Ahmad
NIHR Health Protection Research Unit in Healthcare Associated Infection and Antimicrobial Resistance at Imperial College London, Hammersmith Campus, Du Cane Road, London W12 0NN, UK

Maciej Jáskiewicz, Damian Neubauer and Wojciech Kamysz
Department of Inorganic Chemistry, Faculty of Pharmacy, Medical University of Gda´ nsk, 80-416 Gda´ nsk, Poland

Maria Angeles Argudín, Ariane Deplano, Alaeddine Meghraoui, Magali Dodémont, Amelie Heinrichs, Claire Nonhoff and Sandrine Roisin
National Reference Centre—Staphylococcus aureus, Department of Microbiology, Hôpital Erasme, Université Libre de Bruxelles, Route de Lennik 808, 1070 Brussels, Belgium

Olivier Denis
National Reference Centre—Staphylococcus aureus, Department of Microbiology, Hôpital Erasme, Université Libre de Bruxelles, Route de Lennik 808, 1070 Brussels, Belgium
Ecole de Santé Publique, Université Libre de Bruxelles, Avenue Franklin Roosevelt 50, 1050 Bruxelles, Belgium

Index

www.ingramcontent.com/pod-product-compliance
Lightning Source LLC
Chambersburg PA
CBHW080250230326
41458CB00097B/4196